Incredible Consequences of Brain Injury

Incredible Consequences of Brain Injury: The Ways your Brain can Break explains the acquired brain disorders that can suddenly change a person's life. Underlining the intricate workings of the human brain and the amazing things it does every day, this book examines what happens when the brain stops functioning as it should.

Through the use of case studies and historical examples, this concentrated collection of different neuropsychological conditions provides the reader a glimpse into the lived experiences of each disorder. Each chapter is firmly rooted in relevant neuropsychological literature combined with easy-to-understand explanations and guided reflection. In its essence, this book is a celebration of the human brain and the myriad factors that make it up, serving to maintain hope in recovering from brain conditions, and to marvel at the intricate workings of the brain.

This valuable compendium is essential for anyone who wants to learn more about how the brain functions and dysfunctions and will be equally useful for students, instructors, and healthcare workers. It will further be of use to individuals with brain conditions and their dear ones and for the individuals who are interested in learning more about the human brain.

Alexander R. Toftness, PhD, is a Science Communicator from the Midwestern United States. He hosts the *ARTexplains Science and History* channel on YouTube. Dr. Toftness has taught a variety of biological, cognitive, and educational psychology courses and has presented at numerous science communication events across the country.

Incredible Consequences of Brain Injury

The Ways your Brain can Break

Alexander R. Toftness

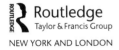

Routledge
Taylor & Francis Group

NEW YORK AND LONDON

Cover image: Alexander R. Toftness

First published 2023
by Routledge
605 Third Avenue, New York, NY 10158

and by Routledge
4 Park Square, Milton Park, Abingdon, Oxon, OX14 4RN

Routledge is an imprint of the Taylor & Francis Group, an informa business

Library of Congress Cataloging-in-Publication Data
Names: Toftness, Alexander R., author.
Title: Incredible consequences of brain injury : the ways your brain can
break / Alexander R. Toftness.
Description: New York, NY : Routledge, 2022. | Includes bibliographical
references and index. |
Identifiers: LCCN 2022023338 (print) | LCCN 2022023339 (ebook) |
ISBN 9781032233673 (hardback) | ISBN 9781032233666 (paperback) |
ISBN 9781003276937 (ebook)
Subjects: LCSH: Brain--Diseases--Popular works. | Brain--Diseases--Case
studies. | Brain--Wounds and injuries--Popular works. | Brain--Wounds
and injuries--Case studies.
Classification: LCC RC386.2 .T64 2022 (print) | LCC RC386.2 (ebook)
| DDC 617.4/81044--dc23/eng/20220802
LC record available at https://lccn.loc.gov/2022023338
LC ebook record available at https://lccn.loc.gov/2022023339

ISBN: 9781032233673 (hbk)
ISBN: 9781032233666 (pbk)
ISBN: 9781003276937 (ebk)

DOI: 10.4324/9781003276937

Typeset in Bembo
by Deanta Global Publishing Services, Chennai, India

Contents

Preface

The intended audience of this book is you. Yes, you. As long as you have a brain—and unless you are reading this in a distant digital future, I'm willing to bet that you do—you'll take something interesting and perhaps even useful away from reading this book. However, depending on who you are, this book can be useful in several different ways.

Are you someone who is interested in brain health? This is a readable guide through neuropsychological disorders that takes complicated topics (including literal brain surgery) and simplifies them while maintaining accuracy. Are you a student of psychology, neuroscience, or any number of the fields that make use of the human brain? This book provides useful summaries and memorable case studies for many dozens of brain disorders, practical for your studies. If you're a fan of learning from videos, you can find a playlist of short educational videos called *The Ways your Brain can Break* that pair with the chapters of this book on my YouTube channel: *ARTexplains Science and History*. Or, if you are an instructor looking for a supplemental text or videos that feature encyclopedic entries and extensive references, perfect for scaffolding your course structure—here you are!

Overall, as a science communicator, my role is translation: sharing stories of interesting brain disorders by putting the published science into more accessible terms. This book came into being because I kept running across stories of people with unforgettable stories about their brain disorders while working toward my PhD in psychology. I asked myself: "why isn't anybody talking about these?" Nobody was talking about them because the science found in medical journals isn't written to be widely read. In the early summer of 2018, I began to collect case studies about the unusual disorders that the human brain can house—such as people who can't see, but think that they can, or people who can't read, but can still write. This project emerged, combining my love of science with my love of science communication.

We can all relate on some level to the stories in this book, because we all have brains. I hope that this book increases your awareness and thankfulness for your own brain. I also hope that this book creates empathy toward those who experience such brain disorders. Not all disabilities are easily noticeable or immediately understandable. Everyone is different, and everyone is someone. I hope you enjoy it!

Dr. Alexander R. Toftness

Acknowledgements

I wrote this book over a span of four years, and throughout that time I am pretty sure that I never stopped talking about it even once. It's strange looking at the final product of literally thousands of hours of work, but here we are. Thank you for reading!

I wish to thank all of those people who have shared their lives with researchers across the centuries as scientists attempted to puzzle together diagnoses for the most mysterious problems of the most mysterious organ. I would also like to thank those who have chosen to speak about their experiences with brain damage in memoirs. The ideas in this book sprung from the minds of countless people and not just from the mind of me, the author. Instead, this book is a remix of old—sometimes *very* old—case studies with new scientific knowledge. I hope that it serves as a bridge between the fantastic true stories contained in the brains of people written down in medical journals across centuries, and the general public with their own questions and stories contained within their respective brains. Telling the stories from science will help people continue to separate science from science fiction.

I would like to thank many people in my life for their guidance and support during the journey of writing this book.

I'd like to thank my incredible partner, Dr. Vanessa Castillo, for being here for me, and for hoodwinking me into the adoption of Sabrina the cat which turned out to be a fantastic decision.

I'd like to thank Lucy Kennedy, my first contact at Routledge, to whom I pitched this book idea. She was enthusiastic and patient throughout the process, and it was a genuine delight working with her.

I'd like to thank the faculty and former faculty of the psychology department at Iowa State University, especially Drs. Eric Cooper, Jon Kelly, Christian Meissner, Jason C. K. Chan, John Grundy, L. Alison Phillips, and Marcus Credé. Thank you to my institutional Interlibrary Loan for miraculously finding many journal articles that I requested from across time and space.

I'd like to thank Christina Meyer for encouragement and many interesting conversations, especially about seizures and pathological déjà vu. Haley Knudsen for creative support and for believing in my project. Sierra Lauber for years of friendship in and out of the lab. Spencer Gjerde for sharing brainwaves. Logan Toftness for being a sister, a friend, and a source of animal photos. Crystal Jewell for her perspective and passion for science communication. Matt Peskar and Rodal Sylte for making me laugh. The members of the cognitive psychology graduate program at Iowa State University, especially Rachel O'Donnell, Taylor Doty, and Jesse Rothweiler, for countless academic and friendly conversations that assisted in keeping me sane in graduate school. My parents, Deb and Rob, and my sister Whitney, for being proud of my weird projects. And everyone at the Iowa State University Writing and Media Center, where I have found a great deal of belonging throughout my time working there as a writing consultant.

I want to thank the wonderful community of educational content creators at WeCreateEdu, especially Sheryl Hosler, Alie & Micah Caldwell, Matt Beat, Tristan Johnson, Aven McMaster, Mark Sundaram, and Jonathan Moore. And, finally, I want to thank my online friends for keeping me going during difficult IRL times, especially the citizens of FunkyTown.

Introduction

My first brain dissection taught me how fragile brains are. Through my too-thin gloves, I held a sheep's brain in its entirety, double-palm up as if I were cupping liquid. As I looked at the optic nerves that could no longer look at me, my own brain was racing. *This*? *How*?

When you examine the brain, you immediately notice that it comes in layers. To truly dissect one, you have to get inside and dismantle it. But, as I found out, a brain doesn't disassemble so gracefully. The layers and sections and structures are not like LEGO bricks, neatly popping free, one off of the other. Instead, the situation almost reminded me of how cotton candy melts away when you touch it with water. Frankly, the fragility is disturbing. I can't help but marvel that the engine powering my own thoughts as I write this (and you, dear reader, as you read this) is made up of the same fats and sugars and fluids that were putting up no resistance whatsoever to my dissection attempts.

In the days before brain dissection was a *careful* science, doctors could make names for themselves in the *creative* ways that they removed the skull and protective layers and revealed the natural structures of the brain. Franz Joseph Gall and his student Johann Spurzheim had quite an impact on the scientific field when they demonstrated their careful and meticulous dissection techniques (Lyons, 2009). So beautiful was their technique of procuring an undamaged brain from a head that perhaps the onlookers were persuaded to not look quite as closely as they would have at the pair's quack theories of phrenology that would rule the anatomy seminars for a while in the 1800s. Later, Spurzheim would be mocked for claiming to know what each part of the brain was for and that the bumps of the skull told stories of the mental abilities contained beneath. Spurzheim was right that specific parts of the brain seem to contribute to specific functions, but his downfall was that he went overboard with how specific the functions were to each part.

This idea that "specific parts do specific things" when it comes to locations and functions in the brain is called "the localization of functions." It is, to put it mildly, a war fought by neuropsychologists and related fields to create an atlas of the human brain that is neither too vague nor too specific. Unfortunately, the human brain continues to hide secrets. Advanced neuroimaging techniques for scanning the brain have lately been revealing that parts of the brain that

DOI: 10.4324/9781003276937-1

we thought we understood were doing *more* than we thought. Similarly, we continue to learn that the brain's parts are connected in additional ways that we didn't suspect. My point is that we are not even close to finishing the atlas of the human brain.

There's a good reason for having an unfinished brain atlas, and that reason is *ethics*. Scientists such as myself can't just go into people's heads and start cutting things out in order to see what happens. Rightly so! For that reason, as bad as it sounds, we researchers are actually somewhat thankful for the fragility of the brain. Why? Because that fragility allows us access to lots of people with different kinds of brain damage, who can be studied by neuropsychologists such as myself, in order to answer questions about how the human brain is organized and how it functions. Thus, neuropsychology unfortunately rests upon a foundation of human suffering, and I won't pretend otherwise. We do what we can to try and *learn* from that suffering.

Especially before the invention of advanced brain scanning techniques, most of what we knew about the functions of the human brain came from *case studies*, which are in-depth descriptions of people after they acquired brain damage. How did they change as people? What abilities did they lose? In the olden days, anatomists clambered at the chance to dissect the brains of people with rare symptoms in the hopes of discovering the secrets of the brain, and, therefore, filling in the brain atlas. Historically, this was done haphazardly, exploitatively, and sometimes even without the knowledge or permission of the person or their loved ones. Medical history is regrettably full of condemnable actions. Like I said, it truly has a foundation of human suffering. Today, researchers are much more respectful and obtain informed consent from the person with the symptoms or their family before writing about their lives.

In this book, we will revisit many of those older case studies, as well as make use of recent case studies and modern-day science, to try and glimpse answers to the mysteries of the brain. We can learn how brains work by comparing differences in damaged and undamaged brains. Thus, we will use brain damage as a lens into the inner workings of this marvelous and fragile organ. But while we are doing this, we must be *thankful*.

That is, please remember as you read about these incredible consequences of brain injury that these stories are about *real people*. I wish for readers to feel wonder while imagining the altered realities within, all while maintaining respect for the duration. I hope that this book showcases what these real people have taught us over the centuries, with respect and thanks. Please also note that they are only a fraction—many others struggle quietly with stories untold.

This book does not center around the *type* of damage to the brain itself, such as the all-too-common problems of strokes or tumors. Instead, I will focus on the *consequences* of the brain damage and remain somewhat agnostic about how it occurred—after all, there are many ways to damage such a fragile organ. Similarly, this book is not explicitly focused on recovering from brain damage. For discussing recovery, I recommend other books, such as *Adjusting to Brain Injury: Reflections from Survivors, Family Members and Clinicians* (Dawson et al., 2020).

Each chapter of this book can be read on its own, much like an encyclopedia entry. Every chapter introduces three or four case studies about people with the disorder, then proceeds to a description of the disorder, and closes out with a more in-depth discussion of the brain pathology (the underlying damage) itself. You'll be asked to imagine what your reality would be like if you had each disorder, and I urge you to think carefully about your own brain as you learn about what's possible.

Please note that I have constrained the topics of this particular book in a few ways. While I do believe that all conditions that a person experiences must necessarily involve the brain, I had to draw boundaries of inclusion and exclusion in order to prevent the number of chapters in this book from reaching infinity. As further described below, lines have been drawn to account for physicality, comorbidity, and consequence.

First, I have restricted the entries to conditions with evidence of *physical* damage. With apologies to neuropsychiatry, this precludes me from including many "mental illnesses," despite the fact that someday soon there may be good evidence of "physical damage" that leads to those so-called "functional" disorders. There is certainly a place for a discussion of mental illnesses and how they relate to the physical brain, but this book is not that place.

However, the observant reader may notice places in this book where the distinction between physical problems resulting from physical damage becomes blurred with problems becoming more functional and psychological in nature. As we will see, there are many blurred lines in the brain, and crossing into some gray areas is a matter of absolute necessity to tell certain stories.

Speaking of gray areas, many of these conditions can occur *comorbidly*, meaning that they can occur in the same brain. Because of the complex distribution of brain functions in adjacent regions of the brain, it is exceedingly rare (and some may argue, nearly impossible) to damage one function of the brain while keeping everything else intact. Classic case studies of patients with brain damage generally reveal multiple issues, and researchers try their best to group these issues into categories. But the categories are mere constructs invented by humans. Disorders of the brain, and natural mechanisms as a whole, do not follow the lines drawn by people; we just do our best to try and draw lines that fit what we see. For an enjoyable analysis of this frustrating aspect of scientific categories and the human condition, I recommend *Why Fish Don't Exist: A Story of Loss, Love, and the Hidden Order of Life* (Miller, 2020).

Therefore, for the sake of readability, I have drawn lines between disorders that are similar and have also grouped together disorders that are perhaps somewhat dissimilar. Again, I do hope that readers will keep in mind that these groupings do not necessarily reflect discrete physical groupings of brain damage but rather reflect the need for humans to pack complex geomorphic issues into well-sorted rectangles.

Additionally, there are disorders of the brain that are relatively well understood by science that are also outside the scope of this book. This is because a further criterion for inclusion in this book is that the entry is an experiential symptom, that is, a *consequence*. For example, Alzheimer disease, Parkinson disease, Lewy Body dementia, and many other neurodegenerative diseases are better understood in this book as the cause of the brain breaking rather than as a consequence of the broken brain itself. As such, some of the possible symptoms of those disorders may appear here (see Amnesia, Ataxia, etc.) but not grouped under their common syndromic name. Again, the lines here are blurry (for example, with Chronic Traumatic Encephalopathy). You could make a case that all neurodegenerative diseases are consequences of brain damage, but for the sake of this book, the line has been drawn just so.

I also want to address why the names of several disorders that are conventionally written with apostrophes have not been written that way (e.g., I have written Bálint syndrome instead of Bálint's syndrome). This is a somewhat philosophical issue that is personal for me; I believe that naming disorders after people (eponyms) should be avoided. Not only is using a person's name to describe a disorder unhelpful for understanding what the disorder actually is, but it can also result in confusion and even medical errors (McNulty et al., 2021). You could also make a pretty good argument that it is unreasonable or even unjust to imply that a person "owns" a disorder. I say this as someone whose own name has been the subject of confusion in the anatomical literature—the "Xander Ligament"—which was humorous at first, but enlightening afterward (Ledger & Toftness, 2020). Unfortunately, many of the eponyms in the neuropsychological literature are so ingrained that I cannot avoid them, although I have tried to reduce their presence by eliminating apostrophes and using some alternative terms. These eponyms, including my own, are something that I do at times elaborate on and even poke fun at within the pages of this book, but I wanted to make my position clear.

Finally, if you have feedback or a story to tell, reach out anytime. There's a good likelihood that there will be another edition of this book released in the future, so I'd love to hear from you. You should be able to find me around the internet pretty easily, especially via my YouTube video series paired with this book called *The Ways your Brain can Break* on my channel: *ARTexplains Science and History*.

References

Dawson, K., Sheikh, A., Hargreaves, K., Archer, M., & Summerill, L. (2020). *Adjusting to brain injury: Reflections from survivors, family members and clinicians*. Routledge.

Ledger, T., & Toftness, A. (2020). The Xander ligament? Caution advised when using online encyclopaedias. *Journal of Anatomy*, *237*(2), 391–391. https://doi.org/gh4hdh

Lyons, S. L. (2009). *Species, serpents, spirits, and skulls: Science at the margins in the Victorian age*. State University of New York Press.

McNulty, M. A., Wisner, R. L., & Meyer, A. J. (2021). NOMENs land: The place of eponyms in the anatomy classroom. *Anatomical Sciences Education, 14*(6), 847–852. https://doi.org/gkqzwr

Miller, L. (2020). *Why fish don't exist: A story of loss, love, and the hidden order of life.* Simon & Schuster.

Achromatopsia

Imagine that you woke up one day to literally find the world in shades of gray. The sunlight is gray, the trees are gray, your breakfast is gray. You find this dullness affects your mood as well as your appetite: who wants to drink gray orange juice or watch a gray sunrise? When you close your eyes, you can't even quite remember what colors used to look like. And when your eyes are open, your friends and loved ones are all ashen-looking, and all of your outfits look dirty and unappealing. You wonder whether the fruit you eat is ripe, because the color won't tell you. You feel like you're living in a period film: black and white and gray all over. But this is more intense than a black and white film, because the gray surrounds you constantly, and even your own body and dreams are affected. Where did the color go?

The Stories

(STORY 1) In a case from 1986, a 65-year-old painter who was known for his use of vivid color was in an auto accident. He lost his ability to see colors, and could no longer remember what color looked like. Colors also vanished from his dreams. At first, this painter found that he could not bear to look at people, such as his wife, because the color of their skin had become so strange-looking. He also refused to eat certain foods because they looked unappetizing without color, and preferred to eat foods that were black or white, such as coffee and yogurt. Eventually, he overcame some of these issues regarding people and food. He also began painting in black and white to match his new perceptions of the world following his *cerebral achromatopsia*. At one point, he created an entire three-dimensional scene including a gray table, gray chairs, and pieces of gray fruit in a room so that other people could get closer to experiencing what the world now looked like to him. He noted that even this did not quite express his condition completely, and that in order to better understand "the observer himself would have to be painted grey, so he would be part of the world, not just observing it" (Sacks, 1995, pp. 10–11). Eventually, he began experimenting with color paintings again, even though he could no longer see the colors (Sacks, 1995; Sacks & Wasserman, 1987).

DOI: 10.4324/9781003276937-2

(STORY 2) A 49-year-old man was giving himself a vigorous neck massage in 1977 when he suddenly felt an electrical prickling sensation in his neck and eyes. Immediately afterwards, he lost the ability to see color in the left half of his visual field. Colors on his right continued to appear colorful, while colors to his left were now only gray. When presented with a brightly colored object on the left, he could not see the color, until it passed over the center of his visual field towards his right, when he suddenly saw the color. When a large red flashlight was held in front of his center of vision, his *hemiachromatopsia* made it so that the right half of the flashlight appeared to be its true red color while the left half looked entirely gray (Damasio et al., 1980, case 1).

(STORY 3) In the year 1875, a 62-year-old man was walking around town when he had a sudden stroke that left him dizzy and seeing darkness—fortunately, he was helped back home and a doctor came to treat him. Nine days later, he went to an eye doctor to complain about changes in his vision. The doctor administered the usual tests and determined that his vision was relatively typical for a man of his age. The doctor wrote in a later case study that he did not understand why the man was complaining about his vision after his stroke because he seemed unimpaired. The doctor was baffled when the patient eventually revealed what was bothering him: he had completely lost the ability to see color ever since the stroke. The doctor tested him by showing him various colors of paper, but the patient reported that it was like trying to distinguish shades of dirty white from shades of gray. The patient had worked as a color printer, and had always had excellent abilities when it came to telling colors apart, so to suddenly lose that ability entirely was an upsetting fate for him. Over the years, he began to be able to tell some of the colors apart when they were very bright and presented against a pure white background—except for, curiously, the color green, which continued to elude him. This case was one of the earliest descriptions of *cerebral achromatopsia* (Steffan, 1881; Zeki, 1990).

The Features

As discussed at length by philosophers through the ages, color is created inside of your brain. That is, color does not exist outside of your head—it is not a part of the real world. What you are experiencing when you see color is just your brain sorting different waves of light into categories. But those categories—red, blue, green—are a product of your own unique brain. There is no real way of knowing if the color that you call red looks the same as the color that I call red (see Synesthesia). So, the next time that someone asks you whether you want white wine or red wine, make sure to reply that "color is a private concept," and recite what you learned in this chapter. This is a good way to change the number of dinner parties that you are invited to.

Because color is made by brains, there are animals that see colors that people will never truly see, such as butterflies and birds. What bonus colors can they see? I wish I could describe them, but I literally can't see them. Within the human color spectrum, the experience of color seems so natural to us that we rarely think about the brain processing necessary for us to truly *see* colors. That is, until the process breaks down.

Before getting into achromatopsia, let's discuss the milder condition of *colorblindness*. Colorblindness occurs when a person can see light but cannot distinguish one or more colors. This condition can begin *within the eyes*, or, more rarely, *within the brain* itself. The colorblindness that the average person is familiar with is the kind that exists in the eyes and is generally genetic. This type of colorblindness, such as common red-green colorblindness, exists from birth and is due to differences in the cells of the eye's *retina*, which is the part of the eye that catches incoming light.

You probably know at least a few people who are colorblind. Most likely they are male due to how common forms of colorblindness are found on the X chromosome. Because males have only one X chromosome, if the chromosome has colorblindness genes then they are stuck with colorblindness—but because females have two X chromosomes, even if one has colorblindness genes, they can compensate with the other chromosome. Colorblind females are therefore more rare because both of their X chromosomes need to carry colorblindness genes in order for them to develop the condition. In extremely rare cases, it is possible for a female with one colorblindness X chromosome to develop colorblindness in only *one eye* (Neitz & Neitz, 2017). This allows her to open and close her eyes one at a time in order to see the world while colorblind or in full color—which in turn allows her to describe to vision researchers what colorblindness actually looks like to someone who isn't colorblind.

There is also a type of complete colorblindness called *congenital achromatopsia*. These people cannot see any colors because their retina doesn't have the type of cells, called *cones*, that are responsible for color vision. In these cases, the person never experiences colors because they were born without the ability to see them. Their eyes are also extremely sensitive to bright light. Congenital achromatopsia is exceedingly rare, but because it is genetic, it can spread through families. Famously, there is an island in Micronesia called Pingelap where about one in 12 people have congenital achromatopsia. This is because a typhoon devastated the island around the year 1775 and greatly reduced the population, and thus, the gene pool. The colorblindness genes multiplied through the descendants of the 20 survivors—Oliver Sacks wrote all about it in his book *The Island of the Colorblind* (Sacks, 1996).

As is more relevant to this book about acquired conditions, it is also possible to be born with typical color vision but then lose it later in life due to brain damage. When severe colorblindness exists due to damage to the brain's cerebral cortex, it is called *cerebral achromatopsia*. In a person with cerebral achromatopsia, their eyes may be no different from a typical person's eyes. That is, the wavelengths of light are entering into their eyes, are turned into signals by the cone cells of the retina, and are sent into the brain. But the brain has forgotten how to turn those signals into perceptions of color. Because of this, these people typically lose the ability to even *imagine* colors (see Aphantasia), but there are exceptions (Bartolomeo et al., 1997).

Adjusting to cerebral achromatopsia takes some getting used to, as indicated by this quote from a person with the condition: "everything appears in various shades of grey. My shirts all look dirty and I can't tell one of them from the other. I have no idea which tie to wear" (Pallis, 1955, p. 219). That experience of colors being changed to look like "shades of grey" is common for people with acquired achromatopsia, but depending on the person and the damage, they may describe it differently, such as "nuances" of "reddish-brown" (Bartolomeo et al., 2014, p. 5).

However, it is not just the experience of what colors look like that may be damaged in a person's brain. A person may also lose *concepts* of colors, such as knowledge about colors or the ability to name colors (Bartolomeo, 2021).

Losing knowledge about colors is called *color agnosia*. In such cases, the person still perceives colors, unlike a person with achromatopsia. For example, they can tell that a shade of red and a shade of green are different from each other. But the person with color agnosia loses the ability to attribute colors to objects, because they have lost the ability to attach their knowledge about color to the object (Bartolomeo et al., 2014). In other words, a person with color agnosia can match and sort colored paper into piles, demonstrating that the colors look different, but they cannot *recognize* those colors (Lhermitte & Beauvois, 1973). Mismatching colors and objects, such as a green giraffe or a red pineapple, may not seem out of place to a person with color agnosia. They can perceive color, but it has been separated from their memories and feelings (Sacks & Wasserman, 1987).

Other disorders of color include *color anomia*, which is an inability to remember the names of colors (Zeki, 1990). When you perceive extra color instead of experiencing the absence of color, such as during a migraine (see Migraine Headaches), that is called *chromatopsia* (Azimova et al., 2016). It is also possible to have cerebral achromatopsia and not realize it (see Anosognosia). That is, you can become colorblind without realizing that you have become colorblind (von Arx et al., 2010). If you'll forgive the pun, I would say that conditions of color perception are quite colorful, and if you take one thing away from this chapter—to share at parties, of course—it's that color perception works a bit differently for everyone.

The Brain Pathology

Thanks to the work of scientists investigating historical cases of cerebral achromatopsia, we have a good idea of where in the brain the damage needs to be in order for this condition to occur (Bartolomeo, 2021). In an analysis of cerebral achromatopsia cases, a large amount of overlap in brain damage was found in an area called the ventral occipital cortex, located near the back and bottom of the brain (Bouvier & Engel, 2006). This region, sometimes called V4, is still being studied in order to determine exactly what its boundaries and subregions are, as well as the exact functions.

What we do know about V4 is that it receives color information from the eyes, and we can actually trace the path that this color information takes from the cones in the retina at the back of your eye, through the lateral geniculate pathway, to the blobs in your primary visual cortex (McIlwain, 1996). Yes, there are groups of cells in your brain to which we have assigned the technical term "blob." The blobs in your primary visual cortex have therefore already done some of the work of segregating color information from other visual information, and then pass that information on to V4 for further processing (Zeki, 1990). Other nearby areas of the brain, which have names like V2 and V8, are also believed to be somewhat involved in color processing (Bartolomeo et al., 2014). In short, when a person sees light, the perception of that light is processed in multiple steps in different places in the brain. It may seem odd, but this makes it possible for a person to have an intact ability to tell apart different wavelengths of light but without the ability to perceive color. This is why a person with cerebral achromatopsia may be able to see *gray tones*, but not color (Sacks & Wasserman, 1987).

Because your brain has one V4 region in each hemisphere, it is also possible for achromatopsia to exist in only part of your visual field. In other words, part of your vision—such as the left or right half—can have intact color vision while the other half has achromatopsia. You might, for example, be unable to tell what color a moving car is as it enters your vision from one side, but as it passes the midpoint, suddenly you are able to realize its color (Bouvier & Engel, 2006). This condition is called *hemiachromatopsia*.

Regardless of our current understanding, cerebral achromatopsia had a controversial history. Many researchers doubted its existence for nearly a century after it was first described in detail in the 1880s (Zeki, 1990). Some scientists weren't ready to believe that there was an area of the brain's cortex that was dedicated specifically to color processing. This was partly because most cases of cerebral achromatopsia occur at the same time as other vision problems, making it difficult to find a "pure" case of achromatopsia (see Visual Object Agnosia). Cerebral achromatopsia cases typically also include partial visual field scotomas (see Hemianopsia), such that the person also experiences partial blindness (Bouvier & Engel, 2006). Other visual recognition issues also commonly occur with cerebral achromatopsia, especially face blindness (see Prosopagnosia), word blindness (see Alexia), and more (Short & Graff-Radford, 2001). This may lead to a complicated constellations of symptoms beyond the fact that your world has been drained of color.

References

Azimova, J. E., Sergeev, A. V., Skorobogatykh, K. V., Klimov, E. A., Tabeeva, G. R., & Rachin, A. P. (2016). Alice-in-wonderland syndrome in patients with migraine. *British Journal of Medicine and Medical Research*, *13*(11), 1–11. https://doi.org/gs4n

Bartolomeo, P. (2021). Color vision deficits. *Current Neurology and Neuroscience Reports*, *21*(10), Article 58. https://doi.org/hgj3

Bartolomeo, P., Bachoud-Lévi, A.-C., & Denes, G. (1997). Preserved imagery for colours in a patient with cerebral achromatopsia. *Cortex, 33*(2), 369–378. https://doi.org/d46w52

Bartolomeo, P., Bachoud-Lévi, A. C., & Thiebaut de Schotten, M. (2014). The anatomy of cerebral achromatopsia: A reappraisal and comparison of two case reports. *Cortex, 56*, 138–144. https://doi.org/f59nm7

Bouvier, S. E., & Engel, S. A. (2006). Behavioral deficits and cortical damage loci in cerebral achromatopsia. *Cerebral Cortex, 16*(2), 183–191. https://doi.org/cqqcv4

Damasio, A., Yamada, T., Damasio, H., Corbett, J., & McKee, J. (1980). Central achromatopsia: Behavioral, anatomic, and physiologic aspects. *Neurology, 30*(10), 1064–1071. https://doi.org/gtht

Lhermitte, F., & Beauvois, M. F. (1973). A visual-speech disconnexion syndrome: Report of a case with optic aphasia, agnosic alexia and colour agnosia. *Brain, 96*(4), 695–714. https://doi.org/djhhwz

McIlwain, J. T. (1996). *An introduction to the biology of vision*. Cambridge University Press.

Neitz, J., & Neitz, M. (2017, May 7–11). *Colorblindness confined to one eye* [Conference session]. ARVO Annual Meeting (Investigative Ophthalmology & Visual Science, 58[8], Article 4298) Baltimore, MD, United States. https://bit.ly/38lj6Kr

Pallis, C. A. (1955). Impaired identification of faces and places with agnosia for colours: report of a case due to cerebral embolism. *Journal of Neurology, Neurosurgery, and Psychiatry, 18*(3), 218–224. https://doi.org/c4v5mb

Sacks, O. (1995). *An anthropologist on Mars*. Knopf.

Sacks, O. (1996). *The island of the colorblind*. Knopf.

Sacks, O., Wasserman, R. (1987, November 19). The case of the colorblind painter. *New York Review of Books, 34*, 25–34.

Short, R. A., & Graff-Radford, N. R. (2001). Localization of hemiachromatopsia. *Neurocase, 7*(4), 331–337. https://doi.org/drmbhh

Steffan, P. (1881). Beitrag zur Pathologie des Farbensinnes. *Albrecht von Græfe's Archiv Für Ophthalmologie, 27*(2), 1–24. https://doi.org/df8bfr

von Arx, S. W., Müri, R. M., Heinemann, D., Hess, C. W., & Nyffeler, T. (2010). Anosognosia for cerebral achromatopsia—A longitudinal case study. *Neuropsychologia, 48*(4), 970–977. https://doi.org/d4vhkk

Zeki, S. (1990). A century of cerebral achromatopsia. *Brain, 113*(6), 1721–1777. https://doi.org/b47g2f

Akinetic Mutism

Imagine that you don't generally move or speak, because you cannot seem to muster up the will to do so. If something happens in the environment around you, it might trigger you to respond, but otherwise you sit still and exist in one spot throughout the day. Perhaps there is a struggle inside of you to try and move or speak, but something else in your head prevents you from actually carrying out that action. Or, perhaps you don't mind either way, as if the acts of moving and speaking don't even occur to you as a possibility. Why has your will vanished?

The Stories

(STORY 1) A 71-year-old man was diagnosed with akinetic mutism following a severe stroke. Over a period of two years, he slowly began to recover, but in that time the medical workers were unsure whether he was refusing to speak to people, or if he had lost most of his ability to do so. Eventually, it became clear that he was capable of speaking in complete sentences, but that he rarely did so. He sometimes expressed his difficulties with *willing* himself to speak, such as when someone said "hello" to him and he replied with "I can't do it, I can't say hello" (p. 238). He had the ability to open his eyes and look at people when they spoke to him, but he rarely responded. Sometimes, he would complete the words to a song that he knew, and there were occasional periods where he would express complex thoughts, such as "something's happened to my brain" (Sinden et al., 2018, p. 239).

(STORY 2) In the case of a 35-year-old man with a severe head injury following a motorbike accident, *mutism* appeared along with occasional signs of impulsive behavior and a lack of emotional responses. His movements were slow, but he could gesture with his head and hands. He could sometimes respond appropriately to verbal commands, such as when told to wiggle his toes, but he did not always respond. The only times his case study noted speaking was when his wife or healthcare worker called him on the telephone. For example, when his psychiatrist asked him over the phone what he had for lunch, the patient responded by saying that he had "some crappy ham sandwich" (p. 610). However, when the psychiatrist then entered the room to try

DOI: 10.4324/9781003276937-3

and continue the conversation in person, the patient fell silent. He eventually began to recover, and was able to speak without the phone, eliminating the dramatic *telephone effect* (Yarns & Quinn, 2013).

(STORY 3) A woman contracted the mysterious illness "encephalitis lethargica" as a teenager in 1918, and slowly developed *akinesia* and almost total *mutism* (p. 67). Over the course of the next several decades, she spent her time in an institution, requiring complete nursing care. She would sit without blinking or moving for many hours at a time, for she was "almost unable to initiate any voluntary motion" (p. 69). She could not speak words but with "great effort" could make faint sounds (p. 68). She experienced total *apathy*, meaning that she was not feeling emotions, even in extreme situations such as when she was verbally or physically abused by other patients in the ward. She could be stood up and walked around with assistance but could not do so on her own. Taking steps on her own "was not only impossible, but somehow seemed *unthinkable*" (p. 69). She began therapy with a drug called L-DOPA in 1969 and experienced a major recovery. She recovered the ability to speak, respond emotionally, and even some fine motor control allowing her to write for the first time in 20 years, which allowed her to express what her experiences had been like. This is why we know about her feelings of effort and apathy. She wrote: "I ceased to have any moods … I forgot what it felt like to be happy or unhappy. Was it good or bad? It was neither. It was nothing" (p. 71). Her recovery is one of those shared in the famous book *Awakenings* by Oliver Sacks (Sacks, 1999, case MB).

The Features

Akinetic mutism describes people who are capable of moving, speaking, and engaging in other *goal-directed behaviors* but rarely choose to do so (Petersen & Posner, 2012). The term can descriptively apply to any person "in no mood for conversation lying quietly in bed,"—and haven't we all had days like that?—but in the realms of neuropsychology it refers to symptoms of brain damage (Segarra, 1970, p. 416). These people may have damaged *centers of motivation* in their brains, and so they do not often spontaneously take actions (Vickers et al., 2018). That is, they tend to spend *most* of their time lying quietly in bed.

Akinetic mutism is a type of *minimally conscious state* (see Coma and Disorders of Consciousness), but the person's ability to react to the environment around them is more intact in akinetic mutism than it is in other disorders of consciousness (Giacino et al., 2014). For example, people with akinetic mutism may respond appropriately to simple commands, they may make eye contact with a person who speaks to them, and they may follow moving objects with their eyes. For example, in describing what akinetic mutism looked like in a child, a team of researchers described that she had:

> an appearance of alertness so incongruous with her silence and general immobility … after urgent and repeated commands, she would make slow

and feeble attempts to carry out the requisite movement … her eyes were easily drawn towards any moving object or sound.

(Cairns et al., 1941, pp. 279–280)

These symptoms are some ways that akinetic mutism can be diagnosed (Rodríguez-Bailón et al., 2012).

Akinetic mutism can be subdivided into *akinesia* and *mutism* as two separate symptoms, although they frequently occur together. Akinesia is the lack of voluntary self-movements. In general, it refers to a person experiencing difficulties with *willing* themselves to move—that is, a difficulty in mustering enough willpower to generate a movement. They haven't lost the ability to move; they've just lost the ability to effectively command their muscles to move. In some cases, a person may not feel the will to move at all. In others, they may experience a curious sensation that whenever they "will" themselves to move, a sort of opposite "counter-will" also rises in them and prevents them from completing the motion (Sacks, 1999).

Mutism is similar in that the person finds it difficult to muster up the will to speak. They are not truly *mute*, however, because the person is still *capable* of speaking. They may experience an internal struggle as if part of them wishes to speak but some other part of them wishes not to. Or, they may show no interest in attempting to speak in the first place. In some people with akinetic mutism, there are situations that can overcome this mutism. One dramatic example of this is the *telephone effect* in which a person with this type of mutism can have a typical, fluid conversation over the phone even though they struggle to hold conversations face-to-face (Giacino et al., 2014).

Additionally, acts of thinking and emotional expression may also be reduced, except in the presence of high-intensity sensations or personally relevant events (Giacino et al., 2014). In other words, if something loud or sufficiently exciting happens, the person may react—and that reaction may be startling to healthcare workers, who may not have known that the person was capable of reacting in that way, such as suddenly moving or speaking after doing neither for extended periods of time.

The Brain Pathology

There are many different possible causes of akinetic mutism, including damage to the frontal lobes, brain stem, and/or thalamus regions, which can occur due to any brain-damaging event such as stroke, tumor, carbon monoxide poisoning, Creutzfeldt-Jakob disease (see Creutzfeldt-Jakob Disease), and many others (Herklots et al., 2016). In the brain, there are loops of communication lines between cells that, by sending signals back and forth to each other, can express a person's motivations to do something through taking action and actually doing that thing. The parts of your brain responsible for generating motivation are mostly located in the frontal lobe, but motivation involves many other brain regions as well (Arnts et al., 2020).

For example, when part of your brain decides that you want to speak, your brain needs to coordinate and send signals to other parts of your brain that control your jaw muscles and to the parts that understand language. Damage to any part of that circuit can result in difficulties with starting and continuing voluntary actions, such as speaking full sentences or standing up and walking (Vickers et al., 2018). More specifically, an area called the anterior cingulate cortex has two-way connections with decision-making regions of the frontal lobes and emotional regions of the limbic system and is thought to use that information for planning behaviors such as moving or talking, so damaging it may produce symptoms of reduced behavior (Arnts et al., 2020). Other regions that combine incoming signals from different places in the brain are the striatum and the thalamus, both of which are often involved in akinetic mutism (Arnts et al., 2020).

What makes akinetic mutism different from other disorders where you can't voluntarily move your muscles (see Locked-In Syndrome) is that in akinetic mutism, commands that come from other people can often *bypass the roadblocks in your brain*. In cases of akinetic mutism, if you are told to speak by someone outside of your brain such as a physician, it's easier for you to speak than if you tried to make it happen on your own. This may be because the connections in your brain that generate internal motivation to move or speak are different from the connections in your brain that relay signals from the outside world that may encourage you to move or speak. External signals like holding a telephone and hearing a voice on the other end may cue the brain to generate a response in a way that the brain cannot generate for itself without that external signal, thus explaining why some people with akinetic mutism experience a dramatic telephone effect (Vickers et al., 2018).

Some cases of akinetic mutism have been successfully treated using a variety of drugs, especially drugs that affect dopamine levels in the brain (Herklots et al., 2016). Over time, such as in other disorders of consciousness, a person may improve somewhat such that the symptoms of akinetic mutism become milder or disappear. However, treatment of akinetic mutism "remains difficult" (Arnts et al., 2020, p. 274). More research is needed in order to find ways to bring back the spark of motivation.

References

Arnts, H., van Erp, W. S., Lavrijsen, J. C. M., van Gaal, S., Groenewegen, H. J., & van den Munckhof, P. (2020). On the pathophysiology and treatment of akinetic mutism. *Neuroscience and Biobehavioral Reviews, 112*, 270–278. https://doi.org/gthv

Cairns, H., Oldfield, R. C., Pennybacker, J. B., & Whitteridge, D. (1941). Akinetic mutism with an epidermoid cyst of the 3rd ventricle. *Brain, 64*(4), 273–290. https://doi.org/bqpd84

Giacino, J. T., Fins, J. J., Laureys, S., & Schiff, N. D. (2014). Disorders of consciousness after acquired brain injury: The state of the science. *Nature Reviews Neurology, 10*(2), 99–114. https://doi.org/f5rqw3

Herklots, M. W., Oldenbeuving, A., Beute, G. N., Roks, G., & Schoonman, G. G. (2016). Lack of motivation: Akinetic mutism after subarachnoid haemorrhage. *Netherlands Journal of Critical Care*, *24*(3), 29–32.

Petersen, S. E., & Posner, M. I. (2012). The attention system of the human brain: 20 years after. *Annual Review of Neuroscience*, *35*, 73–89. https://doi.org/f3j3vw

Rodríguez-Bailón, M., Triviño-Mosquera, M., Ruiz-Pérez, R., & Arnedo-Montoro, M. (2012). Mutismo Acinético: Revisión, propuesta de un protocolo neuropsicológico para el diagnóstico diferencial y su aplicación a un caso. *Anales de Psicología*, *28*(3), 834–841. https://doi.org/gs4q

Sacks, O. (1999). *Awakenings*. Vintage Books.

Sinden, R., Wilson, B. A., Rose, A., & Mistry, N. (2018). Akinetic mutism and the story of David. *Neuropsychological Rehabilitation*, *28*(2), 234–243. https://doi.org/gs4p

Segarra, J. M. (1970). Cerebral vascular disease and behavior: The syndrome of the mesencephalic artery (basilar artery bifurcation). *Archives of Neurology*, *22*(5), 408–418. https://doi.org/dspq7k

Vickers, K. L., Keesler, M. E., Williams, K. S., Charles, J. Y., & Hamilton, R. H. (2018). The telephone effect: Overcoming initiation deficits in two settings. *Rehabilitation Psychology*, *63*(2), 215–220. https://doi.org/gdqmnd

Yarns, B. C., & Quinn, D. K. (2013). Telephone effect in akinetic mutism from traumatic brain injury. *Psychosomatics*, *54*(6), 609–610. https://doi.org/gthw

Akinetopsia

Imagine that you can't perceive movement. Pretend that you are trying to cross the street at a busy intersection full of cars. You can see the cars, and you can hear the cars whizzing by, but you cannot see them moving. Each time you look away and look back, you see a new position for each car. They seem to jump from place to place in surprising ways. Even though you can reasonably guess in which direction each car should be moving based upon its position, you just don't know for sure. Is that car parked, or is it cruising above the speed limit? When you close your eyes and concentrate on the noise, you can imagine where the cars must be. But to your visual brain, the world is standing still.

The Stories

(STORY 1) Drug-induced *akinetopsia* is a temporary but often startling experience. A 47-year-old man taking the drug nefazodone noticed strange things happening in his vision one day in 1997. He would see multiple frozen images of the same object trailing out behind any moving object. While he was walking his dog, he saw an unmoving trail of identical-looking West Highland terriers stretching out behind his dog as it moved. He found driving to be impossible due to seeing multiple images of cars and street signs. When his medications were adjusted, he stopped experiencing akinetopsia (Horton & Trobe, 1999, case 1). Similarly, a 48-year-old woman taking nefazodone noticed akinetopsia while moving her own body one morning in 1998. As she moved her arm, she described seeing multiple fuzzy copies of her limb. When she wasn't moving, her body looked as she expected it to look. The akinetopsia was most noticeable under dim light. The akinetopsia appeared and disappeared over a single day, and her medication was adjusted to prevent future recurrences (Horton & Trobe, 1999, case 2). People have also experienced drug-induced akinetopsia as trails of strange light as opposed to entire duplicated objects. Bright afterimages in the form of light trails may follow objects around, as they did in the case of a 22-year-old woman who was taking nefazodone around 1996. She reported that the light trails lasted for almost a second after the passing of the objects. She did not notice any other side effects, and after an adjustment to her medication, the unusual visual lightshow disappeared (Kraus, 1996).

DOI: 10.4324/9781003276937-4

(STORY 2) Following a stroke, a 37-year-old woman developed problems with seeing motion. She reported seeing "a smear or cloud" around fast-moving objects (p. 514). Yet, she could see some slow-moving objects. A group of researchers administered some visual tests in order to determine the speed of motion at which she struggled. She viewed continuously moving blocks on a computer screen and was able to report the direction of movement—up, down, left, or right—with 100% accuracy when the movement was slow. However, when the moving blocks were sped up to be faster, she began making mistakes. Interestingly, every mistake that she made was in the opposite direction of the true movement of the blocks, suggesting that her brain was correctly detecting at least the axis of movement: up-down or left-right. The researchers suggested in their report that this person may be experiencing a version of the wagon wheel illusion, where the movement of a rotating wheel may be perceived as spinning backward when viewed under a strobe light or filmed at a particular frame rate. Essentially, she may be detecting motion in the opposite direction because her brain is successfully processing some, but not all, of the information coming into her eyes when looking at objects (Heutink et al., 2019).

(STORY 3) In the most classic case of akinetopsia, a woman who suffered a stroke in 1978 reported becoming unable to see motion. She found it exceedingly difficult to cross the street because she could not judge the speed of cars. When looking at a car, it first seemed far away, and then suddenly seemed much closer. She worked around this by using her sense of hearing to try and determine where the cars were and how fast they were moving (Zihl et al., 1983). She could report the color, license plate, and model of each car, showing that motionless visual information was still being processed by her brain. Events such as having a face-to-face conversation with a person felt more like talking to them on the phone, she described, because she could not see their facial expressions as they changed (Ramachandran & Blakeslee, 1998). On days when there were many people at the supermarket, shopping became almost impossible. In situations like that, people would seemingly change position around her so suddenly that she would become confused. She reported that "people, dogs, and cars appear restless, are suddenly here and then there, but disappear in between," and performing activities that involved movement such as cutting bread and using a vacuum cleaner ended up taking her a long time to accomplish (Zihl & Heywood, 2015, p. 4). She also had trouble "pouring tea or coffee into a cup because the fluid appeared to be frozen, like a glacier … she could not stop pouring at the right time since she was unable to perceive the movement in the cup" (Zihl et al., 1983, p. 315). This case was key to our understanding of the neuroscience of how the brain creates movement vision (Zihl & Heywood, 2015).

The Features

The movement that you see around you is created by your brain to help you to navigate and understand the world. Your eyes only pick up small pieces of two-dimensional light patterns—it is your brain's job to stitch them together into a moving picture by capturing light patterns over *time*. This is similar to how a movie is made up of individual still pictures, but with enough frames displayed fast enough, your brain creates movement.

The difference, of course, is that real-world objects do actually move through space while Batman is a series of flat patches of light on a screen— notice that your brain doesn't mind this difference and creates the perception of movement either way. Your brain's job is much harder than it appears, because when the pictures taken in by your eyes reach your visual centers at the back of your brain, the pictures are flat, upside down, and riddled with holes of missing information. The brain usually restores these damaged photos into pristine high-definition three-dimensional footage so seamlessly that you don't even think about it. But, because your brain must actively create the perception of movement, your ability to see movement can be damaged.

Akinetopsia is an extremely rare disorder in which a person loses the ability to perceive movement. This loss of movement perception occurs in all three dimensions: up-down, left-right, and back-forth. Generally, this loss of movement does not depend on whether the person is looking directly at the object or if they are looking somewhere else when the object moves in their peripheral vision. Instead of objects looking like they are smoothly moving from one position to another, unmoving objects may be perceived as *jumping* suddenly from place to place like freeze-frames in a movie (Sakurai et al., 2013). This disorder is probably best illustrated by, perhaps ironically, a video, which is why I have created one over on my *ARTexplains Science and History* YouTube channel (Toftness, 2018).

Quite often, objects will show up multiple times in the vision of a person with akinetopsia, because the brain is tricked into deciding that there are multiple similar-looking objects instead of one moving object. Because of this, the person may see duplicate unmoving images of the same animals, items, or people. People with akinetopsia generally compensate for the loss of movement vision by using touch and hearing, both of which can help them to locate the exact positions of objects (Zihl et al., 1983). For example, objects that make noise such as cars sound louder when they are closer, which can help a person figure out whether they are approaching or moving away.

Similar to akinetopsia is the *Zeitraffer phenomenon*, which is the altered perception of the speed of moving objects (see Alice in Wonderland Syndrome), such as the perception of objects moving more slowly than they are actually moving (Ovsiew, 2014). There also exists a perception distortion that is the opposite of akinetopsia, simply called *kinetopsia*, in which a person perceives movement that is not really happening (Laff et al., 2003).

The Brain Pathology

There have been reports of akinetopsia resulting from a variety of causes, in addition to typical brain lesions such as from strokes (Ardila, 2016). A drug called nefazodone, which has been used to treat depression, has caused temporary akinetopsia in patients, which ends after they stop using the drug (Horton & Trobe, 1999). Akinetopsia has also been reported as occurring as a symptom of epileptic seizures (see Seizures), with the ability to perceive motion returning after the seizure subsides (Sakurai et al., 2013). Additionally, symptoms similar to akinetopsia can result from neurodegenerative diseases such as Alzheimer disease (Tsai & Mendez, 2009).

Unlike many other types of brain damage, researchers have a pretty good idea of which part of the brain can be damaged in order to cause this disorder. In the human brain's visual cortex, located at the back of the brain in the occipital lobe, there is a collection of visual system areas that have been given names such as V1 and V2. One of these regions is called V5, and it seems to be partly responsible for a person's ability to observe motion because it contains cells that react to movement in specific directions (Newsome et al., 1990). The cells of V5 are highly interconnected with other visual regions such as the primary visual cortex, called V1. In situations where brain damage is specific to V5 while sparing surrounding brain tissues such as V1, akinetopsia can occur (Haque et al., 2018). Much of the crucial brain mapping research leading up to these conclusions was performed on monkeys, where researchers were able to selectively damage their brains and observe motion blindness (Zeki, 1991).

One reason that we know that the perception of visual motion depends on how area V5 communicates with area V1 is that we can temporarily disrupt the communication between these areas using a technique called transcranial magnetic stimulation (TMS). When TMS is applied to V5, it interrupts the communication of the brain cells located there, and the person experiences temporary akinetopsia. Anyone can experience motion blindness with the correct application of magnets. It is also possible to cause motion blindness in one half of a person's vision at a time, by using TMS on only one half of the brain (Beckers & Hömberg, 1992).

There are other areas of the brain that play roles in the detection of movement which can help compensate for damage to V5. Because other areas contribute to the perception of motion, akinetopsia is unusual among brain damage in that it is generally not permanent. The amount of time that it takes to recover motion perception after damage to V5 depends on the amount of brain damage. For example, in a stroke, recovery depends on the size of the brain lesion that develops. In cases where damage was done to a large region, the motion blindness can become mostly permanent with only partial recovery (Shipp et al., 1994). In some cases, even after the experience of akinetopsia goes away, there are still detectable abnormalities in the way the person tracks moving objects with their eyes (Cooper et al., 2012). So, the next time that you catch a moving object in your hand, or watch as a movie tricks your brain into seeing movement, spare a moment to think about how hard your brain is working to smooth out those movements.

References

Ardila, A. (2016). Some unusual neuropsychological syndromes: Somatoparaphrenia, akinetopsia, reduplicative paramnesia, autotopagnosia. *Archives of Clinical Neuropsychology*, *31*(5), 456–464. https://doi.org/gkx9s3

Beckers, G., & Hömberg, V. (1992). Cerebral visual motion blindness: transitory akinetopsia induced by transcranial magnetic stimulation of human area V5. *Proceedings of the Royal Society of London B*, *249*(1325), 173–178. https://doi.org/b8cs69

Cooper, S. A., Joshi, A. C., Seenan, P. J., Hadley, D. M., Muir, K. W., Leigh, R. J., & Metcalfe, R. A. (2012). Akinetopsia: Acute presentation and evidence for persisting defects in motion vision. *Journal of Neurology, Neurosurgery & Psychiatry*, *83*(2), 229–230. https://doi.org/chgr7c

Haque, S., Vaphiades, M. S., & Lueck, C. J. (2018). The visual agnosias and related disorders. *Journal of Neuro-Ophthalmology*, *38*(3), 379–392. https://doi.org/gfq3xf

Heutink, J., de Haan, G., Marsman, J. B., van Dijk, M., & Cordes, C. (2019). The effect of target speed on perception of visual motion direction in a patient with akinetopsia. *Cortex*, *119*, 511–518. https://doi.org/gthx

Horton, J. C., & Trobe, J. D. (1999). Akinetopsia from nefazodone toxicity. *American Journal of Ophthalmology*, *128*(4), 530–531. https://doi.org/cwdrcb

Kraus, R. P. (1996). Visual "trails" with nefazodone treatment. *The American Journal of Psychiatry*, *153*(10), 1365–1366. https://doi.org/gthz

Laff, R., Mesad, S., & Devinsky, O. (2003). Epileptic kinetopsia: Ictal illusory motion perception. *Neurology*, *61*(9), 1262–1264. https://doi.org/gs4r

Newsome, W. T., Britten, K. H., Salzman, C. D., & Movshon, J. A. (1990). Neuronal mechanisms of motion perception. *Cold Spring Harbor Symposia on Quantitative Biology*, *55*, 697–705. https://doi.org/fzssjz

Ovsiew, F. (2014). The Zeitraffer phenomenon, akinetopsia, and the visual perception of speed of motion: A case report. *Neurocase*, *20*(3), 269–272. https://doi.org/gs4s

Ramachandran, V. S., & Blakeslee, S. (1998). *Phantoms in the brain: Probing the mysteries of the human mind*. William Morrow.

Sakurai, K., Kurita, T., Takeda, Y., Shiraishi, H., & Kusumi, I. (2013). Akinetopsia as epileptic seizure. *Epilepsy & Behavior Case Reports*, *1*, 74–76. https://doi.org/gs4t

Shipp, S., Jong, B. D., Zihl, J., Frackowiak, R. S. J., & Zeki, S. (1994). The brain activity related to residual motion vision in a patient with bilateral lesions of V5. *Brain*, *117*(5), 1023–1038. https://doi.org/fmzw3c

Toftness, A. R. (2018). *Motion blindness - Akinetopsia. The ways your brain can break* [Video]. https://www.youtube.com/watch?v=2P3cg6St5nM

Tsai, P. H., & Mendez, M. F. (2009). Akinetopsia in the posterior cortical variant of Alzheimer disease. *Neurology*, *73*(9), 731–732. https://doi.org/b53c3r

Zeki, S. (1991). Cerebral akinetopsia (visual motion blindness) a review. *Brain*, *114*(2), 811–824. https://doi.org/dxkt9n

Zihl, J., & Heywood, C. A. (2015). The contribution of LM to the neuroscience of movement vision. *Frontiers in Integrative Neuroscience*, *9*, Article 6. https://doi.org/gs4v

Zihl, J., Von Cramon, D., & Mai, N. (1983). Selective disturbance of movement vision after bilateral brain damage. *Brain*, *106*(2), 313–340. https://doi.org/fjr2bs

Alexia

Imagine if you couldn't read. Duis tristique ex sit amet vulputate lobortis. Duis odio turpis, tempor id leo nec, ullamcorper placerat quam. In egestas elit id eros placerat cursus. Maecenas ipsum nunc, auctor et odio in, imperdiet ultricies turpis. Maecenas accumsan commodo felis, vel vehicula sem semper tristique. Vestibulum facilisis enim eu lobortis semper. Praesent in velit in sapien ultricies scelerisque. Donec in augue eget risus elementum iaculis eget id turpis. Cras pellentesque, sem ac fringilla ullamcorper, eget consequat nisl lectus at leo.

The Stories

(STORY 1) A 67-year-old man who suffered seizures after a stroke lost the ability to read even the simplest of words, a *global alexia*, and also developed complete blindness in the right half of his visual field. However, his ability to write was intact, albeit with some spelling mistakes. He could write down his own thoughts as well as sentences spoken out loud by others. When he was asked to copy over other writings, he did so by carefully reproducing each letter line by line, much like drawing a picture. Curiously, even though he could not tell the difference between the letters of the alphabet—his accuracy in naming them when he saw them was only 46%—he was still able to reliably tell the difference between real letters and fake letters made up of various line segments. It seemed that he could look at a letter and know that it was *a* letter but struggled to determine *which* letter it was (Chanoine et al., 1998).

(STORY 2) A 65-year-old bilingual man lost the ability to read Japanese kanji and kana in 1997, while still having some preserved ability to read in English. His first language was Japanese as he was originally from Japan, meaning that he surprisingly retained the use of his secondary language instead of the one that he had learned first as a child. He had lived in an English-speaking country for more than seven years and had been fluent in both languages since the time of his schooling. He was tested by researchers on a variety of tasks involving the English alphabet and comparable Japanese words using the kana alphabet, revealing a language-dependent *alexia without agraphia* in which he could write in both languages but struggled immensely to read in only one of them (Ohno et al., 2002).

DOI: 10.4324/9781003276937-5

(STORY 3) A medical doctor developed *alexia without agraphia* following a stroke. After a couple of months of recovery, he was able to read single words slowly but continued to struggle with reading in general. For example, longer words were much more challenging for him to read than were shorter words. However, his writing of words was shown to be without error. Nine months after the brain injury, the doctor began training his reading skills at a rehabilitation center for brain injuries. He made some measurable gains in reading speeds across a few weeks of nearly daily effort. He was able to return to his work as a doctor, albeit working reduced hours. The act of reading emails, books, and newspapers was immensely difficult and time-consuming for him. He found that he could still write short messages on the computer and by hand but found difficulties when he later tried to read what he had written (Starrfelt et al., 2010; Wilms, 2015).

The Features

Reading is relatively new to the human repertoire of skills, which makes it an especially interesting brain function. I love all of my brain functions equally, but reading? Reading is special. And I'm not just saying that because I'm a book. Glancing very quickly at a grouping of connected lines, dots, and loops leads to a remarkably fast transfer of information from ink on paper or pixels on a screen into your brain where you can understand a concept written down by someone who could be continents or years removed from your location in space or time. As flabbergasting as this ability is, it should come as no surprise that there are people who cannot successfully do it. But what *may* come as a surprise is that there are people who used to be able to read but lost that ability, despite still being able to *write*.

Alexia is defined as a condition where a person loses the ability to read due to brain damage, and the word literally means "without reading." The word alexia may remind you of a similar word: dyslexia, which means "impaired reading." Technically, the term "acquired dyslexia" is also sometimes used to refer to cases of brain damage that result in reading difficulties, and there is an overlap (Coslett, 2003). For simplicity's sake, this chapter always uses the word alexia. The name of the disorder will become complicated enough once we consider the different subtypes.

Most of the time, the person with alexia also loses their skill of writing. This loss of writing ability is called *agraphia* (see Gerstmann Syndrome). It seems natural for a person to lose the abilities to read and write at the same time when they acquire brain damage; however, these conditions can be independent. When one condition occurs by itself, it is sometimes called *pure agraphia* or *pure alexia*. In order to help with clarifying exactly what the conditions are, sometimes the various forms of the disorder are literally called *alexia with agraphia*, *alexia without agraphia*, and *agraphia without alexia*. Who says neuropsychology names can't be intuitive?

Alexia without agraphia is relatively uncommon, but it is so intriguing to researchers that it has been called the "most studied" of the various acquired reading disorders (Starrfelt & Shallice, 2014, p. 367). Such cases frequently lead to moments where the person can write something down to help themselves remember it, but then they struggle to decipher it later. It gets even more specific. A person with alexia without agraphia usually struggles to *copy* writing by looking at it, but they *are* able to write when dictated to, such as when they are told to write something down, and they can also write spontaneously on their own (Lhermitte & Beauvois, 1973). If they don't overthink it and just let their muscles and brain produce the writing, it can flow like magic, even though technically they have little to no idea what the letters themselves mean.

To get even more nuanced, alexia can affect just the ability to read entire words, or it may also affect the ability to read individual letters. If a person also loses the ability to read individual letters, this is referred to as *global alexia*, which is the most severe type (Hux & Mahrt, 2019). But, more often, people with alexia retain the ability to identify individual letters and symbols while losing the ability to read entire words at once. In the case of kanji characters, which is a system of Japanese writing that can be read in multiple ways, it is possible to lose the ability to read the kanji together (*on* reading) but to retain individual character reading (*kun* reading; Yoshida et al., 2020). The typical person with alexia also has an impairment in the reading of numbers as well (Starrfelt & Behrmann, 2011). Alexia may also include the loss of understanding of symbols such as musical notes and mathematical figures (Joy, 1947).

The telltale sign of alexia without agraphia is increased reading time for longer words. Usually, when a person without alexia reads words, their reading speed does not depend very much on the length of the words because their brain processes words as a whole. So, reading the word "elephant" usually takes roughly the same amount of time to read as the word "bear," even though one is twice as long. In contrast, when a person with alexia without agraphia reads a word, they tend to puzzle through each individual letter slowly and in sequence. They may say the names of the letters out loud as they read, and confuse letters with alike shapes, similar to how a person first learns to read before beginning to recognize whole words (Coslett, 2003). In severe cases, a person with alexia might take a minute to read a single word (Farah, 2004). People with alexia are also slower at reading jumbled up words and nonsense words (Pflugshaupt et al., 2011).

There are also cases where people were capable of reading in multiple languages, but after brain damage, lost the ability to read in one language to a more severe extent when compared to a preserved ability to read in another language (e.g., Hinshelwood, 1902; Ohno et al., 2002). That is, brain damage can selectively reduce your ability to read a *specific* language.

The Brain Pathology

The underlying causes of alexia have been discussed since the 1800s, with a Frenchman named Déjerine reporting two different causes for two different patients: one had alexia with agraphia, and the other had alexia without agraphia (Déjerine, 1891). His theories seem to have been basically correct, although some modern tweaks have been made.

Alexia without agraphia is usually understood as a disconnection between the part of the brain that sees the words as visual input and the part of the brain that understands the words as language. Most notably, there is a region in the middle fusiform gyrus that, when damaged, is a very good predictor of alexia (Martinaud, 2017). That middle fusiform gyrus damage is usually on the left side of the brain, but there are a few cases where damage to this area in the right hemisphere can also cause alexia (Leśniak et al., 2014).

Alexia with agraphia seems to occur due to damage to the language area itself, in the region of the angular gyrus, usually on the left side of the brain (Swanberg et al., 2003). This is an area heavily associated with aphasia (see Aphasia) as well, and so these disorders often occur together, with a person finding difficulty with speaking, reading, and writing.

This seemingly neat division is not the end of the story, however. Other types of underlying damage that cause forms of alexia have also been theorized. Some alexia may be a variant of simultagnosia (see Bálint Syndrome) in which the person has difficulties with seeing more than one letter at the same time (Starrfelt et al., 2010). Some alexia may be due to inattention to the entire visual field (see Hemispatial Neglect) causing the person to miss information from certain parts of the page (Swanberg et al., 2003). Some alexia may also be due to damage to a part of the fusiform area that specifically processes the form of words (see Visual Object Agnosia), which might help account for cases of global alexia in which single letters become extremely difficult to read (Barton, 2011).

Is it possible to recover from alexia? In many cases, some improvements can be made to reading accuracy and reading speed (e.g., Hux & Mahrt, 2019; Wilms, 2015). For people who retain the ability to read individual letters, they may develop a slow strategy of reading words letter by letter in order to regain some reading ability with practice (Martinaud, 2017). People sometimes learn to incorporate alternative senses such as touch and movement—a person may learn to better identify letters by first tracing the letter onto their own skin to feel the shape before identifying it (Starrfelt et al., 2013). Taking it slowly may be the key to reteaching your brain how to turn the squiggles and blots that are letters back into words.

References

Barton, J. J. (2011). Disorder of higher visual function. *Current Opinion In Neurology*, *24*(1), 1–5. https://doi.org/bbnvw3

Chanoine, V., Ferreira, C. T., Demonet, J. F., Nespoulous, J. L., & Poncet, M. (1998). Optic aphasia with pure alexia: A mild form of visual associative agnosia? A case study. *Cortex*, *34*(3), 437–448. https://doi.org/bs6scd

Coslett, H. B. (2003). Acquired dyslexia: A disorder of reading. In M. D'Esposito (Ed.), *Neurological foundations of cognitive neuroscience* (pp. 109–127). MIT Press.

Déjerine, J. (1891). Sur un cas de cécité verbale avec agraphie suivi d'autopsie. *Mémoires de la Société de Biologie*, *3*, 197–201.

Farah, M. J. (2004). *Visual agnosia* (2nd ed.). MIT press.

Hinshelwood, J. (1902). Four cases of word blindness. *The Lancet*, *149*(4093), 358–363. https://doi.org/bdssgc

Hux, K., & Mahrt, T. (2019). Alexia and agraphia intervention following traumatic brain injury: A single case study. *American Journal of Speech-Language Pathology*, *28*(3), 1152–1166. https://doi.org/gth2

Joy, H. H. (1947). Agnostic alexia without agraphia, following trauma. Report of a case. *Transactions of the American Ophthalmological Society*, *45*, 292–312.

Leśniak, M., Soluch, P., Stępień, U., Czepiel, W., & Seniów, J. (2014). Pure alexia after damage to the right fusiform gyrus in a right-handed male. *Neurologia i Neurochirurgia Polska*, *48*(5), 373–377. https://doi.org/gth3

Lhermitte, F., & Beauvois, M. F. (1973). A visual-speech disconnexion syndrome: Report of a case with optic aphasia, agnosic alexia and colour agnosia. *Brain*, *96*(4), 695–714. https://doi.org/djhhwz

Martinaud, O. (2017). Visual agnosia and focal brain injury. *Revue Neurologique*, *173*(7–8), 451–460. https://doi.org/gth4

Ohno, T., Takeda, K., Kato, S., & Hirai, S. (2002). Pure alexia in a Japanese-English bilingual: dissociation between the two languages. *Journal of Neurology*, *249*(1), 105–107. https://doi.org/cs4f47

Pflugshaupt, T., Suchan, J., Mandler, M. A., Sokolov, A. N., Trauzettel-Klosinski, S., & Karnath, H. O. (2011). Do patients with pure alexia suffer from a specific word form processing deficit? Evidence from 'wrods with trasnpsoed letetrs'. *Neuropsychologia*, *49*(5), 1294–1301. https://doi.org/b7cqfn

Starrfelt, R., & Behrmann, M. (2011). Number reading in pure alexia—A review. *Neuropsychologia*, *49*(9), 2283–2298. https://doi.org/bmf5z7

Starrfelt, R., Habekost, T., & Gerlach, C. (2010). Visual processing in pure alexia: A case study. *Cortex*, *46*(2), 242–255. https://doi.org/cvvqdc

Starrfelt, R., Olafsdóttir, R. R., & Arendt, I. M. (2013). Rehabilitation of pure alexia: A review. *Neuropsychological Rehabilitation*, *23*(5), 755–779. https://doi.org/gs4m

Starrfelt, R., & Shallice, T. (2014). What's in a name? The characterization of pure alexia. *Cognitive Neuropsychology*, *31*(5–6), 367–377. https://doi.org/gs4k

Swanberg, M. M., Nasreddine, Z. S., Mendez, M. F., & Cummings, J. L. (2003). Speech and language. In C. G. Goetz (Ed.), *Textbook of clinical neurology* (2nd ed., pp. 77–97). Saunders.

Wilms, I. L. (2015). Case study into the effect of intensive mass training on chronic pure alexia. *International Journal of Neurorehabilitation*, *2*(2), Article 162. https://doi.org/gth5

Yoshida, M., Hayashi, T., Fujii, K., Ishiura, H., Tsuji, S., & Sakurai, Y. (2020). Selective impairment of On-reading (Chinese-style pronunciation) in alexia with agraphia for kanji due to subcortical hemorrhage in the left posterior middle temporal gyrus. *Neurocase*, 1–7. https://doi.org/gth6

Alice in Wonderland Syndrome

Imagine that the size and shape of the objects around you kept changing. One moment, the chair next to you could seem perfectly normal and then suddenly appear as if it had shrunk to the size of an egg. Looking at your outstretched hand, it may well look far off in the distance. Straight lines become waves, and wavy lines straighten out such that you can't tell whether a piece of clothing is wrinkled or not. Your head feels as if it is getting bigger as the room feels smaller and smaller. You rub your eyes and look again, but you still feel too big, out of place, in Wonderland.

The Stories

(STORY 1) In the case of an 11-year-old boy, there were many short instances of Alice in Wonderland syndrome distortions lasting a few minutes at a time. Sometimes they included *time distortions* such as feeling as if everyone was talking too fast, or as if objects around him were moving too fast, or as if he himself was moving too fast. Other times they were *visual distortions* such as feeling as if his body was growing and becoming too large. Other distortions included sometimes feeling like he was holding a heavy object when he wasn't. Because these symptoms occurred just before he got headaches, it seems that the most likely culprit was migraines (Golden, 1979, case 2).

(STORY 2) In a 61-year-old man, Alice in Wonderland syndrome developed after he had a stroke. He began to feel as if the right side of his body was half the length of the left side of his body and that the right side of his body weighed less than the left side. This distortion is specifically known as *microsomatognosia*, when a part of the body is distorted as feeling too small. He also felt that objects, when held in his right hand versus his left hand, weighed less and were smaller. He avoided using the stairs because he was afraid of falling down, because walking with what felt like two different-sized legs was difficult for him (Kawase et al., 2013).

(STORY 3) A 9-year-old boy reported many strange feelings about the shape of his own body, each lasting about 15 minutes. Sometimes he would feel as if his head was too small. He occasionally felt as if he were too tall and too far away from the ground, or otherwise, he felt that he was shrinking. He

DOI: 10.4324/9781003276937-6

also reported feeling that his hand might suddenly grow and feel huge, way too big for his body. He would often feel that sounds were too loud and have terrible headaches. Later, it was found that he was actually experiencing seizures which were triggering the distortions (Kitchener, 2004, case 1).

(STORY 4) A young boy began experiencing Alice in Wonderland syndrome at the age of ten following an infection that caused scarlet fever. One symptom that he regularly experienced was "that he perceived objects as reduced in size but at the correct distance and proportion" (p. 3). These episodes of *micropsia* often lasted longer than 20 minutes and occurred multiple times per day across many months. When he was 12 years old, he was placed in an fMRI scanner during an episode of micropsia. When compared to the brain of a child that was not experiencing micropsia, the scan revealed a reduction of brain activity in some parts of the brain that process visual information and an increase in brain activity elsewhere. The cause of the micropsia was unknown, but some type of migraine was one possible explanation as the child often experienced periods of aversion to sound and light such as many people with migraines experience. He did not, however, have a history of migraine headaches, leaving the case a mystery. As treatment, he began to wear glasses that increased the size of nearby objects during his micropsia episodes, which helped him feel more comfortable but did not prevent the episodes from recurring (Brumm et al., 2010).

The Features

Being able to determine the size of something by looking at it is an amazing ability, but it is generally something that we take for granted. It isn't until we look at an optical illusion that disrupts our ability to tell how big something is, such as a picture of two regular-sized people in a room where one looks huge and the other looks small (the Ames room illusion), that we begin to appreciate the secret work that our brain is doing to help us understand how far away and how large objects are. A lot of that secret work depends on *top-down processing*, which is when your brain uses your knowledge about previous experiences to help inform you about what new information must mean. For example, the size of your hand is (mostly) unchanging, and this is something that you know, so you can use your hand to reasonably guess the size of objects when you can see both your hand and the object at the same time. But in some situations, this process of reasoning through the size of objects is disrupted, leading to some disorienting experiences.

Alice in Wonderland syndrome is an unsettling experience of *distortions* due to events in your brain. More specifically, Alice in Wonderland syndrome refers to a collection of over 60 different distortions, of which a person will experience one or more (Blom et al., 2021).

Distortions are different from hallucinations and illusions. A hallucination is a perception based only on activity in your brain that tricks you into experiencing something that isn't even there at all, like hearing a voice when there are no sound waves. An illusion occurs when a sensation from the environment enters your brain but is misperceived, such as when you look at an unmoving optical illusion but it appears to be moving—your brain is misinterpreting the image. But a distortion, on the flip side, is when a sensation from the environment is *altered* by the brain in a specific way, such as making all straight lines seem wavy. Thus, in Alice in Wonderland syndrome, your brain is responsible for warping the world around you.

As some example distortions, a person with this syndrome might perceive the growing and shrinking of objects, the strange passage of time, feelings of sped-up movement of objects or the self (sometimes called *zooming*), and the distortion of their own body image and the space around them, such that their limbs may seem too big or small or far away (Kitchener, 2004).

The key feature to understand here is that these distortions feel extremely real to the person experiencing them. They may be frightening while they are happening. For example, one 11-year-old girl wrote in her diary that, during an episode, she felt as if she was having a nightmare and tried to go tell her mother, but the journey to her mother's room was bizarre:

> I grabbed my door—it felt about one foot thick… as I went through the hall, it felt as if I was going too fast… I felt like my hands were made out of tiny twigs… I felt like I was holding things.
>
> (Golden, 1979, case 1, p. 517)

Thus, the symptoms can vary wildly and may be altogether disturbing.

Even though many different experiences are possible in Alice in Wonderland syndrome, there are some patterns to the specific distortions. Two of the most common visual distortions of this syndrome are distorting objects as being larger than normal and distorting them as being smaller than normal, which are respectively called *macropsia* and *micropsia* (Blom, 2016). For example, a person with Alice in Wonderland syndrome might perceive a horse to be the size of a cat, or a cat to be the size of a horse. Another common visual distortion is *teleopsia*, in which objects appear further away than they actually are, and this can occur even with the person's own body parts. Less common is *pelopsia*, in which objects appear closer than they actually are.

Interestingly, these visual distortions often occur after the person has already been looking at an object for some time, and then suddenly it looks different. For example, if you were looking at a tree and it looked far away, it might suddenly look like it is much closer to you. A good way to imagine this is with the Necker cube illusion. When you draw a two-dimensional cube by connecting two squares, it looks three-dimensional. But there are two ways that the cube can appear three-dimensional, with either one of the squares appearing to be the front of the cube. As you stare at the cube, your viewpoint may suddenly shift from one viewpoint to the other, but you can only experience one viewpoint at a time. This is similar to how someone with Alice in Wonderland syndrome feels their world suddenly shift as their perception changes.

A variety of other experiences are possible as well. People may experience the world with extra color, or as lacking color (see Achromatopsia). They may experience the feeling of derealization, that things are not real, or they may have the experience of déjà vu (see Pathological Déjà Vu). There may also be an impaired sense of the passage of time (Azimova et al., 2016). These *time distortions* come in different varieties. Time may seem to accelerate in the *quick-motion phenomenon* or decelerate to a crawl in the *slow-motion phenomenon*—or, the person may fail to correctly judge how much time is passing (Blom et al., 2021).

The name "Alice in Wonderland syndrome" comes from the Lewis Carroll story about a young girl who fell down a rabbit hole into a world of zany characters and size-shifting experiences. Throughout the course of her adventures, Alice grows larger and shrinks down to be smaller, which is similar to experiences reported by those with Alice in Wonderland syndrome.

Another reason for the memorable name of this disorder is that it primarily affects children, like the titular character of the story. A systematic review of the known cases involving Alice in Wonderland syndrome found that around 78% of cases occurred in people below the age of 18 years (Blom, 2016). It is unknown how often symptoms such as these occur in children. It is possible that children experience these symptoms more commonly than has previously been believed, due to children underreporting their symptoms to doctors, and parents misunderstanding the experiences that the children are describing (Smith et al., 2015).

The Brain Pathology

The parts of the brain that play the biggest role in Alice in Wonderland symptoms are the areas surrounding the visual centers in the occipital lobe (Brumm et al., 2010). Lesions to the ventral pathway of vision that straddles the occipital and temporal lobes can provoke symptoms such as micropsia—including on just one side of the visual field, in instances where there is a lesion isolated to one hemisphere of the brain (e.g., Kassubek et al., 1999). Overall, because the symptoms of Alice in Wonderland syndrome are many and diverse, many structural or functional "aberrations of the perceptual system" may contribute to the disorder (Blom, 2016, p. 266).

One theory as to why the symptoms are more common in children is that the visual pathways in their brains are not as fully developed as in adults. Specifically, the ventral pathway in the visual cortex, which plays a role in the perception of shapes and colors, is different between children and adults, potentially allowing more excitability of those brain cells in children. During patterns of brain excitement in that region, the children may have more pronounced visual distortions than an adult would have (Azimova et al., 2016).

One common cause of Alice in Wonderland syndrome is the Epstein-Barr virus, which is also the cause of infectious mononucleosis, commonly called "mono" for short. However, there are numerous other potential causes including migraine (see Migraine Headaches), epilepsy (see Seizures), and brain damage, and this syndrome does occur in older adults from time to time as well (Blom, 2016). Preventing migraine attacks in adults seems to also prevent episodes of Alice in Wonderland syndrome for people who have experienced both (Mastria et al., 2021).

Alice in Wonderland syndrome is usually temporary and lasts for less than a single day in some cases. But in rare situations, people experience recurring patterns of these symptoms for much longer periods of time, such as years, unable to find a way to stay out of Wonderland.

References

Azimova, J. E., Sergeev, A. V., Skorobogatykh, K. V., Klimov, E. A., Tabeeva, G. R., & Rachin, A. P. (2016). Alice-in-Wonderland syndrome in patients with migraine. *British Journal of Medicine and Medical Research*, *13*(11), 1–11. https://doi.org/gs4n

Blom, J. D. (2016). Alice in Wonderland syndrome: A systematic review. *Neurology: Clinical Practice*, *6*(3), 259–270. https://doi.org/gfsqwq

Blom, J. D., Nanuashvili, N., & Waters, F. (2021). Time distortions: A systematic review of cases characteristic of Alice in Wonderland syndrome. *Frontiers in Psychiatry*, *12*, Article 668633. https://doi.org/gth7

Brumm, K., Walenski, M., Haist, F., Robbins, S. L., Granet, D. B., & Love, T. (2010). Functional magnetic resonance imaging of a child with Alice in Wonderland syndrome during an episode of micropsia. *Journal of American Association for Pediatric Ophthalmology and Strabismus*, *14*(4), 317–322. https://doi.org/cjktmk

Golden, G. S. (1979). The Alice in Wonderland syndrome in juvenile migraine. *Pediatrics*, *63*(4), 517–519.

Kassubek, J., Otte, M., Wolter, T., Greenlee, M. W., Mergner, T., & Lücking, C. H. (1999). Brain imaging in a patient with hemimicropsia. *Neuropsychologia*, *37*(12), 1327–1334. https://doi.org/cc9p96

Kawase, K., Yamada, M., Satoh, H., Satoh, A., & Tsujihata, M. (2013). Alice in Wonderland syndrome: A case report. *Journal of the Neurological Sciences*, *333*(s1), e181. https://doi.org/f2m3x3

Kitchener, N. (2004). Alice in Wonderland syndrome. *The International Journal of Child Neuropsychiatry*, *1*(1), 107–112.

Mastria, G., Mancini, V., Cesare, M. Di, Puma, M., Alessiani, M., Petolicchio, B., Piero, V. Di, & Vigano, A. (2021). Prevalence and characteristics of Alice in Wonderland Syndrome in adult migraineurs: Perspectives from a tertiary referral headache unit. *Cephalalgia*, *41*(5), 515–524. https://doi.org/gtx9

Smith, R. A., Wright, B., & Bennett, S. (2015). Hallucinations and illusions in migraine in children and the Alice in Wonderland syndrome. *Archives of Disease in Childhood*, *100*, 296–298. https://doi.org/f634dm

Alien Hand Syndrome

Imagine that sometimes your hand does things on its own without you telling it to do so. Pretend that you are trying to wash your hands. After you turn on the faucet, your left hand refuses to let go of the faucet handle. You use your right hand to pry your left hand away, take a breath, and reach for the soap dispenser, where your left hand joyously begins pressing the dispenser button over and over until your right hand is covered in way too much soap. You then successfully bring your hands together and rub them under the running water. Everything seems to be proceeding as expected for a minute as you complete the routine movements of washing your hands. But as you remove your hands from under the water stream, your left hand suddenly jerks out to reach for the soap dispenser again. "No! We've already done that part!" you yell, but your alien hand is not discouraged. How is this possible?

The Stories

(STORY 1) A 54-year-old man with *alien hand syndrome* told his doctor about some of the issues he was experiencing due to his unruly left hand. He reported that once while he was driving his alien hand began grasping and pulling at the steering wheel. He was forced to stop the car in order to try and control his limb. About a week later, he was undressing himself, and as he was taking off his pants, his alien hand swooped in and began to pull the pants back up instead. He struggled against his alien hand using his right hand in *intermanual conflict* for a while but eventually resorted to sitting down and waiting for his alien hand to stop pulling. He was understandably "very distressed and frightened" by these occurrences (p. 789). Fortunately, after brain surgery to remove a mass and some medication, his alien hand symptoms vanished (Leiguarda et al., 1993, case 2).

(STORY 2) A right-handed 61-year-old man lost voluntary control of his left hand after a stroke and experienced extreme *anarchic hand* symptoms. It would often grasp objects such as doorknobs and refuse to let go. Curiously, when someone other than the patient commanded the hand to stop what it was doing, the hand would obey. Most notably in terms of unwanted behavior, when using the bathroom, the left hand would continuously unfurl toilet

DOI: 10.4324/9781003276937-7

paper until directed to stop by the nursing staff. When the medical examiner asked him to grip the examiner's hand using the alien hand, the patient did so but was then unable to let go despite massive effort. It wasn't until the medical examiner commanded him to let go that the alien hand obeyed (Kritikos et al., 2005).

(STORY 3) A case study reported on an 81-year-old woman with an unusually aggressive alien hand that would inflict self-harming behaviors on her against her will. The alien hand, on her left side, would scratch the left side of her face, hit her in the head and shoulder, and reportedly even tried to strangle her. She was forced to use her right hand to defend herself from her left hand. At one point while in the hospital, she tried to protect herself with a pillow to soften the hitting. She displayed the *strange hand sign* when she referred to the alien hand as a "he" and that "someone" was trying to choke her (p. 366). Overall, she reported that she was afraid of her hand because it did not feel as if it were under her control (Ay et al., 1998).

(STORY 4) A 68-year-old woman began to experience alien hand syndrome while recovering from heart bypass surgery. Her family reported that she had been complaining for three days about the "loss of control of her left hand" (p. 803). When she was examined, researchers noted that her left hand was taking unwanted actions, such as unbuttoning her gown and crushing cups that she was given to drink from. She also experienced events where her left hand would fight with the right hand to try and answer the phone, resulting in the necessity of her holding down her left hand. Most alarmingly, it was reported that she would occasionally wake up finding that her left hand was choking her. She described that the sensation was as if someone "from the moon" controlled her left hand (p. 803). Her alien hand symptoms seemed to be due to a stroke that affected her corpus callosum. When she was examined months later, she showed general left-handed clumsiness and weakness and complained that her right hand seemed larger than her left hand, but the alien hand symptoms themselves had vanished (Geschwind et al., 1995).

The Features

Controlling your limbs is something that you learn to do at a very young age. By the time you begin to form permanent memories in childhood, you have generally already started to overcome the hurdle of learning how to coordinate complex tasks with your limbs such as walking, reaching for and grasping things, and pretending to use your foot as a telephone. These complex muscle movements become extremely well learned by your brain so that you barely have to think about how you are accomplishing those tasks by the time you reach adulthood. However, there is a disorder in which you *do not* think about doing those things at all for certain limb movements, to the point that the limb behaves seemingly on its own. In other words, if you have this condition, your limb can do complicated things that you did not tell it to do.

The name of this disorder, *alien hand syndrome*, works well in describing its symptoms. The disorder has also been called Strangelovian hand (or Dr. Strangelove syndrome) after the titular character who had some of the symptoms in the movie *Dr. Strangelove* (Kubrick, 1964). However, the name alien hand syndrome captures the imagination and is the more popular way of referring to the disorder, as it is a memorable name for a memorable diagnosis.

The hand may make movements that seem highly intentional, such as complex coordinated tasks like unbuttoning clothing or grasping and throwing objects—but the person with this disorder reports that those actions were unintentional and performed by the hand's own volition. This symptom of the hand acting on its own is sometimes called *anarchic hand*. A vivid quote about the anarchic hand symptom bluntly states that "the 'alien' hand, seems to act autonomously, carrying out complex movements against the subject's verbally reported will … this is both unpleasant and frightening for him" (Della Sala et al., 1991, p. 1113). For some people with this disorder who have particularly mischievous or violent alien hands, "unpleasant and frightening" is quite the understatement.

They may also feel as though the limb doesn't belong to them, which has been referred to as the *strange hand sign* (see Somatoparaphrenia). They may refer to the hand as "he" or "she" or even by a name. As an example, I've translated a section of an old case study from its original German. In this case, a woman began referring to her own hand as "she/her" (or more accurately, "*sie/ihr*") after it started misbehaving, such as tearing up her bedspread and even trying to strangle her. She claimed that the hand didn't obey her, the patient, but instead "did what *she* wanted … 'I can't do anything with *her* myself; if I drink and *she* takes hold of the cup, *she* doesn't let go and pours it out. I then hit *her* and say: my hand, be still" (Goldstein, 1908, p. 169, translated here with emphasis added).

Much like an alien, the alien hand may interfere with and even attack its human host. People with this syndrome often resort to restraining their alien hand with their other hand and sometimes talk to the hand to try and reason with it. This symptom, when a person's hands act with purposes that are contrary to one another, is sometimes called *intermanual conflict* (Biran & Chatterjee, 2004). In one striking instance, intermanual conflict was noted in a woman who tried to smoke a cigarette with her right hand, but her alien left hand snatched it away—to which the woman remarked: "the left hand 'was trying to keep me from smoking'" (Goldberg & Bloom, 1990, case 1, p. 230).

Different people with alien hand syndrome may experience an anarchic hand, a strange hand sign, and intermanual conflict in different combinations. While an arm is the most commonly affected limb, it is possible to have some alien hand syndrome symptoms in the leg instead, and in rare cases it may occur in multiple limbs of the same person (e.g., Chan et al., 1996; Graff-Radford et al., 2013). When alien hand syndrome is combined with symptoms of neglect (see Hemispatial Neglect), the person may find themselves in a situation where their alien hand is grabbing objects or tearing clothing, and the person does not notice the alien's actions (Assal et al., 2007).

In some cases, the alien hand can be successfully verbally commanded to stop what it is doing by someone *other* than the person with the disorder, such as the doctor examining the patient (Goldberg et al., 1981; Kritikos et al., 2005). In such cases, the doctor can seemingly reason with the person's brain systems that are controlling the alien hand in a way that the person themselves cannot. Oftentimes, a patient will develop a strategy of talking to their alien hand in order to try and alleviate the symptoms, but this doesn't always work (Scepkowski & Cronin-Golomb, 2003). Another strategy that is sometimes adopted is distracting the alien hand by giving it objects to hold such as a cane, or putting it inside of a glove (Hassan & Josephs, 2016).

The Brain Pathology

Of the different brain cell communication pathways that are responsible for the movement of your body, some require more *conscious* input than others. For example, different brain regions contribute when gesticulating—talking with your hands—versus swinging your arms while running in order to balance (Ramachandran & Blakeslee, 1998). When you consciously plan and then make a movement, this is called *volitional movement*.

The key thing to understand is that some muscle movements do not strictly *require* conscious input in the form of volitional movement, meaning that if you do not specifically plan to make the movements, they can still happen anyway. In other words, motor pathways in your brain can send movement commands even without your initial awareness of that movement (Assal et al., 2007).

In alien hand syndrome, the conscious input of volitional movement—the *choice to move* that you have the ability to control—has been cut off from part of your brain that is capable of sending signals that cause you to move your muscles. In theory, this is either due to damage to one of the parts of the brain that generates the signals for volitional movement or because the connections between that part of the brain and the part of the brain that controls the muscles have been damaged (e.g., Hassan & Josephs, 2016; Le et al., 2020). The alien hand has effectively skipped over the usual step of asking your conscious brain for permission to act, and your conscious brain has trouble sending a signal that stops the alien hand from acting. This is why people with this syndrome often fail to let go of objects when they want to or are surprised by their hand's actions, or resort to using their other hand to restrain the alien hand—they fail to send the signals that they want to send to their alien hand's muscles.

Because multiple parts of the brain have roles in movement, alien hand syndrome can result from damage to more than one different brain area. The possibilities are complicated and spread out across the brain. Some possible contributors to alien hand syndrome are damage to the corpus callosum, anterior cingulate cortex, thalamus, and the motor cortex including the anterior prefrontal cortex, posterior parietal cortex, and supplementary motor area

(Schaefer et al., 2016). These areas can become damaged due to neurodegenerative diseases such as corticobasal syndrome and Creutzfeldt-Jakob disease (see Creutzfeldt-Jakob Disease), or because of tumors, strokes, and similar events (Graff-Radford et al., 2013).

Historically, attempts were made to take the somewhat different cases of alien hand syndrome and group them together by symptoms. If you squint a little bit, a pattern of brain damage location emerges that suggests multiple subtypes of alien hand syndrome (e.g., Feinberg et al., 1992; Scepkowski & Cronin-Golomb, 2003). Because of this, some researchers have proposed subtypes of the syndrome based on where the brain damage is located as well as the presenting symptoms (Biran & Chatterjee, 2004). Typically, three subtypes are considered: *frontal*, *posterior*, and *callosal*. We'll discuss those in just a moment.

However, as noted by researchers who compiled over 150 cases, the "individual cases often defy exact classification" and "the quest for an individual clinical definition or neuroanatomic correlate to the alien limb is Sisyphean" (Graff-Radford et al., 2013, p. 1881). That's a splashy way of saying that nature has not drawn a neat boundary in the brain between subtypes of alien hand syndrome, and so any attempt by researchers to do so is going to be at least a little bit wrong. As a result of this and unreliable relationships between symptoms and damage locations, the disorder subtypes are not yet widely agreed upon (Schaefer et al., 2016).

As imprecise as classification may be, the different brain damage locations *do* seem to have a relationship with different abnormal movement patterns of the hand. Damage to the front of the brain commonly leads to "impulsive groping" of objects and a refusal from the hand to let go of objects (anarchic hand), while damage further back in the brain is related to "strong feelings of estrangement" with the alien hand (the strange hand sign)—respectively, these are the *frontal* and *posterior* alien hand syndromes (Hassan & Josephs, 2016, p. 2). It is generally accepted that the movements of the hand in the frontal variant are more complex than movements made in the posterior subtype, with the latter subtype showing simple "involuntary levitating" rather than grabbing or manipulating objects (e.g., Poon & Hsu, 2020).

Besides those two subtypes, another common cause of alien hand syndrome is that the two halves of the brain partially lose communication with one another. This sometimes occurs via damage to a part of the brain called the *corpus callosum*, which is located between the two hemispheres of the brain and is made up of nerve fibers that transfer information back and forth across those hemispheres. This is known as *callosal* alien hand syndrome.

Each half of your brain contributes to controlling the muscles on the opposite half of your body, such that your right brain hemisphere is more in charge of controlling your left arm than is your left hemisphere and vice versa. When the hemispheres of your brain cannot communicate effectively because of a damaged corpus callosum, they may control their own half of the body with less discussion about it with the other hemisphere. For example, "damage to the corpus callosum results in the left [hand] being controlled only by the right hemisphere" without contribution from the left hemisphere (Scepkowski & Cronin-Golomb, 2003, p. 264). This may result in one half of the brain being surprised by the actions taken by the other half of the brain, because one hemisphere did not know what the other hemisphere was planning. Sometimes corpus callosum damage is accidental, but it can be performed intentionally as a treatment for seizures (see Seizures). Callosal alien hand syndrome is strongly associated with intermanual conflict as the two hemispheres of the brain end up disagreeing with one another because of the loss in communication efficiency (Feinberg et al., 1992).

Incidents of alien hand syndrome symptoms may persist for only short amounts of time, measured in minutes (Panikkath et al., 2014). However, they may also last for longer periods that are extremely disruptive to the person's life (Bundick & Spinella, 2000). Many people with alien hand syndrome experience fewer symptoms over time, as they learn how to control the alien attached to their body.

References

Assal, F., Schwartz, S., & Vuilleumier, P. (2007). Moving with or without will: Functional neural correlates of alien hand syndrome. *Annals of Neurology, 62*(3), 301–306. https://doi.org/dhm3db

Ay, H., Buonanno, F. S., Price, B. H., Le, D. A., & Koroshetz, W. J. (1998). Sensory alien hand syndrome: Case report and review of the literature. *Journal of Neurology, Neurosurgery & Psychiatry, 65*(3), 366–369. https://doi.org/d89jtd

Biran, I., & Chatterjee, A. (2004). Alien hand syndrome. *Archives of Neurology, 61*(2), 292–294. https://doi.org/cwg6th

Bundick, T., & Spinella, M. (2000). Subjective experience, involuntary movement, and posterior alien hand syndrome. *Journal of Neurology, Neurosurgery & Psychiatry, 68*(1), 83–85. https://doi.org/dvzxvk

Chan, J. L., Chen, R. S., & Ng, K. K. (1996). Leg manifestation in alien hand syndrome. *Journal of the Formosan Medical Association, 95*(4), 342–346.

Della Sala, S., Marchetti, C., & Spinnler, H. (1991). Right-sided anarchic (alien) hand: A longitudinal study. *Neuropsychologia, 29*(11), 1113–1127. https://doi.org/b85kj3

Feinberg, T. E., Schindler, R. J., Flanagan, N. G., & Haber, L. D. (1992). Two alien hand syndromes. Neurology, 42(1), 19–24. https://doi.org/gjq46q

Geschwind, D. H., Iacoboni, M., Mega, M. S., Zaidel, D. W., Cloughesy, T., & Zaidel, E. (1995). Alien hand syndrome: Interhemispheric motor disconnection due to a lesion in the midbody of the corpus callosum. *Neurology, 45*(4), 802–808. https://doi.org/gs4w

Goldberg, G., & Bloom, K. K. (1990). The alien hand sign. *American Journal of Physical Medicine & Rehabilitation, 69*(5), 228–238. https://doi.org/dpcxnr

Goldberg, G., Mayer, N. H., & Toglia, J. U. (1981). Medial frontal cortex infarction and the alien hand sign. *Archives of Neurology, 38*(11), 683–686. https://doi.org/d4w9p2

Goldstein, K. (1908). Zur Lehre von der motorischen Apraxie. *Journal für Psychologie und Neurologie, 11*, 169–87 and 270–283.

Graff-Radford, J., Rubin, M. N., Jones, D. T., Aksamit, A. J., Ahlskog, J. E., Knopman, D. S., Petersen, R. C., Boeve, B. F., & Josephs, K. A. (2013). The alien limb phenomenon. *Journal of Neurology, 260*(7), 1880–1888. https://doi.org/f434zv

Hassan, A., & Josephs, K. A. (2016). Alien hand syndrome. *Current Neurology and Neuroscience Reports*, *16*, Article 73. https://doi.org/ggb3rw

Kritikos, A., Breen, N., & Mattingley, J. B. (2005). Anarchic hand syndrome: Bimanual coordination and sensitivity to irrelevant information in unimanual reaches. *Cognitive Brain Research*, *24*(3), 634–647. https://doi.org/ckwkss

Kubrick, S. (Director). (1964). *Dr. Strangelove or: How I Learned to Stop Worrying and Love the Bomb* [Film]. Hawk Films.

Le, K., Zhang, C., & Greisman, L. (2020). Alien hand syndrome – A rare presentation of stroke. *Journal of Community Hospital Internal Medicine Perspectives*, *10*(2), 149–150. https://doi.org/gt7z

Leiguarda, R., Starkstein, S., Nogues, M., Berthier, M., & Arbelaiz, R. (1993). Paroxysmal alien hand syndrome. *Journal of Neurology, Neurosurgery & Psychiatry*, *56*(7), 788–792. https://doi.org/fwbqv3

Panikkath, R., Panikkath, D., Mojumder, D., & Nugent, K. (2014). The alien hand syndrome. *Baylor University Medical Center Proceedings*, *27*(3), 219–220. https://doi.org /gs4x

Poon, J., & Hsu, S. (2020). A case of alien hand syndrome. *Proceedings of UCLA Health*, *24*.

Ramachandran, V. S., & Blakeslee, S. (1998). *Phantoms in the brain: Probing the mysteries of the human mind*. William Morrow.

Scepkowski, L. A., & Cronin-Golomb, A. (2003). The alien hand: Cases, categorizations, and anatomical correlates. *Behavioral and Cognitive Neuroscience Reviews*, *2*(4), 261–277. https://doi.org/dtdxmn

Schaefer, M., Denke, C., Apostolova, I., Heinze, H. J., & Galazky, I. (2016). A case of right alien hand syndrome coexisting with right-sided tactile extinction. *Frontiers in Human Neuroscience*, *10*, Article 105. https://doi.org/gtjf

Amnesia

Imagine that you can't remember. And I don't mean trouble with learning names, or forgetting where you put your keys. I'm talking about not knowing important details about yourself because your brain failed to create or retrieve a memory. When you are in the moment, such as when focusing on an activity or conversation, you may not even notice your memory difficulties. But occasionally, something that you don't remember disturbs you. Why does your reflection in the mirror look different, so much older, than expected? Who are these people that are acting so friendly? What happened on that night for which you have no recollection? When someone mentions an event that must have happened, you play along. You don't remember it that way, but you'll just have to take their word for it, even though it doesn't feel real.

The Stories

(STORY 1) After a motorcycle accident in 1981, a man around the age of 30 developed both retrograde and anterograde amnesia. This patient, called KC, was studied extensively by memory researchers. While he had lost his memory for all events experienced over the course of his life, he retained some knowledge about himself, his parents, and other facts. In psychological terms, he had retained some *semantic memory* but had lost his *episodic memory*. KC was described in his original case study as living in the "permanent present" due to losing old memories and his extreme difficulties in forming new ones (p. 14). Video footage of interviews with KC show that he could easily recite his name and date of birth, but he would laugh and ask, "what year is it?" when he was asked how old he was (Tulving et al., 1988).

(STORY 2) A 34-year-old man experienced an unusual bout of amnesia in 2002. Originally from Kazakhstan, this man had been living in Germany since 1993 where he had a wife and two children. In early 2002, he awoke to find himself on a train in Russia, and had no recollection of having traveled to that country. He ended up in a mental ward in a hospital because he had no legal documents with him and could not remember his name. He remained a mysterious case for several months. Eventually, word of the stranger in Russia reached Germany where his family was looking for him, and they retrieved

DOI: 10.4324/9781003276937-8

him from the mental ward to bring him back home. He did not recognize his wife or his brother who claimed him from Russia. His memories did not return spontaneously, so he had to carefully relearn details about his life, and he even had to relearn the German language upon his return (Fujiwara et al., 2008, patient IJ).

(STORY 3) A 67-year-old man finished an interview with two journalists about a historical matter, and the guests had just left his home. Immediately after they left, he turned to his family and began asking questions about who the visitors were and what they had been doing there. Despite his family answering his questions, he continued to repeatedly ask and forget the answers. He was very worried during this event, asking his family the same question many times: "do you see anything wrong with me?" (p. 9). The *transient global amnesia* episode lasted around an hour, during which he couldn't seem to successfully gather his thoughts (Fisher & Adams, 1964, as reported in Larner, 2017, case 1).

(STORY 4) Perhaps the most famous neuropsychological case study of the 20th century concerned a man called HM. In 1953, HM was operated on in order to relieve incapacitating seizures. During the surgery, both *hippocampi* were removed, as well as additional surrounding tissue including both amygdalae and adjacent temporal cortex. The good news was that the surgery did reduce the burden of his seizures. The bad news was that he lost the ability to form certain kinds of new memories. While he was paying attention to something, he could remember new information for a short period of time. However, once he stopped paying attention to that new information, it was lost to him forever because it was not stored as an accessible long-term memory in his brain. For example, he never learned to recognize doctors that he met after his surgery, and when he eventually moved, he was never able to remember his new home address. HM could still remember events from his distant past, but he also forgot the year or so of his life leading up to the surgery (Corkin, 1968; Scoville & Milner, 1957). HM had essentially become stuck in time in 1953 because he was no longer adding new conscious memories to his life story. Very informative psychological tests were performed on HM following the surgery, including experiments showing that he retained the ability to learn and improve at new skills using *procedural memories*, despite being unable to remember that he had learned those skills. Because of his misfortune, scientists learned the importance of the hippocampus in human memory. HM makes an appearance in just about every textbook discussion of how human memory works and is known as "the man who changed the study of memory" (Pinel & Barnes, 2017, p. 273).

The Features

Amnesia is broadly defined as the loss of memories. You have probably heard of it before, as it has become a cliché of television dramas, where a character will get amnesia and then works to figure out what events they forgot such as their evil twin's visit to town. When amnesia happens to people in real life, the consequences are indeed quite interesting for researchers who study memory, but probably not in a way that would make a good soap opera.

There are several kinds of amnesia. To understand them, we should briefly review the different types of memory that may be affected: *episodic*, *semantic*, and *procedural*. Episodic memories are memories of events. An episodic memory is something that happened that you can mentally re-experience to some extent when you remember it, such as re-experiencing smells, sounds, or emotions.

Semantic memories are memories for information, such as names and facts. Unlike episodic memories, semantic memories are not necessarily closely connected to perceptions or emotions. Knowing the name of your hometown is a semantic memory, but re-experiencing the sight of the streets and buildings when you try to remember your childhood is an episodic memory. Other semantic memories include knowing the date of your birthday, your preferences for food, and the names of the countries that you have previously visited. Semantic memories don't include the memory of how you felt on your most recent birthday (joyous? lonely?), the memory of the taste of unique foods (try imagining hot peppers), or memories of the sights or sounds of foreign lands.

And finally, procedural memories are memories for movements performed in order to accomplish a task, such as riding a bicycle or tying your shoes. Procedural memories do not require high levels of thinking because they are rather automatic when performed. As we will discuss, amnesia can disrupt these different types of memory somewhat independently.

There are two main types of amnesia in terms of which part of time is affected: *retrograde amnesia* and *anterograde amnesia*. There are other amnestic disorders, but they do not often map perfectly on to the retrograde/anterograde distinction. One of these amnesia subtypes will also be discussed, called *transient global amnesia*.

Retrograde amnesia is what the average person thinks of when you ask them to describe amnesia. It is a loss of memories for the past, possibly including only a small number of episodic memories in mild cases. In severe cases, a much larger number of episodic memories or an entire lifetime can be forgotten. Sometimes the retrograde forgetting even includes personal information about themselves, called *autobiographical memory*, such as their name and other personal semantic memories (Butters & Cermak, 1986).

When retrograde amnesia impacts only some of a person's memory, it may be limited to memories that were recently created. In other words, in some cases of retrograde amnesia, childhood memories are less likely to be disrupted than recent memories from adulthood. When recent memories are disrupted more than older memories, this is referred to as *temporally graded retrograde amnesia* (Sekeres et al., 2016). In contrast, some people with amnesia lose memories across all life stages, regardless of how far back in time the memories were made (Noulhiane et al., 2007).

Can a person who loses memories due to retrograde amnesia get them back? The answer is yes, they can relearn the forgotten details, but no, they won't be likely to *recover* forgotten memories. People typically do not recover the episodic nature of the lost memories which leaves behind a residual unfamiliarity with their own lives (e.g., Fujiwara et al., 2008; Sellal et al., 2002). That is, the emotions, sights, and sounds typically can no longer be re-experienced as part of the memory, leaving behind only the semantic facts.

Anterograde amnesia, on the other hand, is the inability to create *new* memories. As a person with anterograde amnesia goes about their life, they may act relatively like a person without amnesia, until memory is required, such as when meeting new people or visiting a new location. Medical workers meeting with people with anterograde amnesia must introduce themselves many times to the patient, because they are not remembered.

Interestingly, people with anterograde amnesia retain the ability to learn new procedural memories including new skills and habits (Spiers et al., 2001). For example, if you teach someone with anterograde amnesia how to do a new task, such as tying a knot or solving a puzzle requiring hand movement like tracing lines in a mirror, they can get better at doing that task over time even if they can't remember ever doing it before that moment. Thus, some forms of learning are still possible (Corkin, 1968). There is also evidence that some people with anterograde amnesia can learn new facts with enough exposure, allowing them to add to their general knowledge while bypassing the brain mechanisms typically thought of as essential for memory formation (Sekeres et al., 2016). In other words, not all anterograde amnesia is absolute (e.g., Freed et al., 1987).

It is possible to have both retrograde and anterograde amnesia at the same time. If a person both forgets things that have already happened and also has trouble creating new memories, then they have both. Such people often function perfectly fine in short conversations that make use of preserved autobiographical memories, but after interacting with them for a while, you may realize that they are stuck in a moment called *now*.

Transient global amnesia (TGA) is unusual because the person only *temporarily* loses access to old memories and the ability to form new memories. In other words, an instance of TGA consists of a short episode of defective memory, after which the person does not recall what happened during that period, but regains the ability to create new memories following it (Larner, 2017). During that period, they experience combined temporally graded retrograde amnesia (not knowing information from before the transient episode) as well as anterograde amnesia (not forming new memories during the transient episode), although the anterograde amnesia is usually more noticeable (Jäger et al., 2009). One common symptom during a TGA episode is the repetition of behavior. People often ask questions repeatedly and forget the answers, leading them to ask the questions again in a loop (e.g., Fisher & Adams, 1964).

The Brain Pathology

The way that the brain creates and stores memories have been studied extensively, although there is yet much to learn. We are virtually certain that the storage of memories does not happen within single specific spots in the brain. For example, each brain cell does not hold a different memory, and your core memories are not self-contained spheres as depicted in the movie *Inside Out* (Docter & Del Carmen, 2015). Instead, several researchers have pitched the idea that the brain stores memories using a pattern of many brain cells, sometimes called a *trace* (Nadel & Maurer, 2020). In theory, a trace is a bit like a path of electrochemical activity that follows the connections between neurons, and successful remembering depends upon retracing that path. If the correct cellular path can't be followed, memories may become inaccessible, resulting in amnesia. Cells involved in the trace are believed to mostly be located in the outer temporal lobe, but with the involvement of the hippocampus. Trace-related theories are not completely agreed upon, but the idea of the trace has encouraged much research (Sutherland et al., 2020).

The hippocampus is important for the formation of new episodic memories, and in theory forms a key part of the trace for new memories. Prominent evidence for this comes not only from the case of HM, as discussed near the beginning of this chapter, but also from studies of transient global amnesia. When a person experiences transient global amnesia and temporarily fails to form new memories, it seems to be due to temporary abnormalities in the hippocampus, as revealed by brain scans (Bartsch et al., 2007). Other parts of the brain are also involved in memory storage and retrieval. This is especially true for procedural memories, for which the striatum seems to play an essential function (Perrin & Venance, 2019). This is why hippocampus damage can lead to somewhat specific problems for episodic memory while leaving procedural memory formation, such as learning new skills, more intact.

The even stranger fact about memories is that they are very malleable and change over time. For a memory to stay in the brain long-term, it must go through a process of *consolidation*, in which proteins in the brain help to stabilize the memory so that you can remember it later (Hernandez & Abel, 2008). Over time, memories can become more stable and long-lasting. Consolidation theoretically plays a role in amnesia. For example, many memory researchers believe that a long-term "systems consolidation" process takes place in which the hippocampus becomes less important for retrieving older memories, which might help to explain temporally graded retrograde amnesia when the hippocampus is damaged—older memories rely on the hippocampus less, and so childhood memories are more likely to be preserved in cases of retrograde amnesia (Squire et al., 2015, p. 1).

However, consolidation is not a simple one-way process. Whenever a memory is remembered, it changes a little, and must be *reconsolidated*. Each time that you remember a memory, you remember it a little bit differently at the level of the brain, including the synthesis of new proteins to help stabilize the memory.

While the exact mechanisms of the reconsolidation process remain controversial, it is generally believed that during reconsolidation memories can be strengthened, weakened, or updated, and researchers can reduce memory reconsolidation through the use of chemicals called "inhibitors" (Roesler, 2017). In short, every time a memory is recalled, it is sensitive to being disrupted and overwritten with incorrect details, which can lead to people believing things that are not true (Chan & LaPaglia, 2013). Over time, your memories literally change, probably quite a bit more than you realize. In general, memories tend to change over time from rich episodic memories containing lots of detail (feelings, smells, colors, etc.) into simple semantic memories containing just the facts.

Amnesia may also result from electroconvulsive therapies in which the brain is shocked, thiamine deficiency due to alcohol abuse (see Korsakoff Syndrome), lack of oxygen or blood flow to the brain, encephalitis, or traumatic brain injuries (Squire et al., 2009). Dementia is often associated with amnesia, especially temporally graded amnesia. While certain elements of amnesia can be faked or considered dissociative mental illnesses (see Hacking, 1998), there is enough empirical evidence that memory, something that we hold dear and typically view as a solid foundation of our lives, is much more manipulable and fragile than we'd like to believe.

References

Bartsch, T., Alfke, K., Deuschl, G., & Jansen, O. (2007). Evolution of hippocampal CA-1 diffusion lesions in transient global amnesia. *Annals of Neurology, 62*(5), 475–480. https://doi.org/ccgrp4

Butters, N., & Cermak, L. S. (1986). A case study of the forgetting of autobiographical knowledge: Implications for the study of retrograde amnesia. In D. C. Rubin (Ed.), *Autobiographical memory* (pp. 253–272). Cambridge University Press.

Chan, J. C., & LaPaglia, J. A. (2013). Impairing existing declarative memory in humans by disrupting reconsolidation. *Proceedings of the National Academy of Sciences, 110*(23), 9309–9313. https://doi.org/f43ttv

Corkin, S. (1968). Acquisition of motor skill after bilateral medial temporal-lobe excision. *Neuropsychologia, 6*(3), 255–265. https://doi.org/ckvk4w

Docter, P. & Del Carmen, R. (Director). (2015). *Inside out* [Film]. Pixar Animation Studios & Walt Disney Pictures.

Fisher, C. M., & Adams, R. D. (1964). Transient global amnesia. *Acta Neurologica Scandinavica: Supplementum, 40*.

Freed, D. M., Corkin, S., & Cohen, N. J. (1987). Forgetting in HM: A second look. *Neuropsychologia, 25*(3), 461–471. https://doi.org/bzddg8

Fujiwara, E., Brand, M., Kracht, L., Kessler, J., Diebel, A., Netz, J., & Markowitsch, H. J. (2008). Functional retrograde amnesia: A multiple case study. *Cortex, 44*(1), 29–45. https://doi.org/d9g3q5

Hacking, I. (1998). *Mad travelers: Reflections on the reality of transient mental illnesses.* University of Virginia Press.

Hernandez, P. J., & Abel, T. (2008). The role of protein synthesis in memory consolidation: Progress amid decades of debate. *Neurobiology of Learning and Memory, 89*(3), 293–311. https://doi.org/fr6vhz

Jäger, T., Bäzner, H., Kliegel, M., Szabo, K., & Hennerici, M. G. (2009). The transience and nature of cognitive impairments in transient global amnesia: A meta-analysis. *Journal of Clinical and Experimental Neuropsychology*, *31*(1), 8–19. https://doi.org/d96b3x

Larner, A. J. (2017). *Transient global amnesia: From patient encounter to clinical neuroscience.* Springer. https://doi.org/gt5h

Nadel, L., & Maurer, A. P. (2020). Recalling Lashley and reconsolidating Hebb. *Hippocampus*, *30*(8), 776–793. https://doi.org/ghddbr

Noulhiane, M., Piolino, P., Hasboun, D., Clemenceau, S., Baulac, M., & Samson, S. (2007). Autobiographical memory after temporal lobe resection: Neuropsychological and MRI volumetric findings. *Brain*, *130*(12), 3184–3199. https://doi.org/fbnz5d

Perrin, E., & Venance, L. (2019). Bridging the gap between striatal plasticity and learning. *Current Opinion in Neurobiology*, *54*, 104–112. https://doi.org/gfvmfh

Pinel, J., & Barnes, S. (2017). *Biopsychology* (10th edition). Pearson.

Roesler, R. (2017). Molecular mechanisms controlling protein synthesis in memory reconsolidation. *Neurobiology of Learning and Memory*, *142*, 30–40. https://doi.org/ggzxr8

Scoville, W. B., & Milner, B. (1957). Loss of recent memory after bilateral hippocampal lesions. *Journal of Neurology, Neurosurgery, and Psychiatry*, *20*(11), 11–21. https://doi.org/cfp6bs

Sekeres, M. J., Winocur, G., & Moscovitch, M. (2016). Revisiting Tulving et al.: Priming of semantic autobiographical knowledge: A case study of retrograde amnesia. In B. Kolb & I. Whishaw (Eds.), *Brain and behaviour: Revisiting the classic studies* (pp. 130–154). SAGE Publications. https://doi.org/gtjg

Sellal, F., Manning, L., Seegmuller, C., Scheiber, C., & Schoenfelder, F. (2002). Pure retrograde amnesia following a mild head trauma: A neuropsychological and metabolic study. *Cortex*, *38*(4), 499–509. https://doi.org/fgcc2g

Spiers, H. J., Maguire, E. A., & Burgess, N. (2001). Hippocampal amnesia. *Neurocase*, 7(5), 357–382. https://doi.org/d67bj6

Squire, L. R., Bayley, P. J., Smith, C. N. (2009). Amnesia: Declarative and nondeclarative memory. In L. R. Squire (Ed.) *Encyclopedia of neuroscience* (pp. 289–294). Elsevier.

Squire, L. R., Genzel, L., Wixted, J. T., & Morris, R. G. (2015). Memory consolidation. *Cold Spring Harbor Perspectives in Biology*, 7(8), Article a021766. https://doi.org/gg4g4b

Sutherland, R. J., Lee, J. Q., McDonald, R. J., & Lehmann, H. (2020). Has multiple trace theory been refuted? *Hippocampus*, *30*(8), 842–850. https://doi.org/ghddbt

Tulving, E., Schacter, D. L., McLachlan, D. R., & Moscovitch, M. (1988). Priming of semantic autobiographical knowledge: A case study of retrograde amnesia. *Brain and Cognition*, *8*(1), 3–20. https://doi.org/dq5d3b

Anosognosia

Imagine that you have a problem, but due to brain damage, you are unaware that the problem exists. Pretend that you have lost the ability to walk due to a paralyzed leg and arm. You now use a wheelchair. Despite this, you often ask your friends and family if they'd like to go rock climbing with you sometime soon. They chuckle and think you are joking, but you sure aren't. Eventually, they get fed up with your constant requests to go rock climbing and try to explain to you that it would be impossible for you, because of your paralyzed limbs. "Nonsense," you say, "I could walk out of here and climb a mountain anytime I wanted to, I just choose not to do it today." You believe every word, and nothing they say convinces you otherwise.

The Stories

(STORY 1) Following a stroke, an 85-year-old woman was paralyzed on the left side of her body. Despite this, she insisted that she could walk. When asked to demonstrate that she could do this, she would say that she could do so easily but that it would be better if she rested. When asked if she could move her paralyzed arm, she claimed that she was capable of doing so but that the doctor told her that she needed to rest it. When she was handed an object that required two hands in order to manipulate, including a book and a stethoscope, she became confused and could not explain why she was unable to open the book or use the stethoscope. Her anosognosia persisted for at least two years following the stroke (Venneri & Shanks, 2004).

(STORY 2) A 52-year-old woman who was an artist that specialized in portraits had an aneurysm that led to emergency surgery. She survived but became partially blind and partially paralyzed. She also lost the ability to recognize faces (see Prosopagnosia), but failed to realize that she had this new symptom. When she looked back over her old portraits that she had painted, she could not easily identify who the subjects of the paintings were, even though some were family members. She did not admit that this was unusual. Tests of face recognition showed that she could no longer recognize famous people, for example, but she claimed she could recognize faces as well as she could before the surgery, showing anosognosia for prosopagnosia (Young et al., 1990).

DOI: 10.4324/9781003276937-9

(STORY 3) In the case of an 80-year-old woman who had a severe right-sided stroke in 1996, extreme anosognosia developed for her, resulting in left-sided paralysis. She would frequently *confabulate* by making things up without knowing that she was lying. In one example, she was asked to touch a researcher with her right hand, which she did easily, but when she was asked to touch the researcher with her paralyzed left hand, she first claimed that she was able to do this, and then claimed that she had successfully done it, even though she hadn't. In another example, she was asked to clap her hands. After protesting that she wasn't at "the theatre," she eventually agreed to do this (p. 29). She held her non-paralyzed hand out in front of her and moved it as she would if she were clapping her hands, but her paralyzed left arm remained at her side. She seemed satisfied with her attempt to clap, and when an experimenter asked why there was no clapping noise, she said that she never made noise. Eventually, after about three months, she seemed to have recovered from her anosognosia. She indicated in a brief interview that she remembered having been paralyzed for weeks but did not remember her anosognosia, claiming that she had always told the doctor that her left arm could not move (Berti et al., 1998).

The Features

Here's something that your brain does that you may have never thought about before: it constantly updates itself with information about the *state* of your own body. That is, your brain keeps track of the condition and capabilities that your body currently has, like a spaceship monitoring the integrity of its hull or a treasurer monitoring the balance of their organization's bank account. This is such an automatic function of the brain that it may seem strange to consider it at all, but some people lose this ability to update self-knowledge.

Anosognosia refers to a disorder wherein a person has a problem of some kind, such as an illness, but is unaware that the problem exists or otherwise greatly underestimates the severity of the problem (Nurmi & Jehkonen, 2014). Their brain fails to update their knowledge of themselves with the new problem that they are experiencing, so they do not realize that it is happening. The type of problems that people with anosognosia fail to acknowledge are extremely diverse, and the definition can be broad enough to potentially include all of the other conditions contained in this book. Because anosognosia modifies other conditions, you will see it written as "anosognosia for _____," with the blank filled in by whatever condition the person has but of which they are unaware.

Specific examples include partial paralysis, aspects of cognitive functioning such as memory problems (see Amnesia), and reduced perceptual abilities such as blindness (Orfei et al., 2007). That's right—there are people who believe that they can see despite being unable to see, which is referred to as Anton-Babinski Syndrome (see Cortical Blindness; Carvajal et al., 2012). There are also cases of people *partially* losing vision who then insist that their vision is fine (see Hemianopsia; Celesia et al., 1997). It can also occur in the case of a person who forgets that one side of the world exists, as in neglect patients (see Hemispatial Neglect; Berti et al., 2005). Anosognosia has also been reported in conjunction with color blindness, in which a person did not realize that they had lost the ability to see color (see Achromatopsia; von Arx et al., 2010). There's really no end to the possibilities; there's cases of anosognosia for the loss of the ability to understand speech (see Aphasia), the loss of the ability to recognize faces (see Prosopagnosia), and so on (Gasquoine, 2016).

The degree of anosognosia can vary widely. The person may fail to understand the consequences of their condition; they may be nonchalant or unconcerned with the seriousness of the condition, they may simply be unable to recognize that the condition applies to them, or they may outright deny that anything is wrong with them even if their condition is demonstrated to them such as showing them that their limb is paralyzed (Jenkinson et al., 2011). People with anosognosia may deny that they sustained a brain injury at all, let alone that they may be suffering from persisting symptoms of that injury (Gasquoine, 2016). For example, a woman who was paralyzed on one half of her body was told during a medical consultation that they were going to try electrotherapy to treat her paralysis, but "a few days after the consultation she remarked to her doctor, 'So why do you intend to apply electrical stimulation to me? It is not as if I am paralyzed'" (Babinski, 1914, translation from Langer & Levine, 2014, p. 6).

It is also possible to be aware that you have a brain-related problem but to be unaware of the problem itself—and likewise, it is possible to be aware of the problem itself while being unaware that you are having a brain-related problem. For example, a patient can be in the hospital with the understanding that they are sick but not comprehend that the form of the sickness is that they cannot move. Conversely, a patient may understand that they cannot move but don't realize that it means they have a new condition. These complicated forms of anosognosia are difficult to keep track of, because the person may make them up as they go, continually transmogrifying ways to ignore and explain unexpected changes to their life (Jehkonen et al., 2000).

Anosognosia is important to consider because a person who experiences unawareness of a medical condition may refuse treatment or fail to take appropriate safety precautions (Jenkinson et al., 2011). For example, someone with anosognosia for partial paralysis may refuse to participate in medical exams assessing movement or pain sensitivity because they don't believe that they need to be assessed, or a person with anosognosia for partial blindness may walk into objects because they are confident that they can see. Treatment of patients with anosognosia can be tricky, because they may resist taking medication, completion of therapy, or safety measures, insisting that they do not need those things (Kortte & Hillis, 2009).

A person with anosognosia, when confronted with their condition such as blindness or paralysis, will often resort to something called *confabulation*, which is an unintentional lie. When confabulating, they might insist that they can do something that they are unable to do or make up a fake story to explain a situation. These confabulations are often implausible, such as a paralyzed person insisting that they are sitting in a wheelchair because they were tired and wanted to sit down and that they could stand up and walk if they wanted to. They may claim that they have already done it recently or that they don't feel like doing it right now: "I choose not to walk" versus "I cannot walk." This isn't necessarily the same thing as lying, because they are not *aware* that their story isn't true; they are simply trying to make sense out of a confusing situation. Confabulation is also discussed in the Korsakoff chapter (see Korsakoff Syndrome). The takeaway here is that people with anosognosia often do not want help or do not think that they need help and instead tend to craft a version of reality in which their condition is not a problem.

The Brain Pathology

Anosognosia commonly occurs as the result of a stroke. Importantly, the various conditions affiliated with anosognosia probably result from somewhat different underlying stroke damage (Jenkinson et al., 2011). It is also worth noting that "there is no consensus on the cause of anosognosia" because such a multifaceted condition makes it "probably impossible to find any single comprehensive explanation" (Nurmi & Jehkonen, 2014, p. 44). But let's discuss a typical case.

In a typical anosognosia case, a stroke in the right hemisphere of the brain results in movement problems on the left side of the body, such as muscle weakness called *hemiparesis* or muscle paralysis called *hemiplegia*. Following the stroke, the patient may also exhibit signs of anosognosia, such that they may claim that they can use their frozen arm and walk despite depending on a wheelchair. Anosognosia for movement issues is the most well-studied type of anosognosia, and we will focus on "anosognosia for hemiplegia" when considering brain pathology.

It is difficult to tell how common anosognosia is after a stroke. Estimates for how many people recovering from a stroke also experience anosognosia range from 0% to 100% (Nurmi & Jehkonen, 2014). You have probably noticed that this includes all possible percentages. This is because the answer depends on how long after the stroke the anosognosia diagnostic test was given, which diagnostic test was given, how patients were selected for assessment, and which types of anosognosia were included (e.g., Jenkinson et al., 2011; Nurmi & Jehkonen, 2014; Orfei et al., 2007). Thorough assessment requires specific interviews with the person in order to discover symptoms which are not always obvious. What we can say for sure is that it is a surprisingly common problem for a stroke survivor to be partially or completely unaware of their brain damage-related issues—at least temporarily (Starkstein et al., 2010).

Anosognosia is mysterious. Theories about why it happens tend to discuss that it can be a side effect of brain damage to a variety of brain regions instead of just one specific region, especially in older people and people with multiple strokes or severe strokes (Starkstein et al., 2010). The brain damage in someone with anosognosia is often extensive and located in multiple places such as the frontal and parietal lobes (Pia et al., 2004), or the premotor cortex, somatosensory cortex, and primary motor cortex (Berti et al., 2005). It is also common to discuss the involvement of other brain regions, such as the insula (Jenkinson et al., 2011). Neurodegenerative diseases such as Alzheimer disease may result in anosognosia symptoms that worsen over time, especially relating to a person's overestimating of their abilities (Minati et al., 2009). One relatively consistent detail of the brain pathology is that right-sided strokes more commonly lead to anosognosia than left-sided strokes (Kortte & Hillis, 2009). Overall, it is believed that "no particular lesion location has been consistently associated with anosognosia for any one symptom" (Gasquoine, 2016, p. 267). Therefore, the atlas of the brain isn't particularly useful in these cases.

The way that researchers of anosognosia talk about the disorder typically involves a discussion of *awareness*. It is the impairment of monitoring systems that are supposed to supervise a person's status that leads to this lack of awareness (Vallar & Ronchi, 2006). Specifically, anosognosia seems to disrupt a person's ability to become consciously aware of their problems that they have acquired, and instead the person resorts to "filling in" their problems with plausible explanations such as with confabulations (Venneri & Shanks, 2004, p. 237). In theory, for a person to become aware of a problem with their ability to move, for example, their brain needs to first generate a signal to tell their muscles to move, they need to receive feedback from their muscles regarding how far they moved, and then their brain needs to compare those two signals to see if there is a difference between the expected outcome and the actual outcome. Anosognosia could result from damaging any of the three components of that process: the generation of the intention to move, the feedback from the muscles, or a faulty "comparator" in charge of comparing the two signals (Jenkinson et al., 2011). This theory of a faulty comparison doesn't account for all of the features of anosognosia, but it is a useful illustration of why damage to so many different places in the brain may be important in anosognosia.

Demonstrating the problem to the person with anosognosia may cause them to become temporarily aware of it. But generally, before very long they revert to unawareness and begin to deny the problem again (Cutting, 1978). Eventually, many people who acquired anosognosia through sudden brain damage do become aware of their symptoms. In other words, the anosognosia may only last for a little while immediately after the stroke while the brain is recovering. There are some cases, however, where anosognosia remains permanent (Nurmi & Jehkonen, 2014). It has been theorized that initial damage to the insula is enough to cause temporary anosognosia, but long-lasting unawareness requires damage to additional cortical areas within the parietal, temporal, or frontal cortices (Jenkinson et al., 2011). Those with neurodegenerative diseases such as Alzheimer disease that damage a variety of brain regions are unlikely to overcome anosognosia (Venneri & Shanks, 2004). There is a philosophical discussion to be had here as well: if not knowing about their symptoms prevents them from suffering, then can anosognosia be a positive in some cases? Could the brain be doing itself a favor by failing to detect the brain damage? While that discussion is outside the scope of this chapter, I hope that you'll keep anosognosia in mind as an example the next time that you discuss whether "ignorance is bliss."

References

Babinski, J. (1914). Contribution to the study of mental disorders in organic cerebral hemiplegia (anosognosia). *Rev Neurol (Paris)*, *27*, 845–848.

Berti, A., Bottini, G., Gandola, M., Pia, L., Smania, N., Stracciari, A., Castiglioni, I., Vallar, G., & Paulesu, E. (2005). Shared cortical anatomy for motor awareness and motor control. *Science*, *309*(5733), 488–491. https://doi.org/b4w43t

Berti, A., Làdavas, E., Stracciari, A., Giannarelli, C., Ossola, A. (1998). Anosognosia for motor impairment and dissociations with patients' evaluation of the disorder: Theoretical considerations. *Cognitive Neuropsychiatry*, *3*(1), 21–43.

Carvajal, J. J. R., Cárdenas, A. A. A., Pazmiño, G. Z., & Herrera, P. A. (2012). Visual anosognosia (Anton-Babinski Syndrome): Report of two cases associated with ischemic cerebrovascular disease. *Journal of Behavioral and Brain Science*, *2*(3), 394–398. https://doi.org/gtjh

Celesia, G. G., Brigell, M. G., & Vaphiades, M. S. (1997). Hemianopic anosognosia. *Neurology*, *49*(1), 88–97. https://doi.org/gtjj

Cutting, J. (1978). Study of anosognosia. *Journal of Neurology, Neurosurgery & Psychiatry*, *41*(6), 548–555. https://doi.org/dqngnj

Gasquoine, P. G. (2016). Blissfully unaware: Anosognosia and anosodiaphoria after acquired brain injury. *Neuropsychological Rehabilitation*, *26*(2), 261–285. https://doi.org/g4hh

Jehkonen, M., Ahonen, J. P., Dastidar, P., Laippala, P., & Vilkki, J. (2000). Unawareness of deficits after right hemisphere stroke: Double-dissociations of anosognosias. *Acta Neurologica Scandinavica*, *102*(6), 378–384. https://doi.org/bnn5hv

Jenkinson, P. M., Preston, C., & Ellis, S. J. (2011). Unawareness after stroke: A review and practical guide to understanding, assessing, and managing anosognosia for hemiplegia. *Journal of Clinical and Experimental Neuropsychology*, *33*(10), 1079–1093. https://doi.org/cp7sps

Kortte, K., & Hillis, A. E. (2009). Recent advances in the understanding of neglect and anosognosia following right hemisphere stroke. *Current Neurology and Neuroscience Reports*, *9*(6), 459–465. https://doi.org/b8n9p6

Langer, K. G., & Levine, D. N. (2014). Contribution to the study of the mental disorders in hemiplegia of organic cerebral origin (anosognosia). Translated by KG Langer & DN Levine: Translated from the original Contribution à l'Étude des Troubles Mentaux dans l'Hémiplégie Organique Cérébrale (Anosognosie). *Cortex*, *61*, 5–8. https://doi.org/gc8zdp

Minati, L., Edginton, T., Bruzzone, M., & Giaccone, G. (2009). Current concepts in Alzheimer's disease: A multidisciplinary review. *American Journal of Alzheimer's Disease & Other Dementias*, *24*(2), 95–121. https://doi.org/bfskkw

Nurmi, M. E., & Jehkonen, M. (2014). Assessing anosognosias after stroke: A review of the methods used and developed over the past 35 years. *Cortex*, *61*, 43–63. https://doi.org/f7t4nr

Orfei, M. D., Robinson, R. G., Prigatano, G. P., Starkstein, S., Rüsch, N., Bria, P., Caltagirone, C., & Spalletta, G. (2007). Anosognosia for hemiplegia after stroke is a multifaceted phenomenon: A systematic review of the literature. *Brain, 130*(12), 3075–3090. https://doi.org/ctvb4z

Pia, L., Neppi-Modona, M., Ricci, R., & Berti, A. (2004). The anatomy of anosognosia for hemiplegia: A meta-analysis. *Cortex, 40*(2), 367–377. https://doi.org/d6qczc

Starkstein, S. E., Jorge, R. E., & Robinson, R. G. (2010). The frequency, clinical correlates, and mechanism of anosognosia after stroke. *The Canadian Journal of Psychiatry, 55*(6), 355–361. https://doi.org/gs42

Vallar, G., & Ronchi, R. (2006). Anosognosia for motor and sensory deficits after unilateral brain damage: A review. *Restorative Neurology and Neuroscience, 24*(4–6), 247–257.

Venneri, A., & Shanks, M. F. (2004). Belief and awareness: Reflections on a case of persistent anosognosia. *Neuropsychologia, 42*(2), 230–238. https://doi.org/fm2rtv

von Arx, S. W., Müri, R. M., Heinemann, D., Hess, C. W., & Nyffeler, T. (2010). Anosognosia for cerebral achromatopsia—a longitudinal case study. *Neuropsychologia, 48*(4), 970–977. https://doi.org/d4vhkk

Young, A. W., de Haan, E. H., & Newcombe, F. (1990). Unawareness of impaired face recognition. *Brain and Cognition, 14*(1), 1–18. https://doi.org/b2hcmr

Aphantasia

Imagine that you can't imagine. When most people reflect on a memory that is important to them, they can catch an almost visual glimpse of that place or event with their "mind's eye." If they choose to imagine it, their childhood home presents itself as an image where they can count the windows and perceive the color of the front door. But for you, the person with aphantasia, nothing visual comes to mind. To you, the ability to imagine a color sounds, itself, imaginary. Picturing the face of a loved one in your mind is an impossible feat. Your imagination is dark.

The Stories

(STORY 1) A 65-year-old man who underwent a coronary angioplasty suddenly lost the ability to visualize imagery. He first noticed this in his dreams, when they lost all visual content. He described that he was able to remember which visual details existed. For example, he was able to recite a series of directions that could then be followed to a destination, but he was no longer able to actually picture those visual details in his mind. He had previously worked as a surveyor, and had been able to imagine buildings as part of his job—but no longer. He would sometimes experience visual imagery involuntarily but could not cause himself to experience it at will due to his *acquired aphantasia* (Zeman et al., 2010).

(STORY 2) A woman had a conversation about visualization with her husband during an anniversary dinner at a table for two. He reported that he could imagine people's faces including her mother's face—something that she could not do. Each thought that the other was the strange one. Her husband reported that he could superimpose images on top of real life while his eyes were open, which she declared as abnormal. After more research, she discovered that while most people have the ability to visualize, she was missing that ability and had never realized it before. That was how she discovered her *developmental aphantasia*, and conversations such as this example frequently lead others to discover the condition for themselves, as well (Kendle, 2017, case L, p. 19).

(STORY 3) Following a car accident in 1936, a 36-year-old man was unconscious for eight days. When he was interviewed by a researcher five

DOI: 10.4324/9781003276937-10

years after the accident, he shared that his "picture memory" was gone (p. 289). For example, he was no longer able to mentally picture the faces of his loved ones. The car accident had also resulted in the death of his wife, and he was no longer able to form a mental picture of her face. He also could no longer mentally follow a route to a destination and depended on physical maps to navigate. His career as a builder was disrupted as well, because he could no longer remember what the building plans specified for dimensions without referring back to the written instructions. He also reported that his dreams were now devoid of images. Following up with this individual 15 years after the accident showed his condition unchanged, with the aphantasia continuing to rob him of his mind's eye (Brain, 1954, case 1).

(STORY 4) A man had a stroke at the age of 63, and although he initially suffered from many symptoms such as muscle weakness and difficulty speaking, it was the loss of his mental imagery that was "one of the most painful conse-quences of his brain injury" (p. 436). As part of a battery of tests, a doctor asked him to describe the visual scene of "the Cathedral Square of Milan," a location that he ought to have been able to describe (p. 436). However, the patient failed to add any meaningful description to the visual scene and claimed that he was unable to imagine what the Square looked like. He was able to walk back and forth between the hospital and his house with no trouble, but he was unable to describe what the route itself looked like from his imagination. He also had become unable to visualize faces. The researchers described that "he said he *knew* his wife to be 'small, grey haired, with almond-shaped eyes' but was unable to conjure up a picture of her in his mind" (p. 436). He said that he was also no longer able to imagine smells, tastes, or sounds. He also shared that he used to have vivid images float through his mind at night while lying in bed just before falling asleep—but these images no longer visited, which upset him (Basso et al., 1980).

The Features

Can people *see* things when they imagine those things? That is, if you close your eyes and imagine an object, can you experience an inward seeing of that object? This may seem like a trivial question to someone who regularly experi-ences *mental imagery*. But do not take the ability for granted: as we will discuss, some people do not seem to experience voluntary mental imagery.

Debates have long been fought about whether imagining something actu-ally produces a *picture* of that thing in the brain. The philosophical war was once between *iconophiles* who used and loved mental images and *iconophobes* who denied their very existence (Dennett, 1978). Because mental imagery is such a private experience, each side of the debate frequently accused the other side of exaggerating or misunderstanding mental imagery. Each person was likely to believe that *all* other people had the same experience—or lack of experience—of mental imagery.

The philosophical question has since become a neurological one, which is great, because this is not a philosophy book. To make a very long story short, it was discovered that the brain does in fact produce literal pictures in the brain (Pearson & Kosslyn, 2015). However, there are individual differences in how mental imagery is experienced (or not experienced) depending on the specific person's brain. Actually, it was already suggested over a century ago that it was possible that some people do have mental imagery and others simply do not (Galton, 1880). However, it took until recently for researchers to show this conclusively, which is why the condition of "near or total absence of mental imagery" was not given the name aphantasia until 2015 (Zeman et al., 2015, p. 379).

The name comes from the Greek word "phantasia," which means "imagination." Aphantasia is the diminished or absent ability to mentally visualize using your imagination, which is sometimes called the mind's eye. When you ask the average person to imagine what their own face looks like, most people can do this easily. But a person with aphantasia may be surprised to learn that people *have the ability to do this in the first place.*

There is more than one kind of aphantasia. People who begin life with the ability to see mental images can lose that ability later in life, thanks to brain damage. Such *acquired aphantasia* cases are rare, however. Instead, many people with aphantasia claim to have always had this condition. That is, most people with aphantasia have the type called *developmental aphantasia*, where there is no known brain damage that caused the condition. Many of these people do not discover that their imagination is different from others until they are 20 years old or older (Zeman et al., 2020). Most people with aphantasia learn about it from reading stories about other people who struggle to visualize things or by comparing notes with others about how they imagine. Researchers once thought that developmental aphantasia was rare (e.g., Botez et al., 1985). However, thanks to recent attention on the condition, it has been revealed that many people have this condition (e.g., Faw, 2009).

As typical examples, people with aphantasia do not see a mental picture (imagery) of a car when they try to remember what a car looks like, and they cannot conjure a mental map in order to navigate. Imagining a color such as blue does not cause the generation of a specific shade of blue in their mind. While there are differences between each person with aphantasia, there are some general patterns. People with aphantasia may be less religious and enjoy fictional stories less than people without aphantasia, due to the role that mental pictures can play in those experiences (Toftness, 2022). When reading, they may prefer to skip over lengthy descriptions of scenery, because their imaginations do not generate much to look at while reading those things. Whether or not a person with aphantasia can imagine senses like sounds and smells also depends upon each individual person (Kendle, 2017).

Overall, people with aphantasia report having fewer dreams at night (Dawes et al., 2020). Their dreams may range from having no dreams at all to frequent dreams with vivid imagery and colors (Toftness, 2022). Those who do dream often report that upon waking, the visuals fade quickly, and they cannot re-experience the images when they remember the dream. This highlights an important difference between voluntary and involuntary mental imagery. Some people with aphantasia do not experience much voluntary mental imagery but do experience a lot of involuntary mental imagery, such as when falling asleep, having fevers, while on certain drugs, or during a migraine (Sacks, 2010, p. 221). Others, especially those with acquired aphantasia, report having neither involuntary nor voluntary mental imagery.

People with mental imagery use it quite often to remember the past and plan the future, and this has led researchers to predict that aphantasia may lead to problems with remembering and planning. People with aphantasia report having poorer *autobiographical memory* compared to people without aphantasia, meaning that they remember fewer details about the experiences they have had in life that tell the story of who they are as a person (Zeman et al., 2020). Many people with aphantasia document their lives through photos and videos in order to assist with the absence of visual memories and to prevent forgetting (Watkins, 2018). Some researchers have suggested that aphantasia is also affiliated with depression and feeling like life isn't real, possibly due to their difficulties in imagining the future (de Vito & Bartolomeo, 2016). Because they cannot generate imagery in their minds, they often report problems similar to mild forms of face blindness (see Prosopagnosia) and navigational difficulties (see Topographical Disorientation). There also appear to be some differences in how people with aphantasia complete mental tasks involving remembering pictures compared to people without aphantasia, but the exact nature and extent of those differences is still under investigation (e.g., Pounder et al., 2022; Toftness, 2022).

The experience of a person's imagination is entirely subjective; that is, nobody else can know what you are experiencing—at least, we haven't yet reached that point of the mind-reading future. People with aphantasia typically report that they were under the impression that phrases such as "picture in your mind" were metaphorical and that they were shocked when they discovered other people are capable of seeing images in their minds (Kendle, 2017). People with aphantasia often find that they better understand themselves after learning about their absence of imagery, as it can help to explain life experiences such as difficulties in art class, difficulties in navigation, or preference for science books instead of fantasy novels.

The Brain Pathology

Which parts of the brain are usually affected in cases of acquired aphantasia? If you want a straightforward answer, it has been argued that people with acquired aphantasia usually have damage to their left temporal lobe (Bartolomeo, 2002). However, that explanation is incomplete, because "different types of imagery deficits can be found," typically alongside additional disorders of "visuospatial perception, recognition, or exploration" (Trojano & Grossi, 1994, p. 217).

Most notably, aphantasia seems to occur alongside additional trouble with objects (see Visual Object Agnosia), faces (see Prosopagnosia), and space (see Topographical Disorientation). Indeed, the location and extent of the damage leading up to a person reporting a reduction of their mental imagery ability is different between people and "rarely concerns only one specific brain area" (Dijkstra et al., 2019, p. 425).

There is also evidence that neural representations of both perceived (actually seen) and imagined objects have a large degree of overlap in the brain. As indicated by brain scans, imagery activates some of the same parts of the brain that activate when looking at real objects, especially in the parts of your brain responsible for processing vision in the occipital and temporal cortex (Djikstra et al., 2019). For example, imagining a pattern of lines produces similar brain activation as does actually looking at that same line pattern (Klein et al., 2004). Imagining a bigger and more detailed object activates more visual cortex (Reisberg, 2013). Overall, such findings suggest that seeing objects and imagining objects are very similar at the level of the brain.

Even though imagery and actually seeing objects seem to activate similar areas in the brain, they are different enough that a brain can be more capable of one than the other. This can work in any combination: sighted people can have aphantasia, blind people can have mental imagery (see Cortical Blindness), and it is also possible to never experience mental images or seeing of any kind, such as in people who are blind since birth (e.g., Goldenberg et al., 1995; Meaidi et al., 2014). People who are blinded in life may have a variety of mental imagery experiences, such that some find their mental images faded over time into aphantasia with disuse, but others continued to imagine things visually even after losing sight (Sacks, 2010, p. 203).

In theory, damage to specific layers of the visual cortex that are responsible for either sending out or taking in neural information may lead to these more specific impairments. For example, damaging your "input layer of the visual cortex" coming from the eyes while keeping the input to the visual cortex that comes from your inferior temporal lobes intact might lead to a person losing bottom-up perception (actually seeing objects) while allowing them to retain top-down imagery (imagining the objects)—though much more work is needed to determine such relationships (Djikstra et al., 2019, p. 425).

This gets even more complex when we consider that there is evidence that there are actually at least two types of mental images: visual and spatial (Reisberg, 2013). Visual imagery is used to imagine *what* something looks like, while spatial imagery is used to imagine *where* something is in space. These two types of imagery are not perfectly tied together, meaning that you can be better at one than the other, and they seem to be represented by partially discrete areas in the brain (Farah et al., 1988). Therefore, there may be two forms of aphantasia: visual and spatial (Blazhenkova & Pechenkova, 2019).

There is not currently a formal diagnosis for aphantasia. There are some tests related to visual imagery that a person can take in order to try and determine if they are impaired in this area, such as the Vividness of Visual

Imagery Questionnaire (Marks, 1973). Such tests may also reveal people who are especially gifted in mental imagery: those people are referred to as having *hyperphantasia*. Research is presently underway to more fully develop the ideas surrounding aphantasia and hyperphantasia, and at some point in the future, there may be more standardized tests for these specific conditions. For now, differences in mental imagery are difficult to measure and difficult to understand about each other because mental imagery is such a private experience.

References

Bartolomeo, P. (2002). The relationship between visual perception and visual mental imagery: A reappraisal of the neuropsychological evidence. *Cortex, 38*(3), 357–378. https://doi.org/d5892j

Basso, A., Bisiach, E., & Luzzatti, C. (1980). Loss of mental imagery: A case study. *Neuropsychologia, 18*(4–5), 435–442. https://doi.org/dfzd2j

Blazhenkova, O., & Pechenkova, E. (2019). The two eyes of the blind mind: Object vs. spatial aphantasia? *The Russian Journal of Cognitive Science, 6*(4), 51–62. https://doi.org/gs43

Botez, M. I., Olivier, M., Vézina, J. L., Botez, T., & Kaufman, B. (1985). Defective revisualization: Dissociation between cognitive and imagistic thought case report and short review of the literature. *Cortex, 21*(3), 375–389. https://doi.org/g487

Brain, R. (1954). Loss of visualization. *Proceedings of the Royal Society of Medicine, 47*(4), 288–290.

Dawes, A. J., Keogh, R., Andrillon, T., & Pearson, J. (2020). A cognitive profile of multisensory imagery, memory and dreaming in aphantasia. *Scientific Reports, 10.* Article 10022. https://doi.org/gg3fkf

Dennett, D. C. (1978). *Brainstorms.* Bradford Books.

de Vito, S., & Bartolomeo, P. (2016). Refusing to imagine? On the possibility of psychogenic aphantasia. A commentary on Zeman et al. (2015). *Cortex, 74,* 334–335. https://doi.org/gdf49x

Dijkstra, N., Bosch, S. E., & van Gerven, M. A. (2019). Shared neural mechanisms of visual perception and imagery. *Trends in Cognitive Sciences, 23*(5), 423–434. https://doi.org/gg7jtw

Farah, M. J., Hammond, K. M., Levine, D. N., & Calvanio, R. (1988). Visual and spatial mental imagery: Dissociable systems of representation. *Cognitive Psychology, 20*(4), 439–462. https://doi.org/bzms6f

Faw, B. (2009). Conflicting intuitions may be based on differing abilities: Evidence from mental imaging research. *Journal of Consciousness Studies, 16*(4), 45–68.

Galton, F. (1880). Visualised Numerals. *Nature, 21,* 252–256. https://doi.org/dmsnm8

Goldenberg, G., Müllbacher, W., & Nowak, A. (1995). Imagery without perception—A case study of anosognosia for cortical blindness. *Neuropsychologia, 33*(11), 39–48. https://doi.org/dz3wjx

Kendle, A. (2017). *Aphantasia: Experiences, perceptions, and insights.* Dark River.

Klein, I., Dubois, J., Mangin, J. F., Kherif, F., Flandin, G., Poline, J. B., Denis, M., Kosslyn, S. M., & Le Bihan, D. (2004). Retinotopic organization of visual mental images as revealed by functional magnetic resonance imaging. *Cognitive Brain Research, 22*(1), 26–31. https://doi.org/bnjsr5

Marks, D. F. (1973). Visual imagery differences in the recall of pictures. *British Journal of Psychology, 64*(1), 17–24. https://doi.org/b6v5wv

Meaidi, A., Jennum, P., Ptito, M., & Kupers, R. (2014). The sensory construction of dreams and nightmare frequency in congenitally blind and late blind individuals. *Sleep Medicine, 15*(5), 586–595. https://doi.org/gddnqp

Pearson, J., & Kosslyn, S. M. (2015). The heterogeneity of mental representation: Ending the imagery debate. *Proceedings of the National Academy of Sciences, 112*(33), 10089–10092. https://doi.org/f7pcvd

Pounder, Z., Jacob, J., Evans, S., Loveday, C., Eardley, A. F., & Silvanto, J. (2022). Only minimal differences between individuals with congenital aphantasia and those with typical imagery on neuropsychological tasks that involve imagery. *Cortex.* https://doi.org/hgnw

Reisberg, D. (2013). Mental images. In D. Reisberg (Ed.) *The Oxford handbook of cognitive psychology*, (pp. 374–387). Oxford University Press. https://doi.org/gs44

Sacks, O. (2010). *The mind's eye.* Knopf.

Toftness, A. R. (2022). *Clarifying aphantasia.* [Doctoral dissertation, Iowa State University]. ProQuest Dissertations & Theses Global.

Trojano, L., & Grossi, D. (1994). A critical review of mental imagery defects. *Brain and Cognition, 24*(2), 213–243. https://doi.org/dx82wr

Watkins, N. W. (2018). (A)phantasia and severely deficient autobiographical memory: Scientific and personal perspectives. *Cortex, 105*, 41–52. https://doi.org/gd5m58

Zeman, A. Z., Della Sala, S., Torrens, L. A., Gountouna, V. E., McGonigle, D. J., & Logie, R. H. (2010). Loss of imagery phenomenology with intact visuo-spatial task performance: A case of 'blind imagination'. *Neuropsychologia, 48*(1), 145–155. https://doi.org/cmfgxv

Zeman, A. Z., Dewar, M., & Della Sala, S. (2015). Lives without imagery–Congenital aphantasia. *Cortex, 73*, 378–380. https://doi.org/gdf5hc

Zeman, A., Milton, F., Della Sala, S., Dewar, M., Frayling, T., Gaddum, J., Hattersley, A., Heuerman-Williamson, B., Jones, K., MacKisack, M., & Winlove, C. (2020). Phantasia–The psychological significance of lifelong visual imagery vividness extremes. *Cortex, 130*, 426–440. https://doi.org/ghdxvf

Aphasia

Imagine that you can't use spoken language in quite the way you intend to. Perhaps when you speak, your sentences fill up with nonsense words. Or perhaps you can't quite remember the words you are trying to say and struggle to get a few out at a time. It may be that when you listen to other people speaking, you can't understand most of the words that they are saying. You might have trouble communicating what you want to say, even though you think all of your words are coming out fine. Diminished communication capability because of brain damage is an extremely frustrating situation to be in, and unfortunately, it is all too common.

The Stories

(STORY 1) A case published in 1897 told the story of a 26-year-old woman who developed a variety of language complications following what was described as a "cerebral attack" (p. 1256). For a while, she appeared to be completely deaf, but then she began to show responses to certain sounds such as a closing door or a ticking clock. She did not, however, seem to understand most words spoken to her. She seemed to understand simple written questions and could reply by writing, albeit with some mistakes and extra words. One sentence that she wrote reads: "I two notes and ther is a little nonsense read yes I let me to let you know I would like to a deal to make stronger than I was," seemingly trying to indicate that she knew her communication wasn't great but that she felt she was improving (p. 1257). She would speak words occasionally, but only one or a few at a time. Today, this case would probably be classified as *global aphasia* (Bramwell, 1897, case 11).

(STORY 2) In a case of a 75-year-old woman, *fluent aphasia* was diagnosed following a series of tests demonstrating her tendency to construct sentences that were missing concrete nouns and instead contained extra words that lacked meaning. This difficulty with language extended to all modalities, including speaking and writing. When asked to write down the sentence "he wanted the dog to go home," she instead wrote, "the boys run and the dog is all home" (p. 177). When she was asked to describe a picture, what she said included this sentence: "and that's the boy going to getting with it over there"

DOI: 10.4324/9781003276937-11

(p. 175). Also in line with fluent aphasia, she had difficulties understanding questions asked of her. Other than the language difficulties, she continued to live an independent life (Binder, 2003).

(STORY 3) A military officer with a head injury described the feeling of *nonfluent aphasia*. He expressed himself with a few words at a time, with long pauses in between while he searched for the words he wanted to use. He said: "I sometimes—have to—alter the whole—to alter the sentence—because—I—have—difficulty—in finding—the word" (p. 113). He also frequently substituted colorful expressions in the place of common words in order to get around the problem of being unable to retrieve the exact word that he wanted. He told the physician, "I want to say a word—at the back of my mind—I can't just—dig it up" (p. 113). He also reported that he found silent thought easier than verbal thought, as if the act of verbalizing was messing up his words (Head, 1920, case 17).

The Features

The human ability to verbally communicate has often been credited for the rise of civilization, because it allowed faster sharing of ideas and promoted social bonds through storytelling—presumably the spooky kind—around campfires. However, putting your thoughts into words and the ability to decipher other people's words back into thoughts is enormously complicated, which is why children spend countless hours practicing exactly this. But even once learned, the ability is revocable. Some people have these communication abilities taken away, usually due to strokes.

I want to be clear here that aphasia is a loss of communication abilities but not a loss of intelligence. One of the most frustrating features of this disorder is that a person may be brilliant, but unable to show that brilliance. This was described over a century ago in a useful fashion: "it is easy to ascertain that he is in possession of his intelligence and that the apparent psychical deficiency consists only in his difficulty in understanding others, and in making himself understood" (Lichtheim, 1885, p. 454). Keep this in mind as we explore the specifics.

Aphasia is a disorder with many subtypes. There are subtypes of aphasia in which the afflicted person cannot speak but can still understand speech, types where they cannot understand speech but can still speak, and a severe type in which they can neither speak nor understand speech. In total, there are at least eight subtypes of aphasia, each type being related to the limits of a person's language capabilities (Pedersen et al., 2004). This classification is somewhat arbitrary, and it has been questioned for decades whether the eight subtypes that are commonly used are optimal (e.g., Landrigan et al., 2021; Risser & Spreen, 1985). As with all brain damage-related conditions, sorting people into groups is tricky because brains are complex and differ between people.

The most important distinction between these subtypes of aphasia is the distinction between *fluent* and *nonfluent* aphasias. Fluency is the "flow" of words, or the ease with which they are spoken in sequence, regardless of whether the words themselves are correct in meaning. That is, speaking complete sentences at a rhythmic pace, even if some of the words are nonsense, is considered fluent. In contrast, speaking in incomplete sentences, using one or two words at a time and without typical grammatical structure, is considered nonfluent (Hodges & Patterson, 1996).

The most disruptive subtype of aphasia, and probably the most common subtype, is called *global aphasia* (Pedersen et al., 2004). People with global aphasia lose the ability to speak without great effort, and also lose the ability to understand the speech of others. It is a nonfluent aphasia, with the most severe cases disrupting all language skills to the point that the person can only communicate using facial expressions and gestures. Those who can speak generally have severe deficits of naming, called *anomia*, in which they do not use the appropriate or expected words for things. This anomia can take the form of extra description to avoid the name ("the thing you sit on" instead of chair), as incorrect words (couch instead of chair), or as words with phonetic mistakes (share instead of chair). However, the person with anomia typically still *knows* the object that they are referring to. They may be able to point to it or make a gesture showing what the object does. Thus, people who have an anomia component with their agnosia are generally said to have trouble specifically with *retrieving words*—nouns and verbs, especially, are negatively affected (Mesulam, 2009).

Less severe than global aphasia is a subtype called *Wernicke aphasia*, sometimes simply called *fluent aphasia*, even though it is not the only fluent subtype. In these cases, a person can speak relatively fluently and may use full sentences. However, those sentences often contain extra nonsense words and may lack meaning to a listener. The person with fluent aphasia, however, feels as if they are communicating effectively and are unaware of their errors (Hillis, 2007). This can lead to what is known as *jargon aphasia*, in which the person paraphrases what they are trying to say with many unusual word choices, resulting in long sentences with little meaning (Mesulam, 2009). Additionally, those with fluent aphasia generally cannot understand the meaning behind words when they hear them (see Cortical Deafness) or read them. This can lead to very frustrating situations in which the person with aphasia believes that they are communicating effectively but aren't being understood, and the other person in the conversation may not be able to communicate to the person with aphasia that they do not understand.

Another subtype of aphasia that is somewhat common is *Broca aphasia*, sometimes simply called *nonfluent aphasia*, which is a nonfluent subtype. In these cases, a person struggles with producing fluent sentences when speaking and typically speaks only in short, and often incomplete, sentences. For example, they may shorten sentences into single words in order to avoid the difficulty of mentally retrieving additional words. People with nonfluent aphasia typically retain the ability to respond yes or no to questions and generally have less trouble understanding speech when compared to someone with fluent aphasia (Mesulam, 2009). They also often have "islands of fluent production" where they have an easier time smoothly producing well-learned phrases such as "you know what I mean" when compared to less predetermined speech patterns (Hillis, 2007, p. 201). Additionally, and quite surprisingly, abilities such as singing familiar songs may still be intact and fluent in people with nonfluent aphasia (Ramachandran, 2011).

Interestingly, if a person knows sign language, aphasia may affect that ability in similar ways to verbal speech. For example, they may have trouble using more than a few signs at a time in a case of nonfluent aphasia, or they may use strange sign choices during a long string of signing in a case of fluent aphasia (Hickok et al., 1998). This is evidence that it is not just vocal production or a person's hearing that is affected in aphasia—what is affected is the use of *language* itself. What does damage to language look like in a person's brain?

The Brain Pathology

Aphasia generally results due to damage to the left side of the brain, especially to the temporal lobe. Recently, researchers have successfully used the specific part of the brain that was damaged in order to predict which type of aphasia would develop—now, using a brain scan of each person newly experiencing aphasia, researchers can predict the course of the disorder to some extent (Yourganov et al., 2015). This shows that the subtypes of aphasia are at least somewhat predictably related to damage in different brain areas.

If you've taken certain psychology or anatomy classes, the names Wernicke and Broca may be familiar to you, because they both had places in the brain named after them. Over the course of the 1860s, Broca put the idea together that there was a region in the left hemisphere of the brain that was often damaged in people who had limited or poorly articulated speech—what is now known as Broca's area (Berker et al., 1986; Broca, 1865), which, fortunately, is a lot easier to say than "left posterior inferior frontal cortex" (Hillis, 2007). About a decade later, Wernicke published research about an area of the brain located further back in the left temporal lobe that seemed to be damaged in people who had well-articulated speech but meaningless words—now known as Wernicke's area (Wernicke, 1874). Damage to those respective areas certainly contributes to many cases of Broca aphasia and Wernicke aphasia, respectively, although the reality is more complex than each type of aphasia having one spot in the brain that causes it. Global aphasia, on the other hand, is often described as resulting from "massive lesions" including large swaths of the cortex and the underlying white matter connections between areas of the brain (Pinel & Barnes, 2017, p. 440). This makes sense: if you damage more areas, the aphasia becomes more problematic.

A common set of tests used for sorting people with aphasia into groups is the Western Aphasia Battery (Kang et al., 2010). The person is generally sorted into one of the eight common aphasia categories with tests of writing, reading, speaking, and so on. Because there are so many subtypes of aphasia, each case requires careful testing of language abilities before diagnosis. And, as has been pointed out many times over the years, even if two people end up with the same diagnosis of a particular subtype of aphasia, this does not mean that those two people have the exact same symptoms (Landrigan et al., 2021).

There is evidence that aphasia is not completely permanent. A paper that reviewed many studies that attempted to rehabilitate people with aphasia using speech and language therapy showed that such therapies were effective in restoring some level of reading, writing, and spoken communication abilities (Brady et al., 2016). Over time, aphasia can become milder and can even change classifications. Global aphasia may become fluent aphasia as some fluency is recovered, and nonfluent aphasia may become a milder anomic aphasia (Pedersen et al., 2004). This is good news, because it encourages many people with aphasia to train their brains by communicating in any way they can.

References

Berker, E. A., Berker, A. H., & Smith, A. (1986). Translation of Broca's 1865 report: Localization of speech in the third left frontal convolution. *Archives of Neurology, 43*(10), 1065–1072. https://doi.org/cqst4k (Original work published 1865)

Binder, J. R. (2003). Wernicke aphasia: A disorder of central language processing. In M. D'Esposito (Ed.), *Neurological foundations of cognitive neuroscience* (pp. 175–238). MIT press.

Brady, M. C., Godwin, J., Enderby, P., Kelly, H., & Campbell, P. (2016). Speech and language therapy for aphasia after stroke: An updated systematic review and meta-analyses. *Stroke, 47*(10), e236–e237. https://doi.org/ghsgjd

Bramwell, B. (1897). Illustrative cases of aphasia. *The Lancet, 149*(3845), 1256–1259. https://doi.org/d83zgw

Broca, P. (1865). Sur le siège de la faculté du langage articulé. *Bulletin de la Société d' Anthropologie, 6,* 377–393.

Head, H. (1920). Aphasia and kindred disorders of speech. *Brain, 43,* 87–165. https://doi.org/dzkc5c

Hickok, G., Bellugi, U., & Klima, E. S. (1998). The neural organization of language: Evidence from sign language aphasia. *Trends in Cognitive Sciences, 2*(4), 129–136. https://doi.org/bc9qmc

Hillis, A. E. (2007). Aphasia progress in the last quarter of a century. *Neurology, 69*(2), 200–213. https://doi.org/fhwjc9

Hodges, J. R., & Patterson, K. (1996). Nonfluent progressive aphasia and semantic dementia: A comparative neuropsychological study. *Journal of the International Neuropsychological Society, 2*(6), 511–524. https://doi.org/b9trfv

Kang, E. K., Sohn, H. M., Han, M. K., Kim, W., Han, T. R., & Paik, N. J. (2010). Severity of post-stroke aphasia according to aphasia type and lesion location in Koreans. *Journal of Korean Medical Science, 25*(1), 123–127. https://doi.org/cv4tmb

Landrigan, J. F., Zhang, F., & Mirman, D. (2021). A data-driven approach to post-stroke aphasia classification and lesion-based prediction. *Brain, 144*(5), 1372–1383. https://doi.org/g6kx

Lichtheim, L. (1885). On aphasia. *Brain, 7,* 433–484. https://doi.org/gdj2nm

Mesulam, M. M. (2009). Aphasia: Sudden and progressive. In L. R. Squire (Ed.), *Encyclopedia of neuroscience* (pp. 517–521). Elsevier.

Pedersen, P. M., Vinter, K., & Olsen, T. S. (2004). Aphasia after stroke: Type, severity and prognosis. *Cerebrovascular Diseases*, *17*(1), 35–43. https://doi.org/b742w3

Pinel, J., & Barnes, S. (2017). *Biopsychology* (10th edition). Pearson.

Ramachandran, V. S. (2011). *The tell-tale brain: A neuroscientist's quest for what makes us human*. WW Norton & Company.

Risser, A. H., & Spreen, O. (1985). The western aphasia battery. *Journal Of Clinical And Experimental Neuropsychology*, *7*(4), 463–470. https://doi.org/bg4w3m

Wernicke, C. (1874). *Der aphasische Symptomencomplex: Eine psychologische Studie auf anatomischer Basis*. Cohn & Weigert.

Yourganov, G., Smith, K. G., Fridriksson, J., & Rorden, C. (2015). Predicting aphasia type from brain damage measured with structural MRI. *Cortex*, *73*, 203–215. https://doi.org/f76j2q

Ataxia (and Dysmetria)

Imagine that you can't coordinate the movements of your muscles. Reaching out and grabbing objects is one of the fundamental ways that we interact with the world, so imagine if every time you went to reach, you missed the target. Looking around your environment to search for something is an everyday task, so imagine that you can't get your eyes to look exactly where you want them to. Imagine if, as you walked, you had to focus on each small movement of your legs in order to keep upright and moving. For most, moving a muscle is as simple as a thought. But for some, it is a stressful event that requires careful focus and multiple attempts.

The Stories

(STORY 1) At the Philadelphia Neurological Society's meeting in 1940, one of the case studies discussed was actually a pair of case studies: identical twins, each of whom had died from the same *hereditary ataxia*. The symptoms started at the ages of 33 and 34, with weak muscles in the upper body, including the arms and trunk. Over time, the disease became worse, eventually leading to additional muscle degeneration, partial loss of eyesight, and dementia. They passed away at the ages of 64 and 66 from similar disease complications. When their brains were examined, the damage looked very similar between the two—they had approximately identical neuropathologic changes. Curiously, while they were alive, some of the twin's symptoms were mirror images of one another. One of the twins had worse vision (optic atrophy) on the left side, while the other twin had worse vision on the right side. One of the twins had a neurological sign called hyper-reflexes that was most pronounced on one side of the body, and the other twin had those same hyper-reflexes on the opposite side. Being able to examine the symptoms and brains of identical twins taught the researchers lessons about the hereditary nature of this particular ataxia condition (Wilson & Dean, 1941).

(STORY 2) In the case of a 52-year-old man, he discovered that he was developing ataxia. His eye movements became *dysmetric*, making it difficult to move his eye gaze to a desired place. His voice began to sound different, due to changes in the muscle coordination in his throat. His ability to balance

DOI: 10.4324/9781003276937-12

deteriorated, leading to a wide walking stance with short strides and some staggering. Combined speech therapy and vocal cord injections helped his voice, and physical therapy was suggested as well. Eventually, after some gene sequencing, it was discovered that he had a rare form of a genetic disease called Alexander disease. This was causing the ataxia due to a variant in his genetic code. The researchers were able to pinpoint the exact mutation in his genetic code, showing the power of modern diagnostic medicine (Gass et al., 2017).

(STORY 3) In the 1890s, a 30-year-old man told a physician about the *progressive ataxia* that he had been experiencing for about a decade. He described that he first noticed the problems in his gait around the age of 18, when he began to have trouble coordinating his walking, especially when he was very tired. Over time, his boss thought that he had been drinking on the job due to how unusual his gait was. His coworkers complained that when he leaned on their desks while talking to them, he made them unable to work due to his unsteady wobbling, which shook their desks. He began to notice difficulties in swallowing and speaking as time progressed, which sometimes led to near-choking events. He was unable to reach out quickly to grasp objects and had to slowly and deliberately guide his hand to the object, and even then had to correct his reach by several inches. The coordination of his facial muscles was also affected, leading to uncoordinated facial expressions during conversations. In the final year of his life, he was unable to walk at all. Along with some of his family members, this person donated his brain to the scientific cause of learning more about this form of hereditary ataxia. Because of this, researchers were able to build a family tree showing which family members were affected and unaffected and at which ages the symptoms appeared (Barker, 1903, case xviii).

The Features

Think about all of the specific muscle movements that it takes to walk up to a door, grasp the doorknob with your fingers, twist just enough to one side, push the door open, and walk through. The muscles, large in your legs and small in your wrists, work on specific and coordinated tasks. Fortunately, you usually do not need to think about this beyond "push" or "pull" because your muscles have been well trained to execute these precise movements with little effort. However, the parts of your brain responsible for sending those precise and coordinated orders to your muscles can be damaged, revealing the complexity of such tasks.

Ataxia is the difficulty in coordinating muscle movements. Like a musical conductor keeping an orchestra of instruments organized in timing, it is the job of a conductor in your brain to make sure that muscle movements happen in the correct order and with the intended intensity. Ataxia occurs when that conductor is prevented from doing its job. The resulting lack of coordination may disrupt many kinds of muscle movements. Ataxia may create muscle difficulties in swallowing, called *dysphagia*, and muscle difficulties in speaking, which is called *dysarthria*. Let's focus on a few other important examples.

One important example is balance and walking, which is referred to as a person's *gait*. People with ataxia typically have a specific gait, described as having a broad base wherein the legs are held far apart from one another. This broad base partially makes up for the loss of the natural balance that usually comes from small, coordinated muscle movements, and the person may also lean on canes, walls, or furniture for further assistance. Gaits and other symptoms such as changes in muscle reflexes may differ depending on the underlying neurological problem, which can help with the diagnosis of subtypes of ataxia (Ashizawa & Xia, 2016).

Hand movements are especially challenging for people with ataxia. Because your fingers do not contain muscles for movement, the small movements of your fingers require careful coordination of the muscles in your palms and wrists. Coordinating this orchestration of pulley systems requires especially careful conducting, which is why tasks like writing with a pencil and playing the piano take so much practice. A relatively huge portion of your brain is dedicated to these muscles, but fine movements become incredibly difficult to perform without the conductor in charge of the careful timing and precision of signals sent to and from the muscles.

Your eyes also have several muscles responsible for their movements. Six different muscles control eye position, but because they are plugged into a variety of cranial nerves, they can't directly communicate with each other about what each muscle is planning. Instead, they all send messages to, and receive messages from, your brain. In the brain, it is the conductor's job to calculate exactly when to send signals for each eye muscle to take action. If a signal arrives at the wrong time, or if the signals are incorrect, the eyes won't look at the place where the person intended to look.

These difficulties with planned movement, especially with the hands and eyes, can be described in terms of *dysmetria*. Dysmetria is a difficulty in moving a body part to the intended position. For example, dysmetria may include moving a muscle too far or not moving it enough. Trying to pick up a glass of water may result in knocking the glass over by moving the hand too far. If a person tries to move their eyes to look at something, they may not move their eyes far enough and therefore fail to look at the thing. Moving a muscle too far is called *hypermetria*, while not moving it far enough is called *hypometria* (Timmann & Diener, 2003). The person may need to readjust their hand or eye position multiple times. Dysmetric movements exist both in large movements, such as in the legs, and in small movements, such as in the fingers, and are more inaccurate when movement is attempted quickly (Hore et al., 1991).

The Brain Pathology

Generally, ataxia results from damage in the cerebellum or to the pathways leading into or out of the cerebellum. This is a part of the brain that contributes greatly to *fine motor control*, which is a way of saying "small movements that work together with other small movements." Essentially, the cerebellum receives input from your muscles via your spine and mixes that with input from your brain using a combination of highly interconnected "Purkinje cells" and an incredibly high number of small "granule cells" (Marsden & Harris, 2011). When I say an incredibly high number, I mean it: roughly 80% of the neurons in your brain are located in your cerebellum, and this number is even higher for mammals such as the African elephant, which has about 98% of its neurons located in the cerebellum (Kaas & Herculano-Houzel, 2017). Those extremely numerous cells seem to be essential for maneuvering large bodies in complex ways.

Depending on where exactly the damage is, different areas of the person's body may have more or less pronounced ataxia. For example, if one-half of the cerebellum is disrupted, movement on only one side of the body may be ataxic. If the middle of the cerebellum is damaged, it may lead to *truncal ataxia*, in which a person is unstable while sitting (Ashizawa & Xia, 2016). Depending on the exact nature of the ataxia, there may also be involvement in other areas, including the brain stem and spinal cord (Turk et al., 2018).

Many subtypes of ataxia are known to be inherited genetic disorders that run in families, known as *hereditary ataxias* (Strupp et al., 2007; Turk et al., 2018). There are many kinds of hereditary ataxias, which can be told apart by looking at a person's genetic code or sometimes by their specific symptoms (Ashizawa & Xia, 2016). Oftentimes, ataxia progresses and becomes slowly worse over time, which is referred to as *progressive ataxia*. In severe cases, ataxia progresses to the point that standing and walking are either impossible or require complete assistance (Schmahmann, 2004).

Sometimes a person does not consistently experience ataxia—the symptoms may come and go. In these cases, it is referred to as *episodic ataxia*. Episodic ataxia is also usually hereditary. Depending on the type of episodic ataxia, the episodes may last for just seconds or minutes, or in a more severe type, from hours to days (Ashizawa & Xia, 2016). Episodes may be triggered due to changes in posture, motion, or emotional state, resulting in temporary ataxia symptoms (Strupp et al., 2007). Additionally, episodic ataxia is often associated with symptoms such as sensations of spinning (see Vertigo), migraines (see Migraine Headaches), and seizures (see Seizures), depending on the subtype (Rajakulendran et al., 2007).

However, there are nongenetic reasons that a person might develop ataxia, such as a stroke in the cerebellum, multiple sclerosis, or toxic levels of several substances such as mercury or alcohol. The connection between alcohol and ataxia is especially interesting, because a person with the gait of ataxia may appear to be drunk due to the way they are walking. This is because when a person gets drunk, the alcohol affects their cerebellum in a similar way to how ataxia affects the cerebellum. Most of the time, effects of alcohol wear off, but continued use of alcohol may change the cerebellum and the person's gait permanently (Melgaard & Ahlgren, 1986).

In many cases, ataxia can improve over time with rehabilitation that focuses on balance and coordination exercises (Marquer et al., 2014). Physical therapy seems to be at least somewhat effective for several different types of ataxia (Fonteyn et al., 2014). Recently, promising efforts to rehabilitate have been made using robot-assisted walking devices, immersive virtual reality, and exercise games (Lacorte et al., 2020). Regardless of which method is used, the key to making progress is regular intensive training—enough to convince the brain to rehire the conductor for the delicate symphony of moving your muscles.

References

Ashizawa, T., & Xia, G. (2016). Ataxia. *Continuum, 22*(4), 1208–1226. https://doi.org/ghz8ww

Barker, L. F. (1903). *A description of the brains and spinal cords of two brothers dead of hereditary ataxia.* University of Chicago Press.

Fonteyn, E. M. R., Keus, S. H. J., Verstappen, C. C. P., Schöls, L., De Groot, I. J. M., & Van De Warrenburg, B. P. C. (2014). The effectiveness of allied health care in patients with ataxia: A systematic review. *Journal of Neurology, 261*(2), 251–258. https://doi.org/f5r8pk

Gass, J. M., Cheema, A., Jackson, J., Blackburn, P. R., Van Gerpen, J., & Atwal, P. S. (2017). Novel GFAP variant in adult-onset alexander disease with progressive ataxia and palatal tremor. *The Neurologist, 22*(6), 247–248. https://doi.org/gtjp

Hore, J., Wild, B., & Diener, H. C. (1991). Cerebellar dysmetria at the elbow, wrist, and fingers. *Journal of Neurophysiology, 65*(3), 563–571. https://doi.org/gtjq

Kaas, J. H., & Herculano-Houzel, S. (2017). What makes the human brain special: Key features of brain and neocortex. In I. Opris & M.F. Casanova (Eds.), *The physics of the mind and brain disorders* (pp. 3–22). https://doi.org/g6pm

Lacorte, E., Bellomo, G., Nuovo, S., Corbo, M., Vanacore, N., & Piscopo, P. (2020). The use of new mobile and gaming technologies for the assessment and rehabilitation of people with ataxia: A systematic review and meta-analysis. *Cerebellum.* https://doi.org/gjpm6s

Marquer, A., Barbieri, G., & Pérennou, D. (2014). The assessment and treatment of postural disorders in cerebellar ataxia: A systematic review. *Annals of Physical and Rehabilitation Medicine, 57*(2), 67–78. https://doi.org/gtjs

Marsden, J., & Harris, C. (2011). Cerebellar ataxia: Pathophysiology and rehabilitation. *Clinical Rehabilitation, 25*(3), 195–216. https://doi.org/fsx24k

Melgaard, B., & Ahlgren, P. (1986). Ataxia and cerebellar atrophy in chronic alcoholics. *Journal of Neurology, 233*, 13–15. https://doi.org/bkvcmd

Rajakulendran, S., Schorge, S., Kullmann, D. M., & Hanna, M. G. (2007). Episodic ataxia type 1: A neuronal potassium channelopathy. *Neurotherapeutics, 4*(2), 258–266. https://doi.org/fgnqwr

Schmahmann, J. D. (2004). Disorders of the cerebellum: Ataxia, dysmetria of thought, and the cerebellar cognitive affective syndrome. *The Journal of Neuropsychiatry and Clinical Neurosciences, 16*(3), 367–378. https://doi.org/gtj4

Strupp, M., Zwergal, A., & Brandt, T. (2007). Episodic ataxia type 2. *Neurotherapeutics, 4*(2), 267–273. https://doi.org/d8t4kr

Timmann, D., & Diener, H. C. (2003). Coordination and ataxia. In C. G. Goetz (Ed.), *Textbook of clinical neurology* (2nd ed., pp. 299–315). Saunders.

Turk, K. W., Flanagan, M. E., Josephson, S., Keene, C. D., Jayadev, S., & Bird, T. D. (2018). Psychosis in spinocerebellar ataxias: A case series and study of tyrosine hydroxylase in substantia nigra. *The Cerebellum, 17*(2), 143–151. https://doi.org/gtj5

Wilson, G., & Dean, J. S. (1941). Hereditary ataxia in identical twins affecting the cerebellum and certain of its physiologically related structures: A clinicopathologic study. *Archives of Neurology and Psychiatry, 45*(6), 1044–1046. https://doi.org/g6mw

Bálint Syndrome (including Simultagnosia)

Imagine that you can't see more than one thing at a time. That is, you can't pay attention to more than one object within your vision at the same time. Looking at an aisle in a store to search for the item you wish to buy becomes a lengthy task: rather than scanning the shelves, you have to look at each item in sequence in order to find the one that you want. Reading, too, becomes tricky. Instead of seeing all of the words on the page, which shows you where to start and stop, you find just one word or letter at a time and have difficulty locating the others. What has caused your ability to distribute visual attention to go awry?

The Stories

(STORY 1) A 67-year-old woman complained that "her environment appeared fragmented" following a stroke (p. 1525). She could clearly see individual items but was unable to find the relationships between the items—the objects instead appeared to be isolated in this severe case of *simultagnosia*, and she saw only one object from a scene at a time. She actually found it easier to navigate with her eyes closed when moving through the familiar environment of her home due to the confusing things she saw when her eyes were open. For example, when trying to walk toward her lamp, she tripped when she walked into the dining room table—an object that eluded her detection despite taking up a large area. She no longer enjoyed television because she could only understand one thing on the screen at a time, which meant that programs became confusing quickly. However, she did enjoy listening to the radio. Once, while watching a movie, she was surprised when a character on the screen was sent flying by a punch because she had not seen the character who had done the punching (Coslett & Saffran, 1991).

(STORY 2) A 10-year-old boy was having difficulties at school, especially when it came to reading words. When he was 3 years old, he needed brain surgery, and a side effect of that was now emerging as Bálint syndrome. It turned out that his reading difficulties were mostly stemming from being unable to see all of the letters on the page at once due to simultagnosia. He also had trouble shifting his gaze around the page and fixing it in the desired location due to

DOI: 10.4324/9781003276937-13

ocular apraxia. While walking around, he would reportedly bump into people that he failed to see because he was focusing his visual attention on something else. Over time, he mostly learned to adapt to his difficulties, and he and his parents found it useful to be able to explain exactly what his difficulties were thanks to the diagnosis (Gillen & Dutton, 2003).

(STORY 3) A 30-year-old man was wounded, most likely by a machine gun bullet, in 1918, leading to a coma for a period of several days. The bullet had passed through his brain, entering on the right side above and behind his ear and exiting on the left side above and behind his ear, but somewhat lower than the entry point. He was conscious enough on the sixth day to ask for food, and it seemed at that time that he was capable of seeing, although with partial blindness due to the brain damage. However, in the parts of his visual field that could still see, he developed some symptoms. For example, when he was shown a drawing of a cross drawn inside of a square, he at first only saw the cross. After much hesitation, he was able to change his attention to the surrounding square and finally saw that as well. When a number of coins were placed on a table in front of him, he was unable to accurately count them because, as he reported, "I seem to lose myself when I look from one to the other" (p. 396). However, when the coins were placed close together in a row, he could count them without difficulty. This demonstrated the simultagnosia symptom most associated with Bálint syndrome. When someone spoke to him, he often looked in the wrong direction and kept searching until his line of vision happened across the speaker's face as if by chance. He could write down words correctly but would often place the words irregularly on the paper instead of in sequence, due to his difficulties in his gazing. Another prominent symptom was that his blinking was reduced when objects moved toward his eyes. Specifically, when a doctor would move an object close to his eye, he would fail to blink reflexively. This, along with similar issues with determining how far away objects were located, indicated that he had lost his ability to determine the positions of objects located around him (Holmes & Horrax, 1919).

The Features

Here's something you've probably not thought about recently: how do your eyes figure out what to look at? Sometimes, it is tempting to think of the eyes as windows through which some smaller person inside of your brain is looking. But that isn't true at all. The eyes and the visual systems in your brain work together to *create* the visual world that you see as you look around. Part of that process of building what you see involves deciding which things "out there" end up being given attention "in here"—in your conscious experience of vision within your brain. If you don't pay enough attention to something, you may not see it at all.

You cannot place a basket of fruit in front of someone and expect them to instantly see every detail of every piece of fruit—they must attend to each fruit and construct it from the information that their eyes pick up and their brain merges together. Your brain has a limited capacity for how much stuff it can pay attention to. For example, when you ask people who have been at fault in traffic collisions how the collision happened, one frequent response given is that they "did not even see" the obstacle that they ran into—and such cases are usually under conditions in which the person's visual systems are working typically. In extreme cases, the processes of visual search, pickup, and awareness break down to the point that, despite being *able* to see, the person consistently *doesn't* see objects, even if they are right in front of them.

Visually juggling the many multiples of things competing for our attention is a useful skill, but that skill can diminish or vanish for some people with Bálint syndrome. Sometimes called Bálint-Holmes syndrome, this disorder is characterized by three major symptoms. These symptoms are called a *triad* because of how often they occur together, although they don't all occur together in every case (Chechlacz & Humphreys, 2014). When combined, these three symptoms have such a severe impact on a person's vision that the person may be mistaken for being blind (Heutink et al., 2019).

The first symptom is called *simultagnosia* (also spelled simultanagnosia), which is a visual issue wherein a person can perceive only one object at a time. That is, they are unable to be aware of more than one visually examined object at the same time. Simultagnosia is considered the key feature of Bálint-Holmes syndrome and is the most widely studied symptom (Chechlacz & Humphreys, 2014). Bálint himself wrote of a patient that "independent of how small the object was, his visual field seemed to take in a single object only" (Bálint, 1909, translated in Bálint & Harvey, 1995, p. 270).

For example, when looking at a scene full of objects, such as a desk covered in office supplies, a person with simultagnosia is likely to notice only one thing at a time. This is not limited by the *size* of the object, but rather by the extent of its *form*. If they notice the stapler, they can see the whole stapler's form. On the other hand, if they notice the printer, they can see the form of the whole printer. The person can switch their focus to another form, especially if somebody asks them to switch. Although switching between a complicated group of objects such as letters or shapes may become confusing quickly, which can make tasks like reading very taxing. If given enough time, they can look at each object in turn and eventually see the whole desk in this piecemeal fashion, but they do not experience the objects as being "together" or part of a single scene.

If not given enough time, they will not see everything that a scene has to offer. In a classic example, a person with simultagnosia, when presented with an image of two differently colored triangles arranged to resemble a six-pointed star, will report seeing only one triangle (Luria, 1959). Another commonly used task to assess simultagnosia is Navon letters, which are a bunch of small letters arranged to look like one bigger letter, such as a bunch of letter S's put together to form a larger letter H (Navon, 1977). In general, a person with simultagnosia is unable to identify the larger letter even though they can identify the smaller letter (Rafal & Robertson, 1995).

Because they can only see one object at a time, they struggle to make comparisons between objects. For example, it has been reported that they have trouble determining at a glance whether a person is wearing glasses, because they tend to see either the face or the glasses but not both at the same time (Rafal & Robertson, 1995). One way around this limitation is to group multiple objects in a way that makes them look like single objects. For example, if they are shown a field of red and green circles and are asked whether there are two different colors, it is easier for them to do this if the differently colored circles are connected by lines (resembling the single object of a "barbell"), than if the circles are not connected or if only same color circles are connected (Humphreys & Riddoch, 1993). If the small letters in a Navon letter are placed close enough together, or if the larger letter is made more visible by blurring the smaller letters, the person may be able to perceive the large letter because it looks like one object (Chechlacz & Humphreys, 2014). This is how we know that their vision is not restricted in *space*, but by the limits of the object form.

The second symptom is called *optic ataxia*, which is a difficulty in pointing or reaching toward an object using visual information as a guide. The person has trouble guiding their movements, such as a grabbing motion with the hand, toward their target, such as a cup. If a person with optic ataxia is asked to take a pencil and make a mark in the middle of a circle drawn on a piece of paper, they typically will not be able to do so, and they may even miss the page entirely (Rafal, 2003). However, if the movements do not require the use of visual information to guide the muscles, the person is generally able to make the movements smoothly and quickly, such as pointing to a part of their body, or bringing a cigarette to their mouth (Damasio & Benton, 1979). Optic ataxia can be more severe for one-half of the visual field if brain damage is more severe on one side of the brain, such that reaching is most difficult with one specific hand (Khan et al., 2013).

Optic ataxia has a similar name to ataxia, which is more generally defined as uncoordinated voluntary muscle movements (see Ataxia). But optic ataxia is not really a type of ataxia because it is not a problem with muscle communication. Instead, it seems to be due to your brain *misusing visual information* from your peripheral vision, that is, the corners of your eyes, causing you to misinterpret where an object is located (Rossetti & Pisella, 2018).

The evidence suggests that people with optic ataxia tend to underreach, because their brain has tricked them into thinking that objects in their peripheral vision are closer to the center of their eye than they actually are (Rossetti & Pisella, 2018). For example, Bálint wrote of a patient that "while lighting a cigarette he often lit the middle and not the end" (Bálint, 1909, translated in Bálint & Harvey, 1995, p. 273).

The third symptom of the triad is called *ocular apraxia* (or gaze apraxia), which is when a person has difficulties shifting their gaze to a new visual target. That is, they find it difficult to change their *fixation*—the place at which they are looking—to new objects in their peripheral vision. The person may know where it is that they want to look next but are unable to move their eyes to look there. They may find it difficult to move their fixation away from objects they no longer wish to look at, called *prolonged latency* of eye movements, or they may be unable to maintain a fixation that they do want to keep, called *fixation drift* (Pisella et al., 2021). This was historically called "psychic paralysis" in reference to the difficulties of voluntary eye movements (Bálint & Harvey, 1995). This is not a problem with the muscles or reflexes, and when the visual scene is simple—when there are not very many objects to look at—eye movements may be closer to the movements that the person desires to make (Pisella et al., 2021). Movements of the eyes that depend on other senses may still be possible and effortless, such as when redirecting their gaze toward an unexpected noise or a part of the body that is touched (Rafal, 2003).

Additionally, a person's ability to estimate distance and their depth perception typically both also diminish as a part of Bálint-Holmes syndrome. In combination with simultagnosia, this can lead to the person accidentally tripping over an object because they didn't know it was there or how far away it was. This inability to detect distances may be so severe that the person will forget to blink when an object looms dangerously close to their eyes (Holmes & Horrax, 1919).

The Brain Pathology

As mentioned, the symptoms of Bálint-Holmes don't always occur together—simultagnosia and optic ataxia can happen independently from one another, for example—which means that it doesn't really fit the definition of a syndrome (Rizzo & Vecera, 2002). The symptoms probably occur in the same patients due to the "neuroanatomical proximity" of the brain regions responsible for producing each symptom (Farah, 2004, p. 28). In theory, there are places in the brain that individually produce symptoms of simultagnosia, optic ataxia, ocular apraxia, and loss of depth perception, but those places are located so close together that damaging one often also means that the others have been damaged.

That said, the underlying problems that lead to symptoms of Bálint-Holmes syndrome often occur in a part of the brain called the posterior parietal cortex, near where the occipital lobe and parietal lobe meet (Pisella et al., 2021). Debate continues about the exact function of this part of the parietal cortex. This syndrome, and especially simultagnosia, is sometimes described as a lack of *spatial perception*, but it is also often described as a disorder of *attention*, in which a person cannot pay attention to multiple things at once (French, 2018). Unlike neglect syndromes, in which a person ignores objects and events occurring in specific parts of their visual field such as on the left side of their body (see Hemispatial Neglect), in simultagnosia the location of the object is not as important as the fact that the person is failing to mentally represent multiple locations in space. In other words, this type of brain damage causes a "limitation of visual-spatial attentional resources" (Pisella et al., 2021, p. 245). Although, the line between the conditions can become blurry sometimes, because neglect can also occur together with simultagnosia.

Simultagnosia is often described as an inability to *stop* paying attention to something. That is, the person's attentional system in their brain locks onto an object and refuses to let go, preventing them from then disengaging their attention in order to look at other objects. The degree to which "small and, at times, barely perceptible features" can grab the person's attention and prevent them from seeing other objects has been described as extraordinary—in an example case, a person was unable to see a drawing on a sheet of paper because the watermark on the sheet of paper was too distracting (Rafal & Robertson, 1995, p. 641). Ocular apraxia, too, can potentially be explained in some cases by a failure to disengage attention from an object (Farah, 2004).

Usually, both the left and right sides of the brain need to be damaged in order for all of the symptoms to become pronounced. Damage like this can occur in a few ways, including multiple strokes, "butterfly" tumors that spread from one-half of the brain to the other, and neurodegenerative diseases like Alzheimer disease (Rafal, 2003). However, even though the complete set of Bálint-Holmes symptoms tends to require damage to both sides of the brain, the symptom of optic ataxia only seems to require damage to one side of the brain in the posterior parietal region, which makes it more common that the full syndrome (Kolb & Whishaw, 1996).

Some recovery may be possible for people with Bálint-Holmes syndrome by using training exercises for their eyes in order to overcome their difficulties (Heutink et al., 2019). Overall, more work is needed to determine how brain damage causes these different symptoms and to clarify the interaction between a person's perception of space and their abilities to pay attention to that space. I hope that sounds complicated, because it is, but work will continue toward understanding these symptoms.

References

Bálint, R. (1909). Seelenlähmung des 'Schauens' optische Ataxie, raumliche Storung der Aufmerksamkeit. *Monatsschrift Psychiatrie und Neurologie, 25*, 51–81.

Bálint, R., & Harvey, M. (1995). Psychic paralysis of gaze, optic ataxia, and spatial disorder of attention. *Cognitive Neuropsychology, 12*(3), 265–281. https://doi.org/cz8tq8

Barton, J. J. (2011). Disorder of higher visual function. *Current Opinion In Neurology, 24*(1), 1–5. https://doi.org/bbnvw3

Chechlacz, M., & Humphreys, G. W. (2014). The enigma of Balint's syndrome: Neural substrates and cognitive deficits. *Frontiers in Human Neuroscience, 8*, Article 123. https://doi.org/gtj7

Coslett, H. B., & Saffran, E. (1991). Simultanagnosia: To see but not two see. *Brain, 114*(4), 1523–1545. https://doi.org/drtvg8

Damasio, A. R., & Benton, A. L. (1979). Impairment of hand movements under visual guidance. *Neurology, 29*(2), 170–174. https://doi.org/gk7z85

Farah, M. J. (2004). *Visual agnosia* (2nd ed.). MIT Press.

French, C. (2018). Bálint's syndrome, object seeing, and spatial perception. *Mind & Language*, *33*(3), 221–241. https://doi.org/gtj8

Gillen, J. A., & Dutton, G. N. (2003). Balint's syndrome in a 10-year-old male. *Developmental Medicine and Child Neurology*, *45*(5), 349–352. https://doi.org/dzmxc9

Heutink, J., Indorf, D. L., & Cordes, C. (2019). The neuropsychological rehabilitation of visual agnosia and Balint's syndrome. *Neuropsychological Rehabilitation*, *29*(10), 1489–1508. https://doi.org/gjs4wj

Holmes, G., & Horrax, G. (1919). Disturbances of spatial orientation and visual attention, with loss of stereoscopic vision. *Archives of Neurology and Psychiatry*, *1*(4), 385–407. https://doi.org/gtj9

Humphreys, G. W., & Riddoch, M. J. (1993). Interactions between object and space systems revealed through neuropsychology. In D. E. Meyers & S. Kornblum (Eds.), *Attention and performance XIV: Synergies in experimental psychology, artificial intelligence, and cognitive neuroscience* (pp. 143–162). Erlbaum.

Khan A. Z., Pisella L., Delporte L., Rode G., & Rossetti Y. (2013). Testing for optic ataxia in a blind field. *Frontiers in Human Neuroscience*, 7, Article 399. https://doi.org/gtkb

Kolb, B., & Whishaw, I. Q. (1996). *Fundamentals of human neuropsychology* (4th edition). W. H. Freeman & Company.

Luria, A. R. (1959). Disorders of "simultaneous perception" in a case of bilateral occipito-parietal brain injury. *Brain*, *82*(3), 437–449. https://doi.org/fmh8v9

Navon, D. (1977). Forest before trees: The precedence of global features in visual perception. *Cognitive Psychology*, *9*(3), 353–383.

Pisella, L., Vialatte, A., Zein, A., Rossetti, Y. (2021). Bálint syndrome. *Handbook of Clinical Neurology*, *178*, 233–255. https://doi.org/g69f

Rafal, R. (2003). Bálint's syndrome: A disorder of visual cognition. In M. D'Esposito (Ed.), *Neurological foundations of cognitive neuroscience* (pp. 27–40). MIT press.

Rafal, R., & Robertson, L. (1995). The neurology of visual attention. In M. S. Gazzaniga (Ed.), *The cognitive neurosciences* (pp. 625–648). The MIT Press.

Rizzo, M., & Vecera, S. P. (2002). Psychoanatomical substrates of Bálint's syndrome. *Journal of Neurology Neurosurgery and Psychiatry*, *72*(2), 162–178. https://doi.org/fnk4z4

Rossetti, Y., & Pisella, L. (2018). Optic ataxia: Beyond the dorsal stream cliché. *Handbook of Clinical Neurology*, *151*, 225–247. https://doi.org/gtkc

Bobble-Head Doll Syndrome

Imagine that your head keeps bobbling back and forth like it's on a spring. All day long, it bobbles to and fro with a few bobbles per second. You can stop the bobbling in a few ways, such as by distracting yourself with a difficult math problem, or by focusing your energy on keeping still, but the bobbling always comes back a minute or two later. Fortunately, it disappears when you are asleep, giving your neck a rest. But when you're awake, moving around can be frustrating because of your involuntary bobble. What can you do to stop feeling like a bobble-headed doll?

The Stories

(STORY 1) A 22-year-old man was seen by a neuropsychiatric clinic for what was initially suspected to be mental illness—a tic disorder, a mood disorder, or possibly both. He was making involuntary head movements: nodding four or five times per second and then shaking his head side to side three or four times per second. The movements seemed to be worse when he was under stress, could be reduced when he focused on sitting still, and disappeared while he was asleep. At first, doctors did not give him a brain scan and suspected obsessive-compulsive disorder or perhaps hypomania. As his symptoms worsened, his brain was scanned, revealing a cyst in his third ventricle. He then had surgery to relieve the cyst, and the head-bobbling vanished the next day, showing that the movement was not due to mental illness after all (Hahm et al., 2018).

(STORY 2) A 14-year-old boy with a 3-year-long history of headaches began developing some new symptoms. He began experiencing confusion and "cognitive decline," making tasks like thinking and remembering more difficult (p. 237). Most notably, however, was the head-bobbling. For the past six weeks, he had been experiencing repetitive involuntary motions of his head and upper trunk. Most of the movements of his head were from side to side as if shaking his head "no," although he occasionally moved as if shaking his head "yes." These movements occurred at a rate of about two or three times per second. However, the movements disappeared when resting the back of his head on the bed. He was unable to stand or walk. A brain scan showed a tumor blocking the flow of fluid in his brain. It obstructed the cerebrospinal

DOI: 10.4324/9781003276937-14

fluid aqueduct near the third ventricle. After surgery to correct this, his symptoms of head-bobbling "resolved completely in the recovery room" (p. 237). In follow-up visits months later, the movements did not return. The family allowed the publication of a video showing the head movements and eye exams before and after the surgery to assist with the diagnosis of future cases (Renne et al., 2018, case 1).

(STORY 3) The subject of a case report in 1967 was a 10-year-old boy with an unusually large head and rhythmic head-bobbling. His head size was six standard deviations above average, meaning that his head was bigger than around 99.9999998% of other 10-year-olds' heads. The involuntary head movements were usually from side to side, and only occasionally from front to back. The movements had a rate of about two or three bobs per second and had first started appearing around the age of 9 but had recently become more continuous and seemed to be spreading to the upper trunk of his body. The number of bobs apparently varied depending on the level of attention that he paid to them and vanished entirely when he was sleeping. By asking him a math or spelling problem, the head movements could be temporarily interrupted. However, the movements would resume about a minute later. The symptoms made the doctor suspect hydrocephalus—a buildup of fluid in or around the brain—due to an obstruction that was preventing brain fluids from draining. A valve was placed within the ventricles of his brain to allow the excess fluid to drain. This worked remarkably well: in follow-up visits after his surgical procedures, the head-bobbling movements had stopped entirely (Nellhaus, 1967).

The Features

Bobble-head doll syndrome is a rare neurological disorder that causes involuntary head movements. In the process of naming the disorder, researchers noted that "the movement is reminiscent of that seen in dolls with weighted heads resting on a coiled spring, and thus it is named 'bobble-head doll syndrome'" (Benton et al., 1966, p. 725).

The head movements generally have a frequency of two or three bobs per second (Reddy et al., 2014; Renne et al., 2018). This motion is usually in a forward-back pattern as if nodding the head "yes." Over 80% of reported cases show this "yes" motion (Renne et al., 2018). Other motions can occur as well, such as shaking the head as if to say "no," and there can also be movement in the upper trunk and shoulders while bobbling (Nellhaus, 1967). Walking around often makes the bobbling increase in frequency, which may interfere with coordinated movements, such as climbing stairs.

Generally, this syndrome occurs in children under the age of 10 years old, but cases in adults occasionally occur as well (Olvera-Castro et al., 2017). Children with bobble-head doll syndrome are often reported to have especially large heads, called *macrocephaly* (Guerreiro et al., 2012). Symptoms such as headaches and visual problems may also occur (Renne et al., 2018).

The involuntary movements can occur either continuously or in episodes that start and stop. Such episodes are sometimes called *tics*. These tics are different from the tics seen in disorders such as Tourette syndrome (see Echophenomena and Coprophenomena). The tics disappear when the afflicted person is sleeping or sufficiently engaged in another task, such as a math problem that requires concentration. The movements can also be stopped voluntarily when focusing on sitting still, such as when someone asks the afflicted person to stop moving. They can sit still temporarily, but the bobbling movements eventually return. On the other hand, these movements may increase during strong emotions and stress (Reddy et al., 2014).

The Brain Pathology

The cause of bobble-head doll syndrome is usually traced back to a *cyst* in the brain located in or near the *third ventricle*. A cyst is like a bubble of cell tissue that isn't supposed to be there, and it can potentially form on several surfaces in the brain. The third ventricle, like all ventricles, is not actually a brain structure made up of brain cells such as neurons. Instead, it is an area located between brain structures that is filled with a liquid called *cerebrospinal fluid*. The third ventricle is located deep in the brain, below the corpus callosum, and between the thalami of the brain's hemispheres. Cerebrospinal fluid normally flows through this area, as the third ventricle is part of a series of connected ventricles in the brain. But because a cyst is blocking the connection between the ventricles, the flow of the cerebrospinal fluid is impaired (Hahm et al., 2018). Because of the blockage, pressure builds up in the brain, and the area of the fluid-filled third ventricle expands, resulting in pressure on the other surrounding parts of the brain (Guerreiro et al., 2012). The bobble-head doll syndrome symptoms occur because of this pressure, but exactly *why* this pressure causes head-bobbling is debated.

There are several theories (Renne et al., 2018). One is that the pressure distorts the function of the basal ganglia, which is a brain structure that plays a role in voluntary muscle movements, as evidenced by the fact that the ability to stop the bobbling when concentrating resembles similar problems that arise from basal ganglia damage. Another theory is that head-bobbling is actually a semi-voluntary learned strategy to try and get the pressure to decrease by jostling the cyst and fluid, as evidenced by the improvement of symptoms that can follow after the drainage of fluid from the area.

Thanks to modern brain scanning, finding abnormalities in people's brains near the ventricles is no longer difficult, which is good news for diagnosing cases of bobble-head doll syndrome. Treating this disorder almost always requires minor surgery to relieve the cyst causing the blockage and pressure in the ventricles and sometimes to place a shunt to help with the transfer of the cerebrospinal fluid (Hahm et al., 2018). Improvement is seen in the majority of cases following the surgery, with the best outcomes following surgical interventions that were made early in the progression of the symptoms. The vast majority of cases have happy outcomes, with symptoms disappearing in almost 90% of reported cases following surgical intervention (Renne et al., 2018).

References

Benton, J. W., Nellhaus, G., Huttenlocher, P. R., Ojemann, R. G., & Dodge, P. R. (1966). The bobble-head doll syndrome: Report of a unique truncal tremor associated with third ventricular cyst and hydrocephalus in children. *Neurology*, *16*(8), 725–729. https://doi.org/gtkd

Guerreiro, H., Vlasak, A., Horinek, D., Tichy, M., Lisy, J., Vanek, P., Liby, P., Hoza, D., Beneš, V., & Nimsky, C. (2012). Bobble-head doll syndrome: Therapeutic outcome and long-term follow-up in four children. *Acta Neurochirurgica*, *154*(11), 2043–2049. https://doi.org/f4b8xw

Hahm, M. H., Woo, J., & Kim, K. H. (2018). Hypomania in bobble-head doll syndrome: A case report of surgically treated stereotypy and hypomania. *Psychiatry Investigation*, *15*(5), 546–549. https://doi.org/gdmjdf

Nellhaus, G. (1967). The bobble-head doll syndrome: A "tic" with a neuropathologic basis. *Pediatrics*, *40*(2), 250–253.

Olvera-Castro, J. O., Morales-Briceño, H., Sandoval-Bonilla, B., Gallardo-Ceja, D., Venegas-Cruz, M. A., Estrada-Estrada, E. M., Contreras-Mota, M., Guinto-Balanzar, G., & Garcia-Lopez, R. (2017). Bobble-head doll syndrome in an 80-year-old man, associated with a giant arachnoid cyst of the lamina quadrigemina, treated with endoscopic ventriculocystocisternotomy and cystoperitoneal shunt. *Acta Neurochirurgica*, *159*(8), 1445–1450. https://doi.org/gtkf

Reddy, O. J., Gafoor, J. A., Suresh, B., & Prasad, P. O. (2014). Bobble head doll syndrome: A rare case report. *Journal of Pediatric Neurosciences*, *9*(2), 175–177. https://doi.org/gtkg

Renne, B., Rueckriegel, S., Ramachandran, S., Radic, J., Steinbok, P., & Singhal, A. (2018). Bobble-head doll syndrome: Report of 2 cases and a review of the literature, with video documentation of the clinical phenomenon. *Journal of Neurosurgery: Pediatrics*, *21*(3), 236–246. https://doi.org/gc58k2

Capgras Syndrome (and Other Delusional Misidentification Syndromes)

Imagine that your loved ones all looked unfamiliar to you. Whenever you see their faces, something just *doesn't feel right*. Your brain tells you that it isn't actually *them*, but a stranger, even though they say all of the same words and make all of the same gestures and wear all of the same clothes. Clearly, they have been replaced … with *imposters*. Or, imagine that everyone you meet reminds you of someone else—a specific person that you've seen before, but they are now in disguise, pretending to be this series of strangers. You see them on the street, in restaurants, and everywhere you go. They may change clothing, sex, and age, but you *know* it's the same person. Why are they following you? You might consider yourself to be a pretty reasonable person, but with all of these imposters and disguises, you aren't sure of anything anymore.

The Stories

(STORY 1) A 30-year-old man was in a serious automobile accident that put him into a coma for three weeks. When he awoke, his recovery was going well, but he developed *Capgras syndrome* and began to insist that both of his parents had been replaced by imposters. He was not afraid of these doubles and described them as nice. At one point, his father lied to him and told him that there had been an imposter, but that the imposter had been sent away and that he was now speaking to the real father. As a result, the patient believed that his real father had returned, but only for a week, before returning to his delusion of imposters (Ramachandran & Blakeslee, 1998, chapter 8).

(STORY 2) A 59-year-old man began developing many new symptoms such as difficulties navigating, memory problems, and restlessness. One day, he came home and asked his wife where his wife was. Confused, she told him that she was his wife. He began treating her as someone else, as if she was a different person who happened to have the same voice, name, and appearance as his wife. He was unable to explain why the Capgras double seemed different from his real wife. He would sometimes tell her stories about his past as if she was a brand-new person that he was meeting, and sometimes the stories were about times that they had shared together. At one point, he tried to convince

DOI: 10.4324/9781003276937-15

her to come to the police station with him in order to report his wife as missing (Lucchelli & Spinnler, 2007).

(STORY 3) A 61-year-old man developed *Frégoli syndrome* after acquiring a traumatic brain injury due to falling down the stairs leading to his basement. While in the hospital, he began misidentifying people. He misidentified a person in a wheelchair as his younger son, a boxer on television as his older son, and a social worker as his former boss. He also mistook a professional ice-skater on the television as *himself*—the patient—at one point. Even when the hospital staff pointed out the differences between the person in question and the person that the patient was claiming he was looking at, the patient maintained his delusional misidentifications. He was able to describe the physical differences between the people, for example: "he used to have light blond hair and he always had a big beard"—and yet continued to insist that the two different-looking people shared the same identity (p. 379). He also showed evidence of a *reduplicative paramnesia* such that he claimed to have been to three hospitals, each with the same name but in different places (Feinberg et al., 1999).

(STORY 4) A 66-year-old woman was late to a psychiatric appointment in 1985 because she made a "complicated detour around the town and hospital in order to lose her pursuers" (de Pauw et al., 1987, p. 434). These supposed pursuers were her cousin and a friend of her cousin—but wearing disguises such that they looked like other people. She was not really being pursued but was suffering from the Frégoli delusion such that other people that she encountered reminded her of her cousin and her cousin's friend. She explained that they were disguising themselves with "makeup, wigs, dark glasses, false beards, and different clothes" (de Pauw et al., 1987, p. 434). She sometimes confronted strangers and demanded that they reveal their true identities. She said that she could recognize them by the way they held their heads, the way they walked, and the way they spoke. She reported that "they keep changing their clothes and their hairstyles but I know it's them … they follow the bus when I get into it. They watch me lock my door" (Ellis & Szulecka, 1996, p. 40). She had abnormal brain waves that suggested she may be experiencing epilepsy, and she had suffered at least one stroke. Eventually, her symptoms went away with medication (de Pauw et al., 1987; Ellis & Szulecka, 1996).

The Features

Familiarity is an emotional reaction based on memory. It's what drives the bittersweet feeling of nostalgia and the heartwarming reactions when reunited with someone you haven't seen in a long while. The process of becoming familiar with something may seem automatic, but the following stories will show that it isn't—familiarity is something that your brain must build. There are a few ways in which the process of familiarity can break down, called *delusional misidentification syndromes* as a group, and perhaps the most startling is Capgras syndrome.

Capgras syndrome is a body-snatching science fiction movie turned real for those experiencing it. People with this syndrome become convinced that familiar people have been replaced by imposters. This is sometimes referred to as *doubling*, as in, they accuse people of having been replaced by doubles. Interestingly, they acknowledge that these doubles look exactly like the original, implying that the problem of recognizing is *not* due to misperceiving the person's features—when asked to point out what it is about the person that implies that they are a double, the patient has "great difficulty" explaining themselves (Young, 1999, p. 574).

This pattern often repeats, with the Capgras sufferer accusing the same person multiple times, as if even the doubles are themselves being replaced by additional doubles. They may insist that their loved ones have been replaced an enormous number of times. These accusations typically extend to people that the Capgras sufferer knows well, such as family or medical workers who regularly see the sufferer. In extreme cases, the person may distrust the so-called imposters so much that they resort to violence. One case resulted in a person with Capgras beheading his stepfather in order to look for batteries because he believed that he'd been replaced by a robotic imposter (Blount, 1986). Most cases do not escalate to that extreme, but this case serves to illustrate just how deeply the person can believe their own delusions.

The symptoms of Capgras syndrome are often limited to visual recognition, such that other senses like hearing a person's voice are less likely to trigger the doubling delusion. In other words, if they receive a phone call from a loved one, they may successfully interpret that person as the "original" person. There are, however, cases in which Capgras syndrome can occur non-visually, such as in blind people (Dalgalarrondo et al., 2002). For example, one blind woman began complaining that her cat had been replaced with a duplicate cat and accused the cat's voice and fur of being different—when she was tested on her ability to recognize familiar voices she performed very poorly, indicating that she was experiencing difficulties with auditory recognition (Reid et al., 1993).

Another major delusional misidentification disorder is Frégoli syndrome, which is sort of the opposite of Capgras syndrome (Ardila, 2016). Frégoli syndrome is named after an actor named Léopoldo Frégoli, who performed at music halls in the late 1800s and early 1900s and was known for his ability to quickly change characters (Ellis & Szulecka, 1996). Léopoldo Frégoli had a talent for impersonating other people, which makes his name a good fit for the disorder (Langdon et al., 2014).

In Frégoli syndrome, the brain becomes too easily reminded of a familiar person. Have you ever noticed something about the way that a person moved, talked, or looked that reminded you of some other familiar person? I occasionally meet two people that seem to have the same voice, for example. It's a similar feeling for someone with Frégoli syndrome. But in this syndrome, the feelings of familiarity are strong, and those feelings bombard them when they look at strangers. This results in a situation where it feels like the familiar person is following them around in disguise, because many strangers that they see remind them of that familiar person. That doesn't mean that the person with Frégoli actually thinks the strangers *look* the same as the known person—the people often look wildly different—it just means that something about the stranger reminds them so much of the familiar person that they become suspicious that it is really that familiar person pretending to be someone else.

Those feelings of uncanny familiarity are extremely unnerving and may make the person feel as though they are being *persecuted*, that is, that they are being intentionally harassed. For example, it was written about one patient that she was "at times convinced that people in her entourage are the incarnation of people she knew formerly, powerful persecutors that have returned to torment her. She claims these persecutors are capable of all types of transformation" (Courbon & Fail, 1927, translated in Ellis et al., 1994, p. 134). Thus, the condition may cause extreme discomfort that is disruptive to a person's life.

Other types of delusional misidentification syndrome include duplications of locations, of body parts, and of the self (Joseph, 1986). This duplication is known as *reduplicative paramnesia* (Ardila, 2016). As an example, the person may believe that there are multiple hospitals that they have been admitted to recently, even though there is only one. Another type is called *intermetamorphosis*, which occurs when a person believes that someone has transformed physically into someone else (Joseph, 1986). That is, they believe that a person has actually *become* someone else, as opposed to merely disguising themselves as in Frégoli syndrome.

You may be wondering whether people with these disorders actually *believe* their delusions. One way that we know that these people are truly experiencing their versions of reality is that they continue to show these delusions even when they don't know that they are being watched (Burgess et al., 1996). In some cases, the delusional misidentification syndrome may continue for many years. For example, it was written about one woman that "for about 10 years she has been transforming everyone in her entourage, even those closest to her, such as her husband and daughter, into various and numerous doubles" (Capgras & Reboul-Lachaux, 1923, translated in Ellis et al., 1994, p. 119).

The Brain Pathology

The leading theories that attempt to explain these delusional misidentification syndromes discuss *disconnections* in the brain between regions responsible for emotion, identity, face-processing, and memory. Many different theories have been proposed over the years (Edelstyn & Oyebode, 1999). The majority of research focuses on Capgras syndrome, so I will also focus there, but similar ideas have been floated for other delusional misidentification syndromes.

One theory for where Capgras syndrome and other delusional misidentification syndromes arise is that something has gone wrong in the area of the brain responsible for attaching identities to faces—perhaps a memory disconnection from the "deep right temporo-parieto-occipital junction" (Staton et al., 1982, p. 32). It may be that people with Capgras syndrome have broken this part of their brain responsible for updating and maintaining the link between *seeing* faces and *identifying* people. As a consequence, each time they see what should be a familiar face it doesn't look right when they compare it to their mental representation of the identity of that person. Perhaps they mistakenly create new identities in the brain instead of linking new information to old identities (Ramachandran & Blakeslee, 1998). This would be like if a friend got a haircut and instead of your brain realizing that this was the same person but with different hair, your brain just went ahead and gave this person an entirely new identity. But in a person with Capgras, no haircut or other change is necessary for a new identity to be created.

Additionally, Dr. Capgras himself hypothesized that the claims of imposters stemmed from the emotional systems not behaving as expected when viewing familiar faces (Capgras & Reboul-Lachaux, 1923). In other words, in a person with this disorder, looking at a familiar face creates no emotional warmth, even for a parent or spouse. This suggests a disconnection between *memory* for faces and *emotions*. Supporting this, Capgras syndrome "doubling" often occurs in people with whom the sufferer has close emotional contact—one review found that 85% of cases involved misidentification of family or partners (Bell et al., 2017). Additional evidence comes from skin conductance responses (SCR) which measure unconscious reactions of sweat glands due to emotions. In Capgras syndrome, there are smaller emotional reactions to familiar faces as measured by SCR when compared to people without this syndrome (Ameller et al., 2017). It is as if the part of their brain that should feel good when looking at a familiar face instead feels nothing. In theory, this could lead them to assume that their loved one has been replaced by a double because they don't *feel* emotionally correct.

Both the memory disconnection and emotional disconnection theories could be partly correct or correct within specific individuals. Overall, Capgras syndrome has been investigated by a wide variety of brain scans, which have revealed differences in many brain regions (Thiel et al., 2014). This suggests that Capgras can arise from damage to multiple places rather than a specific part of the brain.

Capgras has been compared to prosopagnosia (see Prosopagnosia) because both involve problems with identifying faces (e.g., Hirstein & Ramachandran, 1997). In prosopagnosia, a person fails to identify familiar faces, but they *can* often retrieve feelings of familiarity, as measured by SCR. In contrast, those with Capgras fail to retrieve feelings of familiarity but can often correctly identify the person because they know who the person is "doubling." Capgras may also occur alongside disorders like schizophrenia, epilepsy (see Seizures), dementia, migraines (see Migraine Headaches), and Parkinson disease (Cannas et al., 2017).

Capgras syndrome has been interpreted as "an interaction of impairments," meaning that damage of more than one kind contributes to the disorder (Reid et al., 1993). It has been proposed that it is not possible to explain the existence of delusional misidentification syndromes without considering both why the person feels differently towards their loved ones and, as a second factor, why they end up with delusional beliefs. In other words, their perceptual experiences combined with unusual reasoning biases about those experiences are what may produce Capgras syndrome (Young, 1999). This may help to explain why Capgras is more common in psychiatric patients—because they are predisposed to believe unusual things (Bell et al., 2017). However, this "two-factor theory" of Capgras has also been challenged and may not be correct (Corlett, 2019). Overall, delusional misidentification syndromes are one of the most mysterious ways that your brain can make mistakes.

References

Ameller, A., Picard, A., D'Hondt, F., Vaiva, G., Thomas, P., & Pins, D. (2017). Implicit recognition of familiar and unfamiliar faces in schizophrenia: A study of the skin conductance response in familiarity disorders. *Frontiers in Psychiatry*, *8*, 181. https://doi .org/gb2zkb

Ardila, A. (2016). Some unusual neuropsychological syndromes: Somatoparaphrenia, akinetopsia, reduplicative paramnesia, autotopagnosia. *Archives of Clinical Neuropsychology*, *31*(5), 456–464. https://doi.org/gkx9s3

Bell, V., Marshall, C., Kanji, Z., Wilkinson, S., Halligan, P., & Deeley, Q. (2017). Uncovering Capgras delusion using a large-scale medical records database. *BJPsych Open*, *3*(4), 179–185. https://doi.org/gtkh

Blount, G. (1986). Dangerousness of patients with Capgras syndrome. *The Nebraska Medical Journal*, 71(6), 207.

Burgess, P. W., Baxter, D., Rose, M., & Alderman, N. (1996). In P. W. Halligan & J. C. Marshall (Eds.), *Method in madness: Case studies in cognitive neuropsychiatry* (pp. 51–78). Psychology Press.

Cannas, A., Meloni, M., Mascia, M. M., Solla, P., Cocco, L., Muroni, A., Floris, G., Di Stefano, F., & Marrosu, F. (2017). Capgras syndrome in Parkinson's disease: Two new cases and literature review. *Neurological Sciences*, *38*(2), 225–231. https://doi.org/f9vkk9

Capgras, J., & Reboul-Lachaux, J. (1923). L'illusion des 'sosies' dans un délire systématisé chronique. *Bulletin de la Société Clinique de Médecine Mentale*, *2*, 6–16.

Corlett, P. R. (2019). Factor one, familiarity and frontal cortex: A challenge to the two-factor theory of delusions. *Cognitive Neuropsychiatry*, *24*(3), 165–177. https://doi.org/ g69g

Courbon, P., & Fail, G. (1927). Syndrome d' "illusion de Frégoli" et schizophrénie. *Bulletin de la Société Clinique de Médecine Mentale*, *20*, 121–125.

Dalgalarrondo, P., Fujisawa, G., & Banzato, C. E. (2002). Capgras syndrome and blindness: Against the prosopagnosia hypothesis. *The Canadian Journal of Psychiatry*, *47*(4), 387–388. https://doi.org/gtkj

de Pauw, K. W., Szulecka, T. K., & Poltock, T. L. (1987). Frégoli syndrome after cerebral infarction. *Journal of Nervous and Mental Disease*, *175*(7), 433–438. https://doi.org/dtv9xp

Edelstyn, N. M. J., & Oyebode, F. (1999). A review of the phenomenology and cognitive neuropsychological origins of the Capgras syndrome. *International Journal of Geriatric Psychiatry*, *14*(1), 48–59. https://doi.org/d6vrfd

Ellis, H. D., & Szulecka, T. K. (1996). The disguised lover: A case of Frégoli delusion. In P. W. Halligan & J. C. Marshall (Eds.), *Method in madness: Case studies in cognitive neuropsychiatry* (pp. 39–50). Psychology Press.

Ellis, H. D., Whitley, J., & Luauté, J. P. (1994). Delusional misidentification: The three original papers on the Capgras, Frégoli and intermetamorphosis delusions. *History of Psychiatry, 5,* 117–146. https://doi.org/cwdfbk

Feinberg, T. E., Eaton, L. A., Roane, D. M., & Giacino, J. T. (1999). Multiple Frégoli delusions after traumatic brain injury. *Cortex, 35*(3), 373–387. https://doi.org/dr4f5p

Hirstein, W., & Ramachandran, V. S. (1997). Capgras syndrome: A novel probe for understanding the neural representation of the identity and familiarity of persons. *Proceedings of the Royal Society of London B: Biological Sciences, 264,* 437–444. https://doi.org/chr4n5

Joseph, A. B. (1986). Focal central nervous system abnormalities in patients with misidentification syndromes. In G. N. Christodoulou (Ed.), *The delusional misidentification syndromes* (pp. 68–79). Karger Publishers.

Langdon, R., Connaughton, E., & Coltheart, M. (2014). The Fregoli delusion: A disorder of person identification and tracking. *Topics in Cognitive Science, 6*(4), 615–631. https://doi.org/f6ndtg

Lucchelli, F., & Spinnler, H. (2007). The case of lost Wilma: A clinical report of Capgras delusion. *Neurological Sciences, 28*(4), 188–195. https://doi.org/cpbmtj

Ramachandran, V. S., & Blakeslee, S. (1998). *Phantoms in the brain: Probing the mysteries of the human mind.* William Morrow.

Reid, I., Young, A. W., & Hellawell, D. J. (1993). Voice recognition impairment in a blind Capgras patient. *Behavioural Neurology, 6*(4), 225–228. https://doi.org/gcd8fs

Staton, R. D., Brumback, R. A., & Wilson, H. (1982). Reduplicative paramnesia: A disconnection syndrome of memory. *Cortex, 18*(1), 23–35. https://doi.org/gtkk

Thiel, C. M., Studte, S., Hildebrandt, H., Huster, R., & Weerda, R. (2014). When a loved one feels unfamiliar: A case study on the neural basis of Capgras delusion. *Cortex, 52,* 75–85. https://doi.org/f5wzb8

Young, A. W. (1999). Delusions. *The Monist, 82*(4), 571–589. https://doi.org/fz8qgm

Charles Bonnet Syndrome

Imagine that you have failing vision, but in addition to seeing less of the real world, you begin to see imaginary things popping up into your field of vision. Images, such as swimming geometric patterns, animals in hats, and small creatures with large faces driving motorcycles, dance in fantastic formations right in front of your eyes. You are well aware that the things you are seeing are not real, but that doesn't mean you can stop seeing them. Strangely, these unreal dancing images are utterly silent.

The Stories

(STORY 1) In 2016, an 81-year-old woman developed some problems with her vision. Specifically, she frequently *pseudohallucinated* visits of white pigeons in the early evening hours. They would appear to sit on top of the television, walk through the room, or even fly around. These pigeons did not scare her, because she knew the pigeons were not real. She would sometimes point out to her husband where the imaginary pigeons were sitting. She did not have any pathological mental problems—she was entirely sane—but she did have cataracts in both eyes and age-related macular degeneration. Thus, her vision was very poor. Her pseudohallucinations began with a frequency of a few times per month but later increased to an occurrence of nearly every day (Stojanov, 2016).

(STORY 2) In the case of a 74-year-old man, a stroke led to partial blindness and symptoms of Charles Bonnet syndrome. He had a right-sided homonymous hemianopsia, meaning that he was mostly blind in the right half of his visual field, but he could still see out of the left half of each eye. Interestingly, he began to experience pseudohallucinations on his right side, in the part of his visual field where he was blind. He reported seeing lions, cats, flocks of birds, packs of hounds, chessboards, and colorful scarves. The images that he saw often repeated themselves and tended to last for several minutes. He was aware that what he was seeing was not real, and reported that when he felt more "animated" in his life such as when talking or laughing, he felt more likely to see pseudohallucinations (Ashwin & Tsaloumas, 2007, p. 184).

DOI: 10.4324/9781003276937-16

(STORY 3) An 82-year-old woman with cataracts obscuring her vision in both eyes began having complex pseudohallucinations, such as a group of four women having a meeting. The women then proceeded to try on clothes and furs. She described the experience as similar to watching television with the volume off. She could see the figures' lips moving but couldn't hear what was being said. When she pseudohallucinated a group of people having a picnic, she was unable to smell the food. When she occasionally tried to touch the pseudohallucinations, her hand touched only air and the pseudohallucinations disappeared. These vivid images happened most frequently in low light, and did not appear in total darkness or when her eyes were closed. She knew that they were not real, and was more curious than frightened. After receiving surgery for her cataracts, the pseudohallucinations stopped occurring (Rosenbaum et al., 1987, case 1).

The Features

Unless you are listening to this chapter rather than reading it, the visual system in your brain is working very hard right now, as it does in most people at most times of the day. If the visual system were an economy, the imports would be blood sugar and information from the light that enters your eyes, and the exports would be the ability to visually experience a vibrant world. But what happens when the eyes send less information, as in old age? You might expect the visual system to produce less vision. But that isn't always what happens. Sometimes, instead of going dark, the visual experience of the world gets stranger, as if your brain was shrugging and saying "well, I might as well do *something* with all of this blood sugar."

In Charles Bonnet syndrome, a person experiences complex and fantastic *pseudohallucinations*. They are called pseudohallucinations because a typical person with Charles Bonnet syndrome realizes that the visions are not real, unlike how people with regularly defined hallucinations typically do *not* realize that the visions are not real. The condition has even been described as "visual hallucinations in sane people" in order to differentiate it from the experience of hallucinations during which sanity is in question (Rosenbaum et al., 1987, p. 66).

The syndrome was named after a Swiss philosopher called, as you would guess, Charles Bonnet (Stojanov, 2016). That's pronounced "bone-ay" kind of like the word "ballet," by the way. In the 1760s, he described how his grandfather, at the age of 90, was a healthy, intelligent, and, by all reports, sane man—but also that his grandfather saw "from time to time, in front of him, figures of men, of women, of birds, of carriages, of buildings… the tapestries in his apartment appear to change suddenly; these tapestries cover themselves with painting displaying different landscapes" (Bonnet, 1769, translated in Hedges, 2007, pp. 112–113). He also mentioned that the apparitions made no noise. As it was the first known case, the condition, as a whole, eventually began to be called by his name.

Besides the fact that the pseudohallucinations are typically silent, there are other characteristics that these images often have, as revealed by surveys (Khan et al., 2008). Most images were "straight-ahead" in front of the person, in color, and were moving in some way. Images often contained people or geometric patterns. Faces, plants, and vehicles were also commonly featured. The average person with Charles Bonnet syndrome had the symptoms once per day, and sometimes at predictable intervals. The pseudohallucinations may differ in duration between people, and may come in intervals of seconds, minutes, or hours.

Some specific examples of pseudohallucinations include "acrobats balancing on bicycles," "an elephant walking down the street with a child on its back," and "people who would pack their belongings and leave" (Carpenter et al., 2019). When they are more simplistic, they may include grid patterns, branching patterns, flashes of light, and repetitive geometric patterns (Jurišic et al., 2018).

This syndrome usually appears as a person ages, and their vision deteriorates. It is most commonly associated with *macular degeneration* or *cataracts*, both of which are normal in aging eyes. Macular degeneration is damage to the cells at the back of the eyeball that leads to lower sensitivity to the light coming into the eye, while cataracts are cloudy lenses in the eye, which lead to less light entering the eyeball in the first place. The consequence is the same either way: a decrease in visual input from the eyes to the brain as the aging person loses their eyesight. Other causes of partial blindness can also lead to this syndrome (see Hemianopsia).

The Brain Pathology

The leading theory about why Charles Bonnet syndrome occurs is that because the visual centers in the brain aren't receiving as much input from the eyes anymore, they begin *making up images instead*. In technical terms, the loss of input to the visual regions of the brain leads these regions to spontaneously generate neuronal discharges that can be interpreted by the person as pseudohallucinations. This is called the "deafferentation theory" by Charles Bonnet syndrome researchers (Stojanov, 2016, p. 883).

Many researchers believe that the cause of Charles Bonnet syndrome may be similar to what causes ringing in the ears (see Tinnitus) and phantom limbs (see Phantom Sensations). In theory, when a person experiences vision loss (in Charles Bonnet syndrome), hearing loss (in tinnitus), or pain in a missing body part (in phantom pain), what is happening is that the brain begins to mistakenly interpret internal signals within the brain as sensational signals coming from the outside world. Those interpretations of internal noise therefore seem like external pictures, external noise, or pain from a body part. But the call is *coming from inside the brain*.

The deafferentation theory is supported by evidence of increased brain activity in the visual centers of people with Charles Bonnet syndrome (Painter et al., 2018). More evidence comes from the fact that the pseudohallucinations are more likely to be triggered when the person is looking around under low light conditions, such as a dimly lit room (Khan et al., 2008). With even less light making it into the brain, more spontaneous neuronal discharges occur, which are interpreted as more wild images. Pseudohallucinations have even been demonstrated in experiments using blindfolds. If people are blindfolded for several days in a row, they will often have visual pseudohallucinations, demonstrating that they are produced by the brain when it has little incoming light to process (Carpenter et al., 2019).

Once thought to be rare, it is increasingly believed that Charles Bonnet syndrome occurs somewhat frequently. It is now believed to occur in more than 10% of people with age-related macular degeneration, although studies have found different percentages depending on the population (Schadlu et al., 2009). The condition seems to be more common in women and becomes increasingly likely in a given person as visual acuity worsens (Niazi et al., 2020).

One reason that researchers once thought the disorder was rare is that people experiencing Charles Bonnet syndrome may be hesitant to share the fact that they are pseudohallucinating with their healthcare provider. Doctors often tell their patients that this syndrome is not a mental illness but just something that can happen in old age as vision declines (Carpenter et al., 2019). Most cases of silent visual pseudohallucinations in older adults turn out to be benign (harmless) symptoms such as in Charles Bonnet syndrome, but it may be important to check them out with a doctor in case they are more serious issues (Schadlu et al., 2009).

There is not yet a standardized test for diagnosing Charles Bonnet syndrome. Instead, doctors rely on ruling out other diagnoses and consider the experiences of the patient, such as whether they are aware that the pseudohallucinations are not real (Painter et al., 2018). The best course of treatment appears to be improving vision via better lighting, removal of cataracts, corrected vision via stronger glasses, or other eye-based treatments (Stojanov, 2016). Overall, people with this condition report that the pseudohallucinations are not that bad to live with, because they aren't dangerous and may even be entertaining.

References

Ashwin, P. T., & Tsaloumas, M. D. (2007). Complex visual hallucinations (Charles Bonnet syndrome) in the hemianopic visual field following occipital infarction. *Journal of the Neurological Sciences, 263*, 184–186. https://doi.org/cvzd8g

Bonnet, C. (1769). *Essai Analytique sur les Facultes de l'Ame* (2nd ed.). Philibert.

Carpenter, K., Jolly, J. K., & Bridge, H. (2019). The elephant in the room: Understanding the pathogenesis of Charles Bonnet syndrome. *Ophthalmic and Physiological Optics, 39*(6), 414–421. https://doi.org/gtkp

Hedges, T. R., Jr. (2007). Charles Bonnet, his life, and his syndrome. *Survey of Ophthalmology, 52*(1), 111–114. https://doi.org/bwvmjm

Jurišic, D., Sesar, I., Cavar, I., Sesar, A., Zivkovic, M., & Curkovic, M. (2018). Hallucinatory experiences in visually impaired individuals: Charles bonnet syndrome – Implications for research and clinical practice. *Psychiatria Danubina*, *30*(2), 122–128. https://doi.org/gtkq

Khan, J. C., Shahid, H., Thurlby, D. A., Yates, J. R., & Moore, A. T. (2008). Charles Bonnet syndrome in age-related macular degeneration: The nature and frequency of images in subjects with end-stage disease. *Ophthalmic Epidemiology*, *15*(3), 202–208. https://doi.org/bxrdfk

Niazi, S., Krogh Nielsen, M., Singh, A., Sørensen, T. L., & Subhi, Y. (2020). Prevalence of Charles Bonnet syndrome in patients with age-related macular degeneration: Systematic review and meta-analysis. *Acta Ophthalmologica*, *98*(2), 121–131. https://doi.org/gjc8gs

Painter, D. R., Dwyer, M. F., Kamke, M. R., & Mattingley, J. B. (2018). Stimulus-driven cortical hyperexcitability in individuals with Charles Bonnet hallucinations. *Current Biology*, *28*, 3475–3480. https://doi.org/gffn6w

Rosenbaum, F., Harati, Y., Rolak, L., & Freedman, M. (1987). Visual hallucinations in sane people: Charles Bonnet syndrome. *Journal of the American Geriatrics Society*, *35*(1), 66–68. https://doi.org/gtkr

Schadlu, A. P., Schadlu, R., & Shepherd, J. B. (2009). Charles Bonnet syndrome: A review. *Current Opinion in Ophthalmology*, *20*(3), 219–222. https://doi.org/bdtb4g

Stojanov, O. (2016). Charles Bonnet syndrome. *Vojnosanitetski Pregled*, *73*(9), 881–884. https://doi.org/gtks

Chronic Traumatic Encephalopathy

Imagine that your memory, mood, and ability to focus all hit rock bottom. You feel sluggish when thinking, speaking, and while attempting to get anything done. You begin having angry outbursts, you feel depressed, and you don't feel like yourself. When you were younger, you were hit in the head many times while pursuing the sport of your choice, but you felt that you recovered from those head blows fairly quickly. But now, many years later, you feel like those concussions have finally caught up with you.

The Stories

(STORY 1) A former professional boxer, now aged 61, developed signs of what would now be called CTE (chronic traumatic encephalopathy). He had fought as a lightweight boxer between 1910 and 1926 and at one point was the flyweight champion of Essex, before taking on new boxing challenges later in life such as competing with "Madame Carpentier, the world's champion lady boxer" (p. 359). Now, as an old man, all of those years of being punched in the head had finally caught up with him. He began noticing a decline in his abilities to concentrate and to remember things. When examined by the doctor, his speech was extremely slurred, and it was noted that he often lost track of what he was saying in conversation and resorted to writing things down to assist his memory. The former boxer said that he would never allow his children to box, insisting that "it ought to be stopped" (Critchley, 1957, case 3, p. 359).

(STORY 2) A 69-year-old former National Football League (NFL) player experienced a cognitive decline over the course of ten years. His gridiron career as a linebacker and offensive lineman—both field positions are high contact and often lead to concussions—lasted from high school, through college, and into the NFL where he played for nine years. After retiring from the NFL, he was a real estate agent but was later forced into retirement due to "poor decision-making and judgment" (p. 14). His wife reported that his abilities to remember and to multitask had been declining for many years. He transitioned from a jovial personality into an aggressive one, with an explosive temper that necessitated his wife calling the police on multiple occasions. His memory declined to the point that he could no longer remember current

DOI: 10.4324/9781003276937-17

events, and when his mental state deteriorated further, he began watching television all day. The researchers noted that he "demonstrated severe episodic memory impairment" and "profoundly impaired performance on most tests of executive function" (p. 14). Because this person was not deceased at the time and diagnosis of CTE requires looking at the brain itself during an autopsy, this person was instead marked as "probable CTE" by the research team (Montenigro et al., 2014, case D, p. 14).

(STORY 3) A 33-year-old man with dwarfism developed CTE, diagnosed at autopsy, as a result of "occupational trauma" (p. 102). He had been working as a circus clown with dangerous routines for around 15 years but was eventually fired due to constant alcohol use. While working at the circus, he was knocked unconscious "dozens of times" and did not receive hospital care following these concussions (p. 102). He was also a "missile" in dwarf-throwing competitions for 8–10 years. He was secretive about the dwarf-throwing and specific injuries were not reported but he was tossed "by strong men as far as possible onto mattresses" and presumably landed in ways that jostled his brain (p. 103). Hospital records revealed that he had shown aggression, poor concentration, panic, and other symptoms that could have been related to the progressive CTE. His brain showed the signature "tau-immunoreactive neurofibrillary tangles" of CTE, as well as additional brain changes due to chronic alcohol use (Williams & Tannenberg, 1996, p. 103).

The Features

Your brain is floating inside of your skull, separated from the bone by a layer of fluid. Getting hit in the head is dangerous because your brain can bounce around, smacking up against that bone. Such hits may result in *concussions*. Concussions are brain injuries that may cause loss of consciousness, confusion, and other symptoms—although not all concussions are obvious. Concussions by themselves can be serious, but when a person regularly suffers from head trauma, even small brain injuries may add up over time to a big problem.

Chronic traumatic encephalopathy, or CTE, is a disorder in which your brain deteriorates over time, usually because of multiple small head traumas (Mariani et al., 2020). The repeated head impacts do not necessarily need to cause symptoms of concussion—that is, they can be repeated milder *subconcussive* impacts (Baugh et al., 2012). It can also develop after a single severe blow to the head (e.g., Bieniek et al., 2021; Omalu & Hammers, 2021). In other words—and of all the facts in this book this one should come as the least surprising—getting hit in the head is bad for your brain.

CTE research has mostly focused on athletes of contact sports in which concussions are likely. Boxing was given early attention, because getting hit in the head is an intended part of the sport (Roberts, 1969). This affiliation with boxing earned CTE a previous name of *punch-drunk syndrome*. I want to emphasize that even though there has been a recent resurgence of concussion research, doctors already suspected how dangerous repeated blows to the head were, even 100 years ago. Illustrative for the time was this cautionary quote from Harrison Martland:

> in punch drunk there is a very definite brain injury due to single or repeated blows on the head… which cause multiple concussion hemorrhages… later replaced by a gliosis or a degenerative progressive lesion… I realize that this theory, while alluring, is quite insusceptible of proof at the present time.
>
> (Martland, 1928, p. 1103)

Notice that Dr. Martland knew that he couldn't prove the theory just yet. Today, we are much better equipped to investigate CTE using advanced brain imaging methods.

But it wasn't just boxing. Other sports in which getting hit in the head is *not* the main objective were also found to be related to CTE. American football (gridiron) was also suspected early on, with much discussion in the 1930s about the dangers of this high-contact sport (Montenigro et al., 2015). Additional sports with players diagnosed with CTE include ice hockey, soccer (football), rugby, mixed martial arts, bull riding, dwarf-throwing, and baseball (Bieniek et al., 2021). Sliding sports like bobsledding and skeleton are also under scrutiny due to repetitive head impacts (Futterman, 2020). People not involved in sports may also develop CTE, such as through physical abuse or through participation in the military (Bieniek et al., 2021).

Before we get into the details, I'll acknowledge that the naming of this disorder is up for some debate right now (e.g., Katz et al., 2021; Omalu & Hammers, 2021). CTE is technically the name of the underlying neuropathy, which describes the state of the brain tissue itself rather than the symptoms that the person shows while alive (Mariani et al., 2020). I will be calling the entire disorder CTE for simplicity, but the symptoms in a living person would probably more accurately be called "CTE syndrome" (Omalu & Hammers, 2021).

CTE primarily consists of *cognitive symptoms* such as difficulties with memory, attention, or executive function (Mariani et al., 2020). Memory problems are an extremely common symptom of CTE (Katz et al., 2021). These memory problems are usually described in the form of deficits to episodic memories, meaning that people begin to forget details about events from their lives that they have experienced (see Amnesia), especially "short-term" memories of recent events (Mez et al., 2017). When it comes to the symptom of lost attention, this is sometimes described as a reduced ability to concentrate on focused tasks. Executive functions, including planning and inhibiting actions, have also been shown to be impaired in those with a history of concussion (Seichepine et al., 2013). In other words, it becomes more difficult to plan ahead for the future or prevent yourself from engaging in behaviors with negative consequences such as overusing drugs or gambling.

Additionally, CTE is often affiliated with *mood symptoms* and *behavioral symptoms*. Most notably of the mood symptoms, CTE is associated with depression.

Depression in aging athletes has been shown to be related to the number of concussions received during their active years (Didehbani et al., 2013). Other mood and behavioral symptoms attributed to this condition include impulsivity, which is acting without thinking it over first, and explosivity, which is being quick to become angry (Katz et al., 2021). It has even been suggested that cases with mood and behavioral symptoms should be considered their own subtype of CTE, separate from people who only show cognitive symptoms (Stern et al., 2013).

There are also frequent mentions of *motor* symptoms in CTE, such as changes in how a person walks, how they talk, or how they make other movements involving muscle coordination (see Ataxia). However, the motor symptoms are less common (Mariani et al., 2020). When motor symptoms occur, they tend to appear later in the condition as it progresses.

That's an unhappy fact about CTE. It is *progressive*, meaning that it slowly becomes worse over time, and this may take entire decades. There is also a delay in showing up, which is one especially nasty fact about CTE. This may be why people used to underestimate the dangers of multiple concussions. While it has long been understood that concussions can cause immediate brain damage, the old conventional wisdom was that if a person recovers from the concussion, then there weren't other long-term effects to worry about—but now it is understood that even mild head injuries can produce changes in the brain (Montenigro et al., 2015). Problematically for diagnosis, CTE can emerge much later in life than any hits to the head that may have helped to produce it, with the first symptoms often emerging around a person's fifties, long after they retired from the sport that produced the head impacts (Seichepine et al., 2013). More exposure to head impacts is associated with worse CTE symptoms later in life (Mariani et al., 2020). Overall, CTE is often associated with the term *dementia* due to the way it slowly causes a person to lose cognitive abilities—CTE even used to be known by the name *dementia pugilistica*.

Much of the recent work in CTE has been a renewed interest in American football players, especially after an impactful case study of a professional player that later influenced the 2015 film *Concussion* (Omalu et al., 2005). Memory-related diseases are disproportionately common in former American football players when compared to other men of the same age (Weir et al., 2009). In a review of 202 brains of former players of American football, CTE was neuropathically diagnosed in 87% of them, including in 99% of the National Football League players, suggesting that CTE is related to participation in American football—but because those brains were specifically donated to be studied, this may be an overestimate of how many players are affected (Mez et al., 2017). Nevertheless, CTE is not rare and should be taken seriously as a risk for any contact sport.

The Brain Pathology

CTE is a type of *tauopathy*, which means that it is a disorder that gets worse over time with the buildup of a protein called *tau* in the brain. Tau is actually a natural protein in the brain, and it serves a useful purpose in stabilizing micro-tubules (Wang et al., 2020). All that you need to know about microtubules for this particular book is that they are tiny tunnel structures that help your brain cells do their jobs. You can think of tau as a protein that hugs around the microtubules, preventing them from falling apart. In CTE, tau stops hug-ging the microtubules and instead collects amongst itself in *tangles*. Because the microtubules fall apart, and because the tangles themselves take up space and damage cells, the person starts experiencing symptoms such as memory loss because the brain cells can no longer effectively send signals to one another. These tangles of tau can be detected under a powerful microscope, but *only* after the person has died because we need to slice up the brain in order to look closely enough at the tissue. I will go into more detail, but if you've finished this paragraph, you already know more about CTE than most people.

Researchers think that one of the big reasons that tau stops hugging microtu-bules is because getting hit in the head damages these tiny structures and causes the tau to become detached (VanItallie, 2019). It's a very literal hypothesis: concussive and subconcussive blows to the head knock tau loose. Sometimes, especially when detached from microtubules, a bunch of phosphate molecules will attach to the tau protein and more or less weigh it down and prevent it from doing its job. When many phosphate molecules are attached to tau, it is known as *hyperphosphorylated tau*, which is generally shortened to *p-tau* (Bieniek et al., 2021). Phosphorylation is also normal in the brain—it is a common way that proteins help to regulate cellular processes. The reason that p-tau gets so much attention is that there appear to be good and evil versions.

The "normal and benign" kind is called *trans p-tau*, while the "abnormal and destructive" type is called *cis p-tau* (VanItallie, 2019, p. 1). Cis p-tau is more likely to be hyperphosphorylated than trans p-tau and therefore isn't as good at doing its job of providing tubular structure and, instead, hyperphosphorylated tau is more likely to clump together and form tangles (Wang et al., 2020). We also know that cis p-tau is toxic because when it is given to nematodes, the nematodes' brains stop working—their neuromuscular synaptic transmissions are disrupted and they can't move around correctly (Zanier et al., 2021).

Where does evil cis p-tau come from? There is almost certainly a genetic component but, interestingly, sometimes the good tau can transform into the evil tau—because they have the same parts, but they are folded differently, like how a sheet of paper can be folded into either a good paper airplane or an evil paper swan. One way that trans p-tau can be turned into cis p-tau is through phosphorylation (Katsumoto et al., 2019). In other words, getting hit in the head may free up the good tau from tubules, then phosphates may attach to it while it floats around freely, and if a phosphate attaches to a particular spot (called site T231), it will turn into evil tau. That's the theory, anyway.

In some severe cases of CTE, there appears to be a relationship between the places in the brain where there is notable p-tau buildup and the symptoms that the person experienced during life—for example, in people with memory loss, p-tau buildup can sometimes be seen in the hippocampus, which would be the expected area for such memory symptoms (Mez et al., 2017). Head injuries appear to produce cis p-tau around the axons of neurons, which has been shown in experiments in which concussions were given to mice (Albayram et al., 2017). I want to make a joke about how the mice should have worn helmets, but I'd rather not think about it.

However, it is believed that symptoms of CTE don't necessarily need to come directly from p-tau buildup, with other underlying pathologies also detected in such brains, including the loss of axons and myelin sheathing (Bieniek et al., 2021). Other possible mechanisms are also under investigation, especially the role of inflammation in the brain (VanItallie, 2019). Also, we can't yet infer that symptoms are direct clinical manifestations of the underlying neuropathology of CTE—we can't say for certain that a person is depressed *because* of tau in their brain (Mariani et al., 2020).

If all of that wasn't enough, it gets even scarier. Cis p-tau can transform trans p-tau into more cis p-tau, thus making healthy brain cells unhealthy and perhaps even killing cells (Clavaguera et al., 2015). In our metaphor, when evil tau interacts with good tau, the good tau is tempted and turns to the dark side, becoming evil itself. This is why CTE gets progressively worse over time: the p-tau is spreading, seemingly from the frontal cortex to deeper parts of the brain (Shively et al., 2021). It is believed that "seeds" of p-tau spread to the limbic system such as the amygdala, where more p-tau is converted into tangles, thus causing cognitive and behavioral symptoms (Kaufman et al., 2021). This is similar to how prion diseases spread in the brain (see Creutzfeldt-Jakob Disease). Thus, cis p-tau can be considered to be a prion.

Intercellular transfer of tau and the resulting spread of the disease is terrifying, and we might not be taking the problem seriously enough. Cis p-tau can spread to other brain regions, including across the other brain hemisphere (Katsumoto et al., 2019). Under specific circumstances, it can spread even further than that. When the abnormal tau resulting from head impacts and associated with CTE months later is injected into the brains of mice, CTE is *transmissible between the mice* (Zanier et al., 2018). In other words, the disease can be spread from animal to animal, including from mouse to mouse and from mouse to nematode (Zanier et al., 2021). If you give a mouse a concussion, wait for a few months, and then grind up their brain and inject into another brain or feed it to another animal, CTE can spread (see Kuru). You might be thinking: "okay, but if it requires a brain injection or eating brains, it doesn't sound that dangerous because I wasn't planning on doing either of those things." But you're not considering brain surgery.

If a person has CTE prions in their brain, and their brain is opened for a surgery, those prions can theoretically escape from that brain by remaining on surgical tools or debris. We know from studies of prion diseases that prions are very difficult to destroy (see Fatal Familial Insomnia). This means that in order to avoid transmission between people we may need to reconsider precautions taken during brain surgeries performed on people who have had brain injuries or have other tauopathies such as Alzheimer disease (Zanier et al., 2018).

Yes, it is believed that everything we have been discussing so far is similar to how Alzheimer disease spreads in the brain. Alzheimer disease is also a tauopathy, meaning that tau is also involved in that disorder. However, the way that the p-tau is distributed around the brain looks different between the two disorders (Katsumoto et al., 2019). Also, the misfolding of the proteins looks different between Alzheimer disease and CTE: the prions appear to literally be folded differently (Falcon et al., 2019). I don't want to live in a world where Alzheimer disease and CTE are theoretically contagious, but here we are.

The diagnosis of CTE is currently only reliable when the person is deceased, because the brain itself needs to be closely looked at for abnormal tangles of p-tau and other reliable indicators of the disease (Bieniek et al., 2021). Despite this, many living American football players report having been diagnosed with CTE, which is problematic because they may be more likely to ignore other possible problems if they prematurely believe that CTE is the culprit responsible for their symptoms (Grashow et al., 2020). We are doing things a bit backward by finding the evidence of CTE in a person's brain and then *going back* and looking at their symptoms while they were alive, even though ideally we would be able to use the symptoms to detect the brain damage (Katz et al., 2021). Many attempts have been made and are currently underway to find ways to detect CTE using clinical evaluations, fluid tests, and brain scans (Mariani et al., 2020).

Diagnosing CTE using symptoms has proved challenging and controversial. Most influential was a set of diagnostic criteria suggested by a 2014 study as a starting point for research (Montenigro et al., 2014). When the criteria were tested, they were found to include too many people that didn't have CTE (Mez et al., 2021). Allowing the diagnosis of CTE based on clinical symptoms has been criticized. It would almost certainly be a mistake to diagnose people with CTE based solely on mood and behavioral symptoms, because too many people fit those definitions, such as people diagnosed with major depressive disorder (Iverson & Gardner, 2021). Meanwhile, the fluid-based CTE tests are "not sufficiently mature to be included in the criteria at this time," and brain-scan-based tests aren't ready either, so, for now, we still rely on autopsy after death before we can call it CTE (Katz et al., 2021, p. 850).

Regardless of whether we can detect it in a living person, there is some promising research into how to fight cis p-tau. One way to do it is with an antibody to target and then break down the troublesome proteins (Albayram et al., 2017). But such therapies may still be a long way off. The moral of the story is: protect your brain because concussions are dangerous. Even if you think that you're fine afterward, that may not be the case decades later.

References

Albayram, O., Kondo, A., Mannix, R., Smith, C., Tsai, C. Y., Li, C., Herbert, M. K., Qiu, J., Monuteaux, M., Driver, J., Yan, S., Gormley, W., Puccio, A. M., Okonkwo, D. O., Lucke-Wold, B., Bailes, J., Meehan, W., Zeidel, M., Lu, K. P., & Zhou, X. Z. (2017).

Cis P-tau is induced in clinical and preclinical brain injury and contributes to post-injury sequelae. *Nature Communications, 8*(1). https://doi.org/gcf6xf

Baugh, C. M., Stamm, J. M., Riley, D. O., Gavett, B. E., Shenton, M. E., Lin, A., Nowinski, C. J., Cantu, R. C., McKee, A. C., & Stern, R. A. (2012). Chronic traumatic encephalopathy: Neurodegeneration following repetitive concussive and subconcussive brain trauma. *Brain Imaging and Behavior, 6*(2), 244–254. https://doi.org/gfb67n

Bieniek, K. F., Cairns, N. J., Crary, J. F., Dickson, D. W., Folkerth, R. D., Keene, C. D., Litvan, I., Perl, D. P., Stein, T. D., Vonsattel, J. P., Stewart, W., Dams-O'Connor, K., Gordon, W. A., Tripodis, Y., Alvarez, V. E., Mez, J., Alosco, M. L., & McKee, A. C. (2021). The second NINDS/NIBIB consensus meeting to define neuropathological criteria for the diagnosis of chronic traumatic encephalopathy. *Journal of Neuropathology and Experimental Neurology, 80*(3), 210–219. https://doi.org/gtkv

Clavaguera, F., Hench, J., Goedert, M., & Tolnay, M. (2015). Prion-like transmission and spreading of tau pathology. Neuropathology and Applied Neurobiology, 41(1), 47–58. https://doi.org/g67q

Critchley, M. (1957). Medical aspects of boxing, particularly from a neurological standpoint. *British Medical Journal, 1,* 357–362. https://doi.org/dzcz39

Didehbani, N., Cullum, C. M., Mansinghani, S., Conover, H., & Hart, J. (2013). Depressive symptoms and concussions in aging retired NFL players. *Archives of Clinical Neuropsychology, 28*(5), 418–424. https://doi.org/f45tsr

Falcon, B., Zivanov, J., Zhang, W., Murzin, A. G., Garringer, H. J., Vidal, R., Crowther, R. A., Newell, K. L., Ghetti, B., Goedert, M., & Scheres, S. H. W. (2019). Novel tau filament fold in chronic traumatic encephalopathy encloses hydrophobic molecules. *Nature, 568*(7752), 420–423. https://doi.org/gfw83k

Futterman, M. (2020, July 26). Sledding athletes are taking their lives: Did brain-rattling rides and high-speed crashes damage their brains? *The New York Times.* https://nyti.ms/3zF8zpt

Grashow, R., Weisskopf, M. G., Baggish, A., Speizer, F. E., Whittington, A. J., Nadler, L., Connor, A., Keske, R., Taylor, H., Zafonte, R., & Pascual-Leone, A. (2020). Premortem chronic traumatic encephalopathy diagnoses in professional football. *Annals of Neurology, 88*(1), 106–112. https://doi.org/gtkw

Iverson, G. L., & Gardner, A. J. (2021). Symptoms of traumatic encephalopathy syndrome are common in the US general population. *Brain Communications, 3*(1), 1–16. https://doi.org/g628

Katsumoto, A., Takeuchi, H., & Tanaka, F. (2019). Tau pathology in chronic traumatic encephalopathy and Alzheimer's disease: Similarities and differences. *Frontiers in Neurology, 10,* Article 980. https://doi.org/g67x

Katz, D. I., Bernick, C., Dodick, D. W., Mez, J., Mariani, M. L., Adler, C. H., Alosco, M. L., Balcer, L. J., Banks, S. J., Barr, W. B., Brody, D. L., Cantu, R. C., Dams-O'Connor, K., Geda, Y. E., Jordan, B. D., McAllister, T. W., Peskind, E. R., Wethe, J. V., Zafonte, R. D., … & Stern, R. A. (2021). National Institute of Neurological Disorders and Stroke consensus diagnostic criteria for traumatic encephalopathy syndrome. *Neurology, 96*(18), 848–863. https://doi.org/g63k

Kaufman, S. K., Svirsky, S., Cherry, J. D., McKee, A. C., & Diamond, M. I. (2021). Tau seeding in chronic traumatic encephalopathy parallels disease severity. *Acta Neuropathologica, 142*(6), 951–960. https://doi.org/g63n

Mariani, M., Alosco, M. L., Mez, J., & Stern, R. A. (2020). Clinical presentation of chronic traumatic encephalopathy. *Seminars in Neurology, 40*(04), 370–383. https://doi.org/g65v

Martland, H. S. (1928) Punch drunk. *Journal of the American Medical Association, 91,* 1103–1107. https://doi.org/bzdrhc

Mez, J., Daneshvar, D. H., Kiernan, P. T., Abdolmohammadi, B., Alvarez, V. E., Huber, B. R., Alosco, M. L., Solomon, T. M., Nowinski, C. J., McHale, L., Cormier, K. A., Kubilus, C. A., Martin, B. M., Murphy, L., Baugh, C. M., Montenigro, P. H., Chaisson, C. E., Tripodis, Y., Kowall, N. W., Weuve, J., ... & McKee, A. C. (2017). Clinicopathological evaluation of chronic traumatic encephalopathy in players of American football. *Journal of the American Medical Association, 318*(4), 360–370. https://doi.org/gtkx

Mez, J., Alosco, M. L., Daneshvar, D. H., Saltiel, N., Baucom, Z., Abdolmohammadi, B., Uretsky, M., Nicks, R., Martin, B. M., Palmisano, J. N., Nowinski, C. J., Montenigro, P., Solomon, T. M., Mahar, I., Cherry, J. D., Alvarez, V. E., Dwyer, B., Goldstein, L. E., Katz, D. I., ... & McKee, A. C. (2021). Validity of the 2014 traumatic encephalopathy syndrome criteria for CTE pathology. *Alzheimer's and Dementia, 17*(10), 1709–1724. https://doi.org/g62g

Montenigro, P. H., Baugh, C. M., Daneshvar, D. H., Mez, J., Budson, A. E., Au, R., Katz, D. I., Cantu, R. C., & Stern, R. A. (2014). Clinical subtypes of chronic traumatic encephalopathy: Literature review and proposed research diagnostic criteria for traumatic encephalopathy syndrome. *Alzheimer's Research & Therapy, 6*(68), 1–17. https://doi.org/gcbsps

Montenigro, P. H., Corp, D. T., Stein, T. D., Cantu, R. C., & Stern, R. A. (2015). Chronic traumatic encephalopathy: Historical origins and current perspective. *Annual Review of Clinical Psychology, 11,* 309–330. https://doi.org/ggfnnh

Omalu, B. I., DeKosky, S. T., Minster, R. L., Kamboh, M. I., Hamilton, R. L., & Wecht, C. H. (2005). Chronic traumatic encephalopathy in a National Football League player. *Neurosurgery, 57*(1), 128–134. https://doi.org/b237kw

Omalu, B., & Hammers, J. (2021). Letter: Traumatic encephalopathy syndrome [TES] is not chronic traumatic encephalopathy [CTE]: CTE is only a subtype of TES. *Neurosurgery, 89*(3), E205–E206. https://doi.org/g63j

Roberts, A. H. (1969). *Brain damage in boxers: A study of the prevalence of traumatic encephalopathy among ex-professional boxers.* Pitman Medical & Scientific Publishing.

Seichepine, D. R., Stamm, J. M., Daneshvar, D. H., Riley, D. O., Baugh, C. M., Gavett, B. E., Tripodis, Y., Martin, B., Chaisson, C., McKee, A. C., Cantu, R. C., Nowinski, C. J., & Stern, R. A. (2013). Profile of self-reported problems with executive functioning in college and professional football players. *Journal of Neurotrauma, 30*(14), 1299–1304. https://doi.org/f435fx

Shively, S. B., Priemer, D. S., Stein, M. B., & Perl, D. P. (2021). Pathophysiology of traumatic brain injury, chronic traumatic encephalopathy, and neuropsychiatric clinical expression. *Psychiatric Clinics of North America, 44*(3), 443–458. https://doi.org/g63p

Stern, R. A., Daneshvar, D. H., Baugh, C. M., Seichepine, D. R., Montenigro, P. H., Riley, D. O., Fritts, N. G., Stamm, J. M., Robbins, C. A., McHale, L., Simkin, I., Stein, T. D., Alvarez, V. E., Goldstein, L. E., Budson, A. E., Kowall, N. W., Nowinski, C. J., Cantu, R. C., & McKee, A. C. (2013). Clinical presentation of chronic traumatic encephalopathy. *Neurology, 81*(13), 1122–1129. https://doi.org/f5q6sz

VanItallie, T. B. (2019). Traumatic brain injury (TBI) in collision sports: Possible mechanisms of transformation into chronic traumatic encephalopathy (CTE). *Metabolism: Clinical and Experimental, 100,* 1–6. https://doi.org/g63q

Wang, L., Zhou, Y., Chen, D., & Lee, T. H. (2020). Peptidyl-prolyl cis/trans isomerase Pin1 and Alzheimer's disease. *Frontiers in Cell and Developmental Biology, 8,* Article 355. https://doi.org/g65z

Weir, D. R., Jackson, J. S., & Sonnega, A. (2009). *National football league player care foundation study of retired NFL players*. University of Michigan Institute for Social Research. http://ns.umich.edu/Releases/2009/Sep09/FinalReport.pdf

Williams, D. J., & Tannenberg, A. E. G. (1996). Dementia pugilistica in an alcoholic achondroplastic dwarf. *Pathology*, *28*(1), 102–104. https://doi.org/fhgxjs

Zanier, E. R., Bertani, I., Sammali, E., Pischiutta, F., Chiaravalloti, M. A., Vegliante, G., Masone, A., Corbelli, A., Smith, D. H., Menon, D. K., Stocchetti, N., Fiordaliso, F., De Simoni, M. G., Stewart, W., & Chiesa, R. (2018). Induction of a transmissible tau pathology by traumatic brain injury. *Brain*, *141*(9), 2685–2699. https://doi.org/gd2qg6

Zanier, E. R., Barzago, M. M., Vegliante, G., Romeo, M., Restelli, E., Bertani, I., Natale, C., Colnaghi, L., Colombo, L., Russo, L., Micotti, E., Fioriti, L., Chiesa, R., & Diomede, L. (2021). *C. elegans* detects toxicity of traumatic brain injury generated tau. *Neurobiology of Disease*, *153*, Article 105330. https://doi.org/g69m

Cluster Headaches

Imagine that you regularly get headaches so severe that you cannot conceive of anything more painful. You can't do anything while it is occurring except wish for the pain to stop. These are no ordinary headaches, but you have no way of communicating just how terrible the pain is to someone who has never felt such a thing. The headaches come at semi-reliable times, almost predictably. But just as suddenly as they begin, they vanish, and you feel like yourself again. You hope that it was the last one, but for the rest of your life you'll be dreading another.

The Stories

(STORY 1) A 48-year-old man reported that during the nighttime, he experienced regular shooting pains above his right eyebrow that radiated to his skull. The "violent shooting pain" followed a somewhat predictable pattern, lasted between 30 and 45 minutes, and usually began abruptly around 1 AM. He became used to being awakened in the middle of the night by pain in that same location, and the attacks never happened during the day. The attacks would occur once each night for five or six weeks and then stop completely for six months, after which they would return for another five or six weeks— these active-headache and *remission* periods continued in such a pattern for about 10 years. Through trial and error, a medication was found that he could administer himself before bedtime that helped diminish the attacks. However, over the course of about seven years, the attack patterns shifted, sometimes occurring during the day or in new locations on his head, such that relief was not guaranteed (Symonds, 1956, case 5).

(STORY 2) A head injury in a 31-year-old woman was thought to have led to cluster headaches. This woman had been in a minor car accident six days before her cluster headache symptoms began. She had no history of headaches before the minor head trauma from the car accident. The pain was located around the area of her right eye and lasted for 30–45 minutes each time. During the attacks, she would often intentionally bang her head on objects in response to the pain. Pain pills such as oxycodone and acetaminophen were not helping enough with the headaches, which she described as a spike through her

DOI: 10.4324/9781003276937-18

right eye. Eventually, after several unsuccessful treatments, doctors were able to relieve the pain using a combination of drugs (Turkewitz et al., 1992).

(STORY 3) A 39-year-old man had been experiencing cluster headaches for about 5 years. He had two–five attacks each day. During these, he suffered excruciating pain for between 30 minutes and four hours, and his face swelled up around the eyes. To address the pain, several treatments were attempted. Medications were tried but did not produce any "worthwhile" benefit (p. 1428). Surgery was then turned to as an option. First, nerves were permanently numbed on the right side of his face, but after this treatment he experienced worsening cluster headaches on the left side of his face. Eventually, an electrode was implanted into his brain in his hypothalamus. The electrode continuously produced electrical stimulation in the area, which led to the disappearance of the headaches. However, when the electricity was shut off, the pain returned (Leone et al., 2001).

The Features

There are few medical maladies more relatable than the humble headache. The spectrum of headaches includes those from hangovers, ice cream, caffeine withdrawal, stress, and others. But the pain caused by each of these is absolutely blown out of the water by one type of headache that, mercifully, most people will never experience.

Cluster headaches are reportedly among the most painful disorders possible. In comparison to another severe headache, the migraine, cluster headaches are more rare and more painful (see Migraine Headaches). One influential cluster headache researcher wrote that:

> pain is the outstanding complaint. It is constant, excruciating, burning, and boring; it involves the eye, the temple, the neck and often the face. So severe and frequent are the attacks of pain (as often as twenty times a week) that practically every patient has contemplated suicide.
>
> (Horton, 1941, p. 377)

By "influential cluster headache researcher," I mean that at one point cluster headaches were called "Horton's headache" (Mainardi et al., 2009). I'm not a big fan of that name, so I'm glad it was changed.

Indeed, cluster headaches are sometimes called *suicide headaches* because of just how painful they are. I'm not a big fan of that name, either. It is true, though, that sufferers often threaten, but rarely attempt, suicide (Kudrow, 1980). Female sufferers have reported that each cluster headache is more painful than childbirth, although males are more likely to experience cluster headaches than females (May, 2005). The pain has been described as "boring, piercing, or burning in nature" with a concentration behind the eye, but with radiation to the rest of the head, and even the neck and shoulders (Silberstein & Young, 2003, p. 1196).

During an attack, a person with a cluster headache will have this extreme pain on one side of the head. Usually, the person has attacks on the same side of the head every time (e.g., always on the left), but, in some people, there may be an attack on either side or, even more rarely, the pain may switch sides *during the attack* (Kudrow, 1980). These single-sided attacks are known as *unilateral* attacks and are a standard feature in almost all cases.

In an attempt to get relief from the pain, sufferers may have trouble sitting still, and may pace around, rock back and forth, and put pressure on the areas where the pain is, such as by pressing on their eye (May, 2005). The pain is so severe that sitting still seems to become almost impossible, leading to the person moving around and trying to find comfort or distractions—up to and including some patients fracturing their hands by striking the floor or the wall (Kudrow, 1980). The pain is more than enough to deal with, but pain is not the only symptom.

Before and after the pain, people may have feelings of restlessness, difficulties in concentration, and changes in energy or mood (Snoer et al., 2018). More noticeably, they may also show *autonomic* signs. This means that they are associated with *automatic* and more or less uncontrollable bodily processes. These autonomic signs may include a stream of tears, constriction of the pupil into a small point, a drooping eyelid, a runny nose, and so on (May et al., 2006). The autonomic symptoms are usually also unilateral and typically appear *only* on the same side of the head as the cluster headache. Therefore, the person may cry from one eye or sweat excessively above one eyebrow. Such unilateral autonomic signs are another standard cluster headache feature.

One attack generally lasts between 15 and 180 minutes. There usually is not just one attack, however. Attacks may occur multiple times per day or follow a semi-regular pattern over multiple days. This pattern of *clustered attacks* is where the name cluster headache comes from (Kunkle et al., 1954).

There are two subtypes of cluster headaches, and the difference lies in how often they attack. The first type are *episodic* cluster headaches. These are the preferable of the two types, but still seriously terrible. The episodic subtype is characterized by intermittent *active* periods in which headaches occur, and *remission* periods of complete relief during which headaches, thankfully, do not occur. These remission periods typically last anywhere from one month to over 12 months (May et al., 2006). After that, the headaches return for a period of weeks or months, with headaches occurring every other day or even more frequently (Rizzoli, 2017). This cycle continues from active to remission to active to remission and, as will be discussed, it often occurs with a consistent pattern.

The second type are *chronic* cluster headaches, in which there are either no remission periods or the remissions do not last long (Torelli et al., 2006). A typical person with the chronic subtype will have multiple cluster headaches every single day. Nobody deserves cluster headaches, but *absolutely nobody* deserves chronic cluster headaches.

The Brain Pathology

In the early days of cluster headache investigations, the combination of excruciating pain and patterned attacks baffled researchers. In terms of the disorder's cause, it was written in the 1950s that "almost as many theories exist as authors who described the syndrome" (Friedman & Mikropoulos, 1958, p. 654). Over time, the picture became clearer.

One important clue is how cluster headaches sometimes follow patterns, allowing some people to predict when they have attacks. Attacks may be associated with a specific time of day, time of year, and details of a person's sleep cycle. Notably, attacks most commonly occur during the nighttime (Pergolizzi et al., 2020). Cluster headaches become more likely to happen following the beginning or ending of daylight saving time when some people have to adjust their internal clocks forwards or backward by an hour (Silberstein & Young, 2003). Other changes to a person's sleep schedule that cause sleep loss may also trigger attacks.

The part of the brain most implicated in these patterns that follow the rhythm of time is the *hypothalamus*. While some of the sleep research that scientists wish to do is hindered by the fact that people typically do not sit still enough to measure of brain activity during cluster headache attacks, researchers have been able to show that there is increased activity in the hypothalamus during attacks (Pergolizzi et al., 2020). And while the details are still unknown, "that the hypothalamus is involved, at least in primary cluster headache, seems indisputable" (May, 2005, p. 846). The fact that more men are affected than women may be partially explained by the fact that young men are more likely to damage or disrupt their hypothalamus and related brain areas due to "excessive drinking, sleep deprivation, drug use, and other potentially damaging experiences" (Kudrow, 1980, p. 119).

We don't yet know exactly what triggers the pain, but one current avenue of research is on a particular kind of *vasodilator* called calcitonin gene-related peptide, which can be found in the hypothalamus (Carmine Belin et al., 2020). A vasodilator is a chemical that widens blood vessels. It may be this widening, along with *neuroinflammation* causing additional swelling, that causes the pain behind the person's eye. Infusing calcitonin gene-related peptides into a person who is currently experiencing an active cluster can trigger a headache but infusing them during their remission period does not trigger such an attack (Vollesen et al., 2018). It has also been shown that there are places in a person's genetic code that make them vulnerable to cluster headaches, and those genes seem to be associated with neuroinflammation (O'Connor et al., 2021). Indeed, cluster headaches run in families, where relatives are more likely to experience attacks (Waung et al., 2020).

There's more to the story than genetics, however. People who experience cluster headaches often have a history of head trauma, usually with delays between the trauma and the first cluster headache (Turkewitz et al., 1992). Sometimes, a person doesn't experience their first cluster attack until late into their adult life (Friedman & Mikropoulos, 1958). That suggests that events in people's lives can cause the development of cluster headaches in at least some cases, although over such a long period of time it is almost impossible to prove what caused the disorder in any one particular case. Unfortunately, "cluster headache is almost always idiopathic," which means that we don't know why a specific person developed the disorder (Taub et al., 1995, p. 319)

There are, however, cases of people developing cluster headaches soon after traumatic events such as head injuries (Lambru et al., 2009), brain surgeries (Rahmann et al., 2003), and surgeries on parts of their heads with many nerve endings including the teeth (Sörös et al., 2001). We don't exactly understand why this is, but according to one account: "stimulation of nociceptive sensory afferents caused by trauma or a structural lesion theoretically may produce a reorganization phenomena of the trigeminal nerve system and the hypo-thalamus that leads to the onset of a symptomatic cluster headache syndrome" (Rahmann et al., 2003, p. 131). That's a fancy way of saying that if enough pain signals are sent into the brain, the brain changes in response, and cluster headaches may begin to appear.

Complicating matters, headaches that closely mimic cluster headaches may result from brain abnormalities including tumors, and these are called *cluster-like headaches*. It's possible for a person with cluster-like headaches such as these to *stop* having those headaches upon the removal of a tumor in their brain (Taub et al., 1995). These are important to consider, because if the headache is due to an underlying cause, it is important to treat that problem instead of merely treating the headache itself (Mainardi et al., 2009).

There are no clear-cut treatments for *preventing* cluster headache attacks, although steroids and a few other drugs may be effective in some cases (Greener, 2021). In lieu of prevention, pain may be *reduced* during an attack using a variety of treatments. Two of the more effective techniques are breathing from an oxygen tank and the use of nasal spray or injections containing serotonin-affecting drugs called *triptans* (Pearson et al., 2019). There are also several less effective methods, such as using caffeine or using capsaicin. Capsaicin is a component of hot peppers that gives them their spiciness. Putting a component of hot sauce in the nose first causes burning, as you might imagine, but in some cases then leads to a reduction in pain (Fusco et al., 1994). One type of medication that doesn't seem to work well at all is traditional opioid-based painkillers like morphine (Pearson et al., 2019).

An exciting area of research is deep brain stimulation, where stimulating the hypothalamus with electrodes may relieve some headaches (Akram et al., 2017). Other stimulation techniques, such as noninvasive vagus nerve stimulation in which an electronic device is pressed against the neck, are also being researched and may be promising (Lai et al., 2020). In order to find a treatment that works for one particular person, there is usually a large amount of trial and error that must be gone through, so it is often up to the sufferer to hold on and keep exploring options until relief is finally found.

References

Akram, H., Miller, S., Lagrata, S., Hariz, M., Ashburner, J., Behrens, T., Matharu, M., & Zrinzo, L. (2017). Optimal deep brain stimulation site and target connectivity for chronic cluster headache. *Neurology, 89*(20), 2083–2091. https://doi.org/gcq3kf

Carmine Belin, A., Ran, C., & Edvinsson, L. (2020). Calcitonin gene-related peptide (CGRP) and cluster headache. *Brain Sciences, 10*(1), 1–16. https://doi.org/ghz9b3

Friedman, A. P., & Mikropoulos, H. E. (1958). Cluster headaches. *Neurology, 8*(9), 653–663. https://doi.org/g7zb

Fusco, B. M., Marabini, S., Maggi, C. A., Fiore, G., & Geppetti, P. (1994). Preventative effect of repeated nasal applications of capsaicin in cluster headache. *Pain, 59*(3), 321–325. https://doi.org/b8w5tv

Greener, M. (2021). Understanding the enigma of cluster headaches. *British Journal of Neuroscience Nursing, 17*(1), 21–23. https://doi.org/gtmd

Horton, B. T. (1941). The use of histamine in the treatment of specific types of headaches. *Journal of the American Medical Association, 116*(5), 377–383. https://doi.org/dg47gs

Kudrow, L. (1980). *Cluster headaches: Mechanisms and management.* Oxford University Press.

Kunkle, E. C., Pfeifer, J. J., Wilhoit, W. M., & Hamrick, J. L. (1954). Recurrent brief headache in cluster pattern. *North Carolina Medical Journal, 15*(10), 510–512.

Lai, Y. H., Huang, Y. C., Huang, L. T., Chen, R. M., & Chen, C. (2020). Cervical noninvasive vagus nerve stimulation for migraine and cluster headache: A systematic review and meta-analysis. *Neuromodulation, 23*(6), 721–731. https://doi.org/gtmg

Lambru, G., Castellini, P., Manzoni, G. C., & Torelli, P. (2009). Post-traumatic cluster headache: From the periphery to the central nervous system? *Headache, 49*(7), 1059–1061. https://doi.org/b883wt

Leone, M., Franzini, A., & Bussone, G. (2001). Stereotactic stimulation of posterior hypothalamic gray matter in a patient with intractable cluster headache. *New England Journal of Medicine, 345*(19), 1428–1429. https://doi.org/bsdksh

Mainardi, F., Trucco, M., Maggioni, F., Palestini, C., Dainese, F., & Zanchin, G. (2009). Cluster-like headache: A comprehensive reappraisal. *Cephalalgia, 30*(4), 399–412. https://doi.org/b4tdm8

May, A. (2005). Cluster headache: Pathogenesis, diagnosis, and management. *The Lancet, 366*(9488), 843–855. https://doi.org/d4g4pj

May, A., Leone, M., Afra, J., Linde, M., Sandor, P. S., Evers, S., & Goadsby, P. J. (2006). EFNS guidelines on the treatment of cluster headache and other trigeminal-autonomic cephalalgias. *European Journal of Neurology, 13*(10), 1066–1077. https://doi.org/dqwnh3

O'Connor, E., Fourier, C., Ran, C., Sivakumar, P., Liesecke, F., Southgate, L., Harder, A. V. E., Vijfhuizen, L. S., Yip, J., Giffin, N., Silver, N., Ahmed, F., Hostettler, I. C., Davies, B., Cader, M. Z., Simpson, B. S., Sullivan, R., Efthymiou, S., Adebimpe, J., … Belin, A. C. (2021). Genome-Wide association study identifies risk loci for cluster headache. *Annals of Neurology, 90*(2), 193–202. https://doi.org/gmjcbb

Pearson, S. M., Burish, M. J., Shapiro, R. E., Yan, Y., & Schor, L. I. (2019). Effectiveness of oxygen and other acute treatments for cluster headache: Results from the cluster headache questionnaire, an international survey. *Headache, 59*(2), 235–249. https://doi.org/gtmm

Pergolizzi, J. V., Jr., Magnusson, P., LeQuang, J. A., Wollmuth, C., Taylor, R., Jr., & Breve, F. (2020). Exploring the connection between sleep and cluster headache: A narrative review. Pain and Therapy, 9(2), 359–371. https://doi.org/gh9m7p

Rahmann, A., Husstedt, I. W., & Evers, S. (2003). Cluster headache after removal of a subarachnoid cyst: A case report. *Headache, 43*(2), 130–131. https://doi.org/fs6g4r

Rizzoli, P. (2017). Cluster headaches. In R. Yong, M. Nguyen, E. Nelson & R. Urman (Eds.), *Pain medicine* (pp. 527–529). Springer. https://doi.org/gtmn

Silberstein, S. D., & Young, W. B. (2003). Headache and facial pain. In C. G. Goetz (Ed.), *Textbook of clinical neurology* (2nd ed., pp. 1187–1205). Saunders.

Snoer, A., Lund, N., Beske, R., Hagedorn, A., Jensen, R. H., & Barloese, M. (2018). Cluster headache beyond the pain phase: A prospective study of 500 attacks. *Neurology, 91*(9), e822–e831. https://doi.org/gtmp

Sörös, P., Frese, A., Husstedt, I. W., & Evers, S. (2001). Cluster headache after dental extraction: Implications for the pathogenesis of cluster headache? *Cephalalgia, 21*(5), 619–622. https://doi.org/d7f9ch

Symonds, C. (1956). A particular variety of headache. *Brain, 79*(2), 217–232. https://doi.org/bzdz5d

Taub, E., Argoff, C. E., Winterkorn, J. M. S., & Milhorat, T. H. (1995). Resolution of chronic cluster headache after resection of a tentorial meningioma. *Neurosurgery, 37*(2), 319–322. https://doi.org/fmd9tr

Torelli, P., Castellini, P., Cucurachi, L., Devetak, M., Lambru, G., & Manzoni, G. C. (2006). Cluster headache prevalence: Methodological considerations. A review of the literature. *Acta Bio-Medica: Atenei Parmensis, 77*(1), 4–9.

Turkewitz, L. J., Wirth, O., Dawson, G. A., & Casaly, J. S. (1992). Cluster headache following head injury: A case report and review of the literature. *Headache: The Journal of Head and Face Pain, 32*(10), 504–506. https://doi.org/dkbxjm

Vollesen, A. L. H., Snoer, A., Beske, R. P., Guo, S., Hoffmann, J., Jensen, R. H., & Ashina, M. (2018). Effect of infusion of calcitonin gene-related peptide on cluster headache attacks: a randomized clinical trial. *JAMA Neurology, 75*(10), 1187–1197. https://doi.org/gkqpff

Waung, M. W., Taylor, A., Qualmann, K. J., & Burish, M. J. (2020). Family history of cluster headache: A systematic review. *JAMA Neurology, 77*(7), 887–896. https://doi.org/ghzc5z

Coma and Disorders of Consciousness

Imagine that you were unconscious for a long time. As you sleep, the world continues without you. Perhaps you awaken one day, and everything has changed. Maybe you have some vague and unquieting memories about your unconscious times, about lights and sounds and feelings. Or maybe, the entire time is a cold and blank slate without a single trace of memory. It feels like flirting with nonexistence: the comatose state.

The Stories

(STORY 1) A 9-year-old boy was struck by a car and fell into a coma. While treating him, medical workers regularly monitored pupil dilation and other bodily responses. At first, he had only slow reactions of his pupils to light, which was a very bad sign. He did not speak or react to inflicted pain. However, he slowly began to improve. Seventy-five days into the coma, he began to react to pain. After around 90 days in a mostly comatose state, the boy began to respond more. By day 100, he was following the commands of the medical staff. Over the course of the next several months, he underwent intense physical and occupational therapies, and he made good progress. At age 12, he remained paralyzed on the left side of his body and may have developed a slight learning disability as a result of the brain damage, but otherwise was in remarkably good shape considering the lengthy comatose state (Mahoney et al., 1983, case 1).

(STORY 2) A 50-year-old woman lost oxygen flow to her brain and entered a coma for about three weeks. Upon awakening from the coma, she showed very few signs of communication, attention, and movement. After several months, she was taken home to be cared for by her family. Most of the time she remained nonverbal, but she did occasionally speak to her family, perhaps once every month or two. With the hope that she may yet recover, they began working with a rehabilitation center. When examined, she met the criteria for a *minimally conscious state* based on her ability to make eye contact, occasionally speak, and respond to sound. Healthcare workers tried an experimental drug treatment, which had an immediate positive effect. She was temporarily able to do many things that she had been unable to do for many

DOI: 10.4324/9781003276937-19

months. She could speak in short sentences, recognize loved ones, read, do math, feed herself, laugh, and express affection. She was even able to, with assistance, stand up and take a couple of steps. Unfortunately, within hours, she returned to a minimally conscious state and those abilities vanished. However, repeated uses of the drug were also successful, allowing the family to "have their family member back, even if only for a few hours a day" (Shames & Ring, 2008, p. 387).

(STORY 3) A car accident led to a coma in an 18-year-old man, and he seemed unlikely to recover. His score on a scale used to assess coma severity was so low that his survival was "very unlikely," but his family kept him on life support with the hope that he would improve (p. 62). And he did—against the odds, he slowly improved. By the end of the second month, he was no longer on ventilation to assist his breathing. By the third month, he had improved to a *minimally conscious state* and began to groan in response to painful stimuli. At around seven months, he began "situation-independent screaming," meaning that he would, at seemingly random times, begin screaming (p. 63). This unfortunate symptom lasted for around four weeks, and painkillers did not seem to help. At eight months, he could close his eyes when asked to do so, and at nine months he began to be able to communicate via blinking and then nodding or shaking his head. He was then able to go home, where he continued intense rehabilitation efforts. He often participated in several hours per week of therapies for speech and movement. Around 18 months after the accident, he had made major improvements in cognitive functions such as memory, although he continued to have difficulties with some other types of tests. Ten years following the accident he still showed some signs of slowed speech and reduced memory but, otherwise, he was living an independent life with a nearly full recovery (Steppacher et al., 2016).

The Features

It is difficult to conceive of living your life without *awareness* of your life. Consciousness, in which your mind is aware of events and the passage of time, may seem to be the most essential element of human existence. Yet, our conscious awareness is just as much a part of our brains as everything else that makes up the human experience. Awareness is not a necessary component of a living creature, and you can prove this to yourself every day by falling asleep, and even more so if you or your roommate is a sleepwalker. Besides sleep, there are pathological ways to lose consciousness. Ways from which a person may never truly wake, and yet continue to live.

The most well-known disorder of consciousness is the *coma*, where a person loses responsiveness to the world around them as if they were in a deep sleep. But there are also disorders of consciousness where certain elements of responsiveness are retained, such as *unresponsive wakefulness syndrome* (UWS) and the *minimally conscious state* (MCS).

Because disorders of consciousness are notoriously different for each person, physicians rely on *scales* to grade the responsiveness of the patient. They do this by assigning number ratings to tests of awareness, including calling the patient's name to see if they open their eyes, causing pain to the skin and noting the reaction of the patient, and observing reflexes and movements. These numbers can then be compared to other patients to try and determine the likely outcome of the disorder as well as the best treatments (Bordini et al., 2010). The disorders in order from least to most indicators of consciousness are coma, UWS, and then MCS.

Coma is a state of nonconsciousness in which both *movement* as a response to the world around you and *psychological responses* have completely disappeared (Plum & Posner, 1966). In other words, someone in a coma entirely loses responsiveness to everything that the external environment can throw at them: light, sounds, touch, and everything else. In some comas certain reflexes remain, such as pupil dilation in the eyes or posturing reflexes in response to pain. In deeper comas even those basic reflexes disappear. Comas that are not severe usually improve within a few weeks into either consciousness or UWS (Georgiopoulos et al., 2010). When you read about people in long-term comas lasting months or years those are often UWS cases and not actually proper comas.

Unresponsive wakefulness syndrome (UWS) is a condition in which a person is awake but unaware. UWS was formerly called a "vegetative state," but, because the name seemed insensitive and is less descriptive than the name UWS, it was changed (Laureys et al., 2010). One noticeable difference between a person in a coma and a person with UWS is that in UWS the person has the ability to open their eyes—that is what the term "wakefulness" refers to. However, they are not conscious and the movements are just reflexes. People with UWS tend to have some additional preserved reflexes in the eyes, as well as coughing and swallowing (Multi-Society Task Force on Persistent Vegetative State, 1994). However, no intentional actions are made—they do not consciously plan to do something and then do it, like deciding to open their eyes and look at the clock to see what time it is. People with UWS may show some surprising behaviors such as smiling, crying, and even moaning or speaking single words, but these behaviors do not reflect what is happening around them and are instead "random" events (Schnakers & Majerus, 2018).

It is important to monitor people with UWS, especially their eye movements, for indications that the person is conscious but unable to move, such as in locked-in syndrome (see Locked-In Syndrome). Unfortunately, because the diagnosis of UWS requires careful assessment over time, misdiagnosis is common. This results in some people being treated as if they were in a lower state of consciousness than they actually are (Andrews et al., 1996). Plus, people can improve, so re-evaluation is often needed. When a person with UWS improves, they typically enter an MCS.

Minimally conscious state (MCS) is "a condition of severely altered consciousness" where the person shows a small amount of awareness for themselves or their environment (Giacino et al., 2014, p. 100). They may be considered partially conscious, but their ability to follow commands of doctors is inconsistent. In other words, they can do some things that a conscious person can do, but not always. These behaviors include watching moving objects with their eyes, reaching for and holding objects, and communicating by gesture or even voice (Giacino et al., 2002). Most people in an MCS that eventually recover full consciousness do so within a year of entering the MCS. Some continue to improve even beyond a year, but usually with some leftover disabilities (Estraneo & Trojano, 2018). One subtype of MCS is akinetic mutism (see Akinetic Mutism), where the *will* to perform actions is diminished, rather than there being damage to consciousness systems (Giacino et al., 2014). As the person begins to reliably communicate, they are classified as having "emerged" from the MCS (Schnakers & Majerus, 2018). Thus, they have returned to being both awake and aware.

The Brain Pathology

For a person to be conscious—awake and aware—communication between widely spread out brain areas is needed. Because such a wide area of the brain is involved, many kinds of damage can be disruptive to consciousness. Comas and disorders of consciousness can result from a wide variety of issues, including drugs or poisons, lack of oxygen, strokes, traumatic brain injuries, degenerative diseases, and many others (Multi-Society Task Force on Persistent Vegetative State, 1994). The brain damage for people with different disorders of consciousness may vary widely, but an overall description of what the brain is experiencing is reduced *intracortical modulation*. What this means is that brain cells are not exciting and inhibiting each other in the typical way that brain cells communicate (Bagnato et al., 2012). The brain is less active in disorders of consciousness, and brain activity doesn't spread or follow patterns like it usually does. Both wakefulness and awareness depend on the interaction between the cerebral cortex and the reticular system (Bleck, 2003).

We can get a bit more specific. Comas usually result from damage to the reticular activating system in the brain stem or from "global brain dysfunction" such that there is extensive damage in many parts of the brain and they are unable to effectively communicate with one another (Schnakers & Majerus, 2018, p. 3). In contrast, UWS indicates an intact reticular formation, but damage has disrupted "the flow of information from the midbrain to the cortex" (Bleck, 2003). Such damage may be to the underlying white matter of the brain or to the thalamus in each of the brain's hemispheres (Schnakers & Majerus, 2018).

Some people with UWS retain isolated pockets of cognitive function, such as a limited ability to process speech (Coleman et al., 2007). Specifically, we can scan the person's brain and show that certain areas, especially language centers (see Aphasia), become more active when the person hears words versus when they hear nonsense sounds—their brain can "listen" and tell the difference between the noises. These are known as *implicit language abilities*, and they are somewhat frequently detected in UWS and even more frequently in MCS (Aubinet et al., 2022). This is evidence that some people with severe disorders of consciousness really are hearing and mentally processing what is going on around them, but this is *not* necessarily evidence that they are consciously experiencing the words or that they will remember them (see Amnesia).

The prognosis in disorders of consciousness can be predicted somewhat based on how the patient scored on the coma scale, with those receiving higher scores more likely to improve. However, improvement from disorders of consciousness is notoriously difficult to predict, with some patients making unpredicted recoveries while others suddenly deteriorate. When it comes to predicting whether someone in a coma will ever regain consciousness, uncertainty abounds.

Despite the difficulties, there are some useful predictors of outcome. In general, the longer a person is in an unconscious or partially conscious state, the less likely they are to recover, and the less likely they are to make a complete recovery (Andrews, 1993). If a person loses or does not regain their most fundamental reflexes—those of the eye's pupil—a poor outcome is reliably predicted (Zandbergen, 2008). Additionally, the older a person is, the less likely they are to recover (Estraneo & Trojano, 2018). In theory, brain scans can also be used to predict improvement by detecting brain activity that is not expressed as behavior—for example, the person may be asked to imagine playing tennis or to imagine navigating rooms of a house, and then their brain activity may indicate that they are doing so—and people who show this difference seem more likely to recover than people in which this brain activity is not as pronounced (Stender et al., 2014).

It is uncommon, but recovery into full awareness is still possible after long periods of time such as multiple years (Andrews, 1993). However, improvements in these long-term cases are usually minimal and generally accompanied by disabilities that last a lifetime (Estraneo & Trojano, 2018). In younger people, recovery from disorders of consciousness is certainly possible and may be enhanced by intensive rehabilitation programs (Eilander et al., 2005).

In some cases, there has been improvement after the administration of certain medications. The recovery of some patients thanks to medications supports a theory of *neurotransmitter depletion*, in which adding chemicals to the brain can help it recover (Clauss, 2010). In other words, some people may experience disorders of consciousness due to a depletion of chemicals in the brain, and replenishing those chemicals may be enough to improve their condition.

Additionally, *neuromodulation* may offer new treatment options for disorders of consciousness, including the use of deep brain stimulation, which can be used to target areas of the brain for inhibition or excitation (Thibaut & Schiff, 2018). That is, electrical pulses can be delivered to parts of the brain in the hope that this will improve the symptoms of the patient towards conscious awareness (Giacino et al., 2014). After learning about the disorders of consciousness, I hope that you feel more aware of the science of awareness in your brain.

References

Andrews, K. (1993). Recovery of patients after four months or more in the persistent vegetative state. *British Medical Journal*, *306*(6892), 1597–1600. https://doi.org/cbvjd5

Andrews, K., Murphy, L., Munday, R., & Littlewood, C. (1996). Misdiagnosis of the vegetative state: Retrospective study in a rehabilitation unit. *British Medical Journal*, *313*(7048), 13–16. https://doi.org/d4j5f9

Aubinet, C., Chatelle, C., Gosseries, O., Carri, M., Laureys, S., & Majerus, S. (2022). Residual implicit and explicit language abilities in patients with disorders of consciousness: A systematic review. *Neuroscience and Biobehavioral Reviews*, *132*, 391–409. https://doi.org/g86d

Bagnato, S., Boccagni, C., Sant'Angelo, A., Prestandrea, C., Rizzo, S., & Galardi, G. (2012). Patients in a vegetative state following traumatic brain injury display a reduced intracortical modulation. *Clinical Neurophysiology*, *123*(10), 1937–1941. https://doi.org/gtms

Bleck, T. P. (2003). Levels of consciousness and attention. In C. G. Goetz (Ed.), *Textbook of clinical neurology* (2nd ed., pp. 3–18). Saunders.

Bordini, A. L., Luiz, T. F., Fernandes, M., Arruda, W. O., & Teive, H. A. (2010). Coma scales: A historical review. *Arquivos de Neuro-psiquiatria*, *68*(6), 930–937. https://doi.org/bg3vjc

Clauss, R. P. (2010). Neurotransmitters in coma, vegetative and minimally conscious states, pharmacological interventions. *Medical Hypotheses*, *75*(3), 287–290. https://doi.org/dnngd2

Coleman, M. R., Rodd, J. M., Davis, M. H., Johnsrude, I. S., Menon, D. K., Pickard, J. D., & Owen, A. M. (2007). Do vegetative patients retain aspects of language comprehension? Evidence from fMRI. *Brain*, *130*(10), 2494–2507. https://doi.org/dc694b

Eilander, H. J., Wijnen, V. J. M., Scheirs, J. G. M., De Kort, P. L. M., & Prevo, A. J. H. (2005). Children and young adults in a prolonged unconscious state due to severe brain injury: Outcome after an early intensive neurorehabilitation programme. *Brain Injury*, *19*(6), 425–436. https://doi.org/bc5wzz

Estraneo, A., & Trojano, L. (2018). Prognosis in disorders of consciousness. In C. Schnakers & S. Laureys (Eds.), *Coma and disorders of consciousness* (pp. 17–36). Springer International Publishing. https://doi.org/gtmv

Georgiopoulos, M., Katsakiori, P., Kefalopoulou, Z., Ellul, J., Chroni, E., & Constantoyannis, C. (2010). Vegetative state and minimally conscious state: A review of the therapeutic interventions. *Stereotactic and Functional Neurosurgery*, *88*(4), 199–207. https://doi.org/d4x8cm

Giacino, J. T., Ashwal, S., Childs, N., Cranford, R., Jennett, B., Katz, D. I., Kelly, J. P., Rosenberg, J. H., Whyte, J., Zafonte, R. D., & Zasler, N. D. (2002). The minimally conscious state: Definition and diagnostic criteria. *Neurology*, *58*(3), 349–353. https://doi.org/gcsf4s

Giacino, J. T., Fins, J. J., Laureys, S., & Schiff, N. D. (2014). Disorders of consciousness after acquired brain injury: The state of the science. *Nature Reviews Neurology*, *10*(2), 99–114. https://doi.org/f5rqw3

Laureys, S., Celesia, G. G., Cohadon, F., Lavrijsen, J., León-Carrión, J., Sannita, W. G., Sazbon, L., Schmutzhard, E., von Wild, K. R., Zeman, A., & Dolce, G. (2010). Unresponsive wakefulness syndrome: A new name for the vegetative state or apallic syndrome. *BMC Medicine*, *8*, Article 68. https://doi.org/cwzww5

Mahoney, W. J., D'Souza, B. J., Haller, J. A., Rogers, M. C., Epstein, M. H., & Freeman, J. M. (1983). Long-term outcome of children with severe head trauma and prolonged coma. *Pediatrics*, *71*(5), 756–762.

Multi-Society Task Force on Persistent Vegetative State (1994). Medical aspects of the persistent vegetative state. *New England Journal of Medicine*, *330*, 1499–1508. https://doi .org/fp3bm8

Plum, F., & Posner, J. B. (1966). *The diagnosis of stupor and coma*. FA Davis Co.

Schnakers, C., & Majerus, S. (2018). Behavioral assessment and diagnosis of disorders of consciousness. In C. Schnakers & S. Laureys (Eds.), *Coma and disorders of consciousness* (pp. 1–16). Springer International Publishing. https://doi.org/gtmw

Shames, J. L., & Ring, H. (2008). Transient reversal of anoxic brain injury-related minimally conscious state after zolpidem administration: A case report. *Archives of Physical Medicine and Rehabilitation*, *89*(2), 386–388. https://doi.org/ft4m2g

Stender, J., Gosseries, O., Bruno, M. A., Charland-Verville, V., Vanhaudenhuyse, A., Demertzi, A., Chatelle, C., Thonnard, M., Thibaut, A., Heine, L., Soddu, A., Boly, M., Schnakers, C., Gjedde, A., & Laureys, S. (2014). Diagnostic precision of PET imaging and functional MRI in disorders of consciousness: A clinical validation study. *The Lancet*, *384*(9942), 514–522. https://doi.org/sdq

Steppacher, I., Kaps, M., & Kissler, J. (2016). Against the odds: A case study of recovery from coma after devastating prognosis. *Annals of Clinical and Translational Neurology*, *3*(1), 61–65. https://doi.org/gtmz

Thibaut, A., & Schiff, N. D. (2018). New therapeutic options for the treatment of patients with disorders of consciousness: The field of neuromodulation. In C. Schnakers & S. Laureys (Eds.), *Coma and disorders of consciousness* (pp. 207–223). Springer International Publishing. https://doi.org/gtm2

Zandbergen, E. G. J. (2008). Postanoxic coma: How (long) should we treat? *European Journal of Anaesthesiology*, *25*(S42), 39–42. https://doi.org/d8nxf6

Cortical Blindness (Plus Anton-Babinski Syndrome, Blindsight, & Riddoch Syndrome)

Imagine that you lost the ability to see, even though your eyes were completely unharmed. Perhaps you hit your head in the wrong way, or a stroke damaged your brain. Suddenly, the information sent by your eyes into your brain can no longer be interpreted. But blindness may not be the whole story of your new disorder—syndromes of vision loss are complex. Imagine that you were blind but believed that you could see. Imagine that you thought you were blind, but when guessing what was happening in front of you, you were often correct, suggesting that you could, in fact, see. Imagine that you couldn't see objects, but you could still see movement, even without form, color, or size. How does your brain make these things possible?

The Stories

(STORY 1) A 96-year-old man was brought to the emergency room with a severe headache, and when his eyes were examined he was found to have "severe vision loss" (p. 394). Despite this, he continued to claim that he could see perfectly fine and began confabulating details about the world around him. He tried to convince the medical staff that he could see by describing the color of a tie that one of them appeared to be wearing, but unfortunately for the patient, the doctor was not wearing a tie. He also commented on the landscape that he claimed he could see from the window. This occurred while he was in a room without any windows. His denial of his own blindness was a clear case of *Anton-Babinski syndrome* (Romero Carvajal et al., 2012, case 1).

(STORY 2) A woman in her thirties developed brain damage in both hemispheres of her primary visual cortex. As a result, she acquired *blindsight*. She reported that she did not possess any vision, but there were exceptions to this. She could name the colors of moving objects in front of her and could mimic hand gestures made by others, all without feeling like she was truly seeing. She could see the movement of her daughter's ponytail swaying from side to side while she was walking but could not see her daughter. She also had some ability to navigate around obstacles when walking, which surprised her. She developed a strategy with the help of her healthcare providers where she sat in a rocking chair and used the motion of her body to enhance her vision,

DOI: 10.4324/9781003276937-20

because she better perceived moving objects, and from the chair it seemed that the world was moving. She said that her visual experiences were as if looking "down at a stream—the way water flows around with the current" (Arcaro et al., 2019, p. 152). She was so proficient at detecting movement, despite being mostly blind, that she was able to catch moving balls (Arcaro et al., 2019; Dutton, 2003).

(STORY 3) A man who acquired extensive brain damage in a car accident around the age of 7, developed blindness in roughly one-half of his visual field. But even though he could not see to his right, he could still sometimes detect movement in that area. This was a case of *Riddoch syndrome*. He said that he could feel when something was moving in that blind area, even though he could not see it nor describe the features of the moving item. When he was forced to guess whether something was moving toward or away from him on his blind side, he responded accurately much of the time, despite often reporting very low confidence in his guess. In other words, he was often correct even when he was seemingly unaware of the movement and when he felt like he was guessing. He sometimes did feel aware of the movement, however, describing it as "a black shadow moving on a black background" (Zeki & ffytche, 1998, p. 30). Overall, his ability to guess correctly was related to his level of awareness, but his accuracy and awareness were sometimes wildly out of sync (Barbur et al., 1993; Weiskrantz, 1990; Zeki & ffytche, 1998).

The Features

If you can see, you have probably built most of the activities of your life around that fact. A useful sense, vision is perhaps the most complicated thing for which your brain is responsible. The visual system of the brain takes up a huge amount of space, especially in the occipital lobe at the very back of your head and the regions in the temporal and parietal lobes that are immediately adjacent. There are many ways in which damage to the brain can disrupt the myriad processes necessary for this large region to function properly. Because of this, there are many startling ways that it can break. As a start, when a person loses the ability to see due to brain damage to this area, it is called cortical blindness.

You may think that blindness is, well, *complete* blindness, and these people must experience total darkness. But that's not always the case. For example, a person who becomes cortically blind may or may not retain the ability to imagine pictures—that is, visualize images in their mind's eye (see Aphantasia)—depending on how extensive the brain damage is (Bartolomeo, 2002). Some people who *can imagine* but *can't see* may replace much of the visual world with internal imagery, allowing them to navigate complex environments by using mental maps that they can "see" without seeing (Sacks, 2010). As another example, a mostly cortically blind person was reported to suffer from extremely vivid nightmares with "striking visual character," which demonstrates the power of the brain in generating its own images (Brown, 1972, case 12, pp. 208–209). Despite no longer consciously receiving information about the world from their eyes, they may nonetheless use visual images to interact with the world. They are therefore really only partially blind, at least by that definition. And it is such cases of partial blindness, where the person retains some abilities or knowledge in the face of lost vision, that create especially notable case studies. Three types are *Anton-Babinski syndrome*, *blindsight*, and *Riddoch syndrome.*

Anton-Babinski syndrome, sometimes simply called *Anton syndrome*, is one of the most unusual disorders, full stop. This disorder occurs when blindness or partial blindness is combined with anosognosia, or the absence of knowledge about one's own disorder (see Anosognosia). Or, as Anton himself wrote it: "the symptom that we must emphasize in consideration of the following case was the fact that the patient was not conscious of her blindness" (Anton, 1899, translated in Forde & Wallesch, 2003, p. 203). In these cases, the person insists that they can see despite clear evidence that they cannot (Chen et al., 2015). For example, they may walk into walls, trip over furniture, and describe objects that they claim to see but in reality are not there (Maddula et al., 2009). These people may reportedly offer excuses for why they cannot seem to see, such as the room being too dark, or they may even try—and fail—to *prove* that they can see (Galetović et al., 2005).

People with Anton-Babinski syndrome replace real vision with fake vision. They do this with visual imagery that is generated *inside* of the brain, but the person is not aware that these are mental images and not real images. This process of mistakenly believing that the mental images are vision is a type of *confabulation*, when a person lies without meaning to do so. Even if you try to convince someone with Anton-Babinski syndrome that they cannot see, you probably will not succeed, because the brain damage makes the conscious awareness of their blindness more difficult, plus they feel as if they are experiencing sight.

If people with Anton-Babinski syndrome believe that they *are* seeing when they actually are *not*, are there people who believe that they are *not* seeing when they actually *are*? Yes, and that condition is known aptly as *blindsight*.

In blindsight, a person loses the ability to consciously use visual information, but they can still use it nonconsciously. In other words, if you ask them whether they are blind, they will say yes, but if you test their blindness, they will perform better than chance on tasks where they have to visually identify things like object position and movement, and they might report feelings similar to seeing that are not seeing (Overgaard, 2011). In blindsight, people can often successfully detect color and orientations of lines, and sometimes they can detect shapes, but they generally cannot detect more complex things such as identities of faces (Ajina & Bridge, 2017). These scenes can be remarkable— for example, cortically blind children with blindsight being fed by caregivers can detect a spoon approaching their mouths if the spoon is moved in a particular way (Boyle et al., 2005).

There are also cases where a person has cortical blindness but is able to consciously experience *movement*, called *Riddoch syndrome* after George Riddoch, who described it in a case series presented in 1916 (Riddoch, 1917b). Specifically, people with Riddoch syndrome report being able to see movement but are unable to see objects that are not moving. This is just the impression of movement—it typically has neither shape nor color (Riddoch, 1917a). This disorder may be considered the opposite of akinetopsia (see Akinetopsia), wherein a person loses the ability to see movement but can still see shapes and color (Zihl et al., 1983).

The Brain Pathology

There are degrees of cortical blindness, with partial cortical blindness much more common than complete cortical blindness (Melnick et al., 2016). Two important types of partial blindness are hemianopsia and scotoma, which are discussed in a separate chapter (see Hemianopsia). Complete cortical blindness requires the destruction of a large area on both sides of the brain, which makes it impossible for the person to process visual information in certain ways. As a dramatic example, people who are blind because of problems with their *eyes* can still "see" letters when they are *drawn directly onto their brain* using electrical patterns, similar to how you could use your finger to draw a letter in the palm of their hand (Beauchamp et al., 2020). People with cortical blindness cannot do this because their brain has been damaged to the point that they no longer *have* the place where the letter would be drawn, analogous to them not having a hand and therefore making it impossible to trace the letter onto their palm. That is to say that people who are cortically blind are much more blind than people who are blind because of problems with their eyes. This is *brain* blindness that I am talking about.

There are a few theories that try to explain what is happening in the brain to cause Anton-Babinski syndrome, but it is still quite mysterious (Celesia & Brigell, 2005). One idea is that, in such people, there are preserved islands of brain cells in the visual cortex that were not destroyed, and so they are able to generate mental images that *feel* like real seeing (Goldenberg et al., 1995). In theory, both true visual perception and visual mental imagery happen at the same stage in the brain, in the *primary visual cortex*. That is, there is an overlap between truly perceived pictures that are created from light entering into a person's eyes and imagined pictures generated by the brain, but, usually, a person is able to tell the difference between the two (Dijkstra et al., 2019). However, if true visual perception is disrupted by brain damage, but visual mental imagery is able to continue, then it becomes harder to tell the difference between the two, leading to possible hallucinations or Anton-Babinski syndrome (Heilman, 1991). This has been called the "release phenomenon," in which mental images are misinterpreted as real (Celesia & Brigell, 2005, p. 435).

The leading theory for both blindsight and Riddoch syndrome is that there are paths that information from the eyes can take to the parts of the brain that detect features of objects or motion *without* passing through the part of the brain thought to be responsible for the perceptual *experience* of "seeing" (Ajina & Bridge, 2017). In these people their primary visual cortex is typically severely damaged, but other connections leading from their eyes into their brain remain intact (Weiskrantz, 1996). Essentially, their brain is still using information from the eyes for things other than typical conscious sight. This leads to a situation where a person is capable of "looking, pointing, detecting and discriminating without seeing" (Cowey & Stoerig, 1991, p. 140). Many connections bring information from the eyes into different places in the brain, and the pattern of surviving connections seems to determine what type of blindsight or Riddoch syndrome develops (Arcaro et al., 2019). This arrangement is similar to disorders of central hearing (see Cortical Deafness).

Cortical blindness may be permanent, but it may also be partially or completely recovered from (Bharati et al., 2017). The best outcomes seem to occur for younger people, especially those under the age of 40 (Aldrich et al., 1987). Overall, cortical blindness, whether partial or complete, can be startling at first, but the majority of people with disorders such as these find clever ways to adapt.

References

Ajina, S., & Bridge, H. (2017). Blindsight and unconscious vision: What they teach us about the human visual system. *Neuroscientist, 23*(5), 529–541. https://doi.org/gb2wr4

Aldrich, M. S., Alessi, A. G., Beck, R. W., & Gilman, S. (1987). Cortical blindness: Etiology, diagnosis, and prognosis. *Annals of Neurology, 21*(2), 149–158. https://doi.org/b7b3bh

Anton, G. (1899). Ueber die Selbstwahrnehmung der Herderkrankungen des Gehirns durch den Kranken bei Rindenblindheit und Bindentaubheit. *Archiv für Psychiatrie und Nervenkrankheiten, 32*(1), 86–127.

Arcaro, M. J., Thaler, L., Quinlan, D. J., Monaco, S., Khan, S., Valyear, K. F., Goebel, R., Dutton, G. N., Goodale, M. A., Kastner, S., & Culham, J. C. (2019). Psychophysical and neuroimaging responses to moving stimuli in a patient with the Riddoch phenomenon due to bilateral visual cortex lesions. *Neuropsychologia, 128*, 150–165. https://doi.org/cvmb

Barbur, J. L., Watson, J. D. G., Frackowiak, R. S. J., & Zeki, S. (1993). Conscious visual perception without V1. *Brain, 116*(6), 1293–1302. https://doi.org/drmdvh

Bartolomeo, P. (2002). The relationship between visual perception and visual imagery: A reappraisal of the neuropsychological evidence. *Cortex, 38*(3), 357–378. https://doi.org/d5892j

Beauchamp, M. S., Oswalt, D., Sun, P., Foster, B. L., Magnotti, J. F., Niketeghad, S., Pouratian, N., Bosking, W. H., & Yoshor, D. (2020). Dynamic stimulation of visual cortex produces form vision in sighted and blind humans. *Cell, 181*(4), 774–783. https://doi.org/dvs6

Bharati, S., Sharma, M. K., Chattopadhay, A., & Das, D. (2017). Transient cortical blindness following intracardiac repair of congenital heart disease in an 11-year-old boy. *Annals of Cardiac Anaesthesia, 20*(2), 256. https://doi.org/f92mq2

Boyle, N. J., Jones, D. H., Hamilton, R., Spowart, K. M., & Dutton, G. N. (2005). Blindsight in children: Does it exist and can it be used to help the child? Observations on a case series. *Developmental Medicine & Child Neurology, 47*(10), 699–702. https://doi .org/bgpftw

Brown, J. W. (1972). *Aphasia, apraxia, and agnosia: Clinical and theoretical aspects.* CC Thomas.

Celesia, G. & Brigell, M. (2005). Cortical blindness and visual anosognosia. In G. Celesia (Ed.), *Handbook of clinical neurophysiology: Disorders of visual processing* (pp. 429–440). Elsevier. https://doi.org/fqs4sz

Chen, J. J., Chang, H. F., Hsu, Y. C., & Chen, D. L. (2015). Anton–Babinski syndrome in an old patient: A case report and literature review. *Psychogeriatrics, 15*(1), 58–61. https:// doi.org/gtm3

Cowey, A., & Stoerig, P. (1991). The neurobiology of blindsight. *Trends in Neurosciences, 14*(4), 140–145. https://doi.org/cpj69k

Dijkstra, N., Bosch, S. E., & van Gerven, M. A. J. (2019). Shared neural mechanisms of visual perception and imagery. *Trends in Cognitive Sciences, 23*(5), 423–434. https://doi .org/gg7jtw

Dutton, G. N. (2003). Cognitive vision, its disorders and differential diagnosis in adults and children: Knowing where and what things are. *Eye, 17*(3), 289–304. https://doi.org/ dsj87d

Forde, E., & Wallesch, C. W. (2003). 'Mind-blind for blindness': A psychological review of Anton's syndrome. In C. Code, C. W. Wallesch, Y. Joanette, & A. R. Lecours (Eds.), *Classic cases in neuropsychology* (Vol. 2, pp. 199–222). Psychology Press.

Galetović, D., Karlica, D., Bojić, L., & Znaor, L. (2005). Bilateral cortical blindness - Anton syndrome: Case report. *Collegium Antropologicum, 29*(SUPPL. 1), 145–147.

Goldenberg, G., Müllbacher, W., & Nowak, A. (1995). Imagery without perception—A case study of anosognosia for cortical blindness. *Neuropsychologia, 33*(11), 1373–1382. https://doi.org/dz3wjx

Heilman, K. M. (1991). Anosognosia: Possible neuropsychological mechanisms. In G. Prigatano & D. Sacher (Eds.), *Awareness of defect after brain injury* (pp. 429–440). Oxford University Press.

Maddula, M., Lutton, S., & Keegan, B. (2009). Anton's syndrome due to cerebrovascular disease: A case report. *Journal of Medical Case Reports, 3*(9028). https://doi.org/d8xc7b

Melnick, M. D., Tadin, D., & Huxlin, K. R. (2016). Relearning to see in cortical blindness. *Neuroscientist, 22*(2), 199–212. https://doi.org/f8ft75

Overgaard, M. (2011). Visual experience and blindsight: A methodological review. *Experimental Brain Research, 209*(4), 473–479. https://doi.org/ck2kt2

Riddoch, G. (1917a). Dissociation of visual perceptions due to occipital injuries, with especial reference to appreception of movement. *Brain, 40*(1), 15–57. https://doi.org /fvww93w

Riddoch, G. (1917b). On the relative perceptions of movement and a stationary object in certain visual disturbances due to occipital injuries. *Proceedings of the Royal Society of Medicine, 10*, 13–34.

Romero Carvajal, J. J., Arias Cárdenas, A. A., Pazmiño, G. Z., & Herrera, P. A. (2012). Visual anosognosia (Anton-Babinski Syndrome): Report of two cases associated with ischemic cerebrovascular disease. *Journal of Behavioral and Brain Science, 2*(3), 394–398. https://doi.org/gtjh

Sacks, O. (2010). *The mind's eye.* Knopf.

Weiskrantz, L. (1990). The Ferrier Lecture, 1989: Outlooks for blindsight: Explicit methodologies for implicit processes. *Proceedings of the Royal Society of London. B. Biological Sciences, 239*(1296), 247–278. https://doi.org/cv2z3m

Weiskrantz, L. (1996). Blindsight revisited. *Current Opinion in Neurobiology*, *6*(2), 215–220. https://doi.org/d4m4hm

Zeki, S., & ffytche, D. H. (1998). The Riddoch syndrome: Insights into the neurobiology of conscious vision. *Brain*, *121*(1), 25–45. https://doi.org/b9smh8

Zihl, J., Von Cramon, D., & Mai, N. (1983). Selective disturbance of movement vision after bilateral brain damage. *Brain*, *106*(2), 313–340. https://doi.org/fjr2bs

Cortical Deafness (Plus Other Central Hearing Disorders)

Imagine that the way you hear things isn't quite what it used to be. The ability to hear can be damaged in numerous ways, and you might have acquired any number of symptoms. Perhaps you can no longer tell one sound apart from another. Perhaps you can no longer enjoy the nuances of music. Or perhaps there are parts of your brain that can still react reflexively to sounds, but you yourself are unable to "hear" anything. Where in your brain have the meanings of these sounds become lost?

The Stories

(STORY 1) A 56-year-old woman had one stroke in 2008, and then another stroke in 2009. After the first one, she developed some problems typical of stroke aftermath such as slurring her speech, but her hearing abilities were typical. However, after the second stroke, she suddenly and profoundly lost the ability to hear all sounds, with the exception of severe tinnitus such that she could hear a phantom ringing all of the time. Her ears were examined and were shown to be intact and functioning; it was damage to the processing regions of her brain that caused the cortical deafness. Interestingly, this sudden onset of deafness was not due entirely to the 2009 stroke. The 2008 stroke had knocked out a large part of her brain responsible for hearing, but the other half of her brain had compensated so well for the damage that she wasn't even aware of a difference to her hearing until the second stroke removed her remaining ability to hear. The patient showed poor volume control of her voice following the second stroke but could speak fluently (Brody et al., 2013).

(STORY 2) A 46-year-old woman was admitted to a hospital many years after first beginning to suffer from *pure word deafness*. She originally developed the condition because of a hemorrhage or stroke in her brain but continued to live for 15 years after this original incident. It was only spoken words that she could no longer understand, and she was said to still enjoy music and sounds of various sorts. For example, she could hear knocking at her front door and come down from upstairs in order to let a person inside. She seemed able to read and understand what she was reading but occasionally mixed up words when speaking or writing. Eventually, a second stroke robbed her of her ability

DOI: 10.4324/9781003276937-21

to hear other sounds as well, presumably because lesions in her temporal lobes continued to spread. By the end, the doctor wrote that she was testing as deaf. Her cortical deafness was believed to be caused entirely by internal damage to her brain, but this all occurred before brain scanning technology was available, so it is impossible to be certain (Mills, 1891).

(STORY 3) A 62-year-old woman who worked as a professional singer had a stroke in 2002 that left her with an unfortunate set of symptoms for her profession. She reported that she had lost the ability to sing in tune and that musical instruments had lost their unique "timbre" such that they all sounded dull to her "as if they were being heard from a great distance" (p. 480). As a result of her condition of *amusia*, she lost much of her enjoyment that she had previously gained from music. She was still able to recognize songs and music but no longer dared to sing aloud in public (Terao et al., 2006).

The Features

The ability to interpret sound is absolutely incredible from a physical stand-point. You've probably heard the term "sound wave" before, but let's take a moment to explore it. In order to hear something, you first need a vibrating object. In the case of a guitar, it's the string wiggling back and forth. Next, the guitar string smacks air molecules around in a particular pattern, causing those air molecules to bump into other molecules which continue the pattern. This causes the molecules to bunch up close together in some places and spread out away from each other in the places in between, creating *pressure*. Because the molecules are *moving*, there is *change in pressure over time*. When this whole assembly of moving pressure thwaps up against the inside of the ear, what has essentially happened is that the vibration from the guitar has jumped into the tiny *bones* inside of your head, specifically the inner ear bones called *ossicles*. Your ear bones then turn that vibration into waves of fluid which travel into a circular structure in your inner ear called the *cochlea*. The cochlea converts the fluid waves into tiny amounts of electricity depending on the change in pressure over time. All of that is the *easy* part of hearing sound.

Hearing gets complicated quickly because hearing sound is almost never a simple matter of listening to one guitar string vibrating. Usually, there are multiple sound waves happening at the same time, and they are coming from different places in your environment. Your brain has to take all of that confusing molecular movement and turn it into the perception of a 40-piece orchestra, or birdsong by a waterfall, or dogs barking at a garbage truck at six in the morning.

There are many ways to damage that first part of hearing with the ear bones and the cochlea and the conversion into tiny amounts of electricity which make up the *peripheral auditory system* (Hain, 2007). But for the purposes of this chapter, we are going to pretend that we've made it past those first remarkable steps and are already on our way into the *central auditory system* in the brain itself. Damage to the central auditory system may result in a variety of *central hearing disorders*, beginning with *cortical deafness*.

Cortical deafness occurs when a person cannot hear due to brain damage, but has a healthy peripheral auditory system. That is, your ears are fine but you cannot hear. *Partial* hearing loss is common after strokes, but *complete* cortical deafness is much rarer (Bamiou, 2015). In other words, while it is extremely easy to partially damage a person's ability to hear, it is extremely difficult to completely take hearing away, for reasons that will be discussed later.

Other central hearing disorders are more common than complete cortical deafness, because they require a smaller portion of the brain to be damaged. These other central hearing disorders include *auditory agnosia, pure word deafness, word meaning deafness, nonverbal auditory agnosia*, and *amusia*.

A person with *auditory agnosia* is still able to hear some sounds. However, the sounds that they hear become confusing and difficult to comprehend such that they don't know *what* the noises are. For example, they may have trouble recognizing the sound of a telephone (Hain, 2007). Or, the noise of their dog barking may suddenly sound different (Michel et al., 1980). One sound that someone with auditory agnosia may hear better than a person with cortical deafness is a *pure tone*—single, consistent sound waves—although not always for every possible tone (Poliva, 2014). Auditory agnosia and cortical deafness are similar enough that it is difficult to "choose one terminology over the other," although in theory the underlying damage is different such that cortical deafness refers to more extensive brain damage (Michel et al., 1980, p. 368).

Pure word deafness is a disorder in which a person can still hear sounds, but they don't understand words. Instead, words start to sound a bit like a foreign language. They have the ability to hear, the ability to read, and the ability to speak, but not the ability to understand what other people are saying. Language sounds like nonsense to them. Despite this, a person with pure word deafness can understand other sounds. For example, they may hear and respond to music or knocks on the door (Mills, 1891). Pure word deafness may be a mild version of auditory agnosia, where the problem is with understanding short and quick speech sounds but they can still understand longer, repeated, and slower sounds of music or from nature (Phillips & Farmer, 1990). That is, musical and natural sounds may be easier for the brain to understand because they are simply more distinct, and more predictably repetitive, than language (Pinard et al., 2002).

A similar sounding but different disorder is *word meaning deafness*. A person who has word meaning deafness can hear spoken language, but they cannot attach meaning to the words. They can *repeat* a word that is said to them without knowing what it means. Sometimes a person with word meaning deafness will write down the sounds that they hear, and then read them, in order to figure out what they mean (Kohn & Friedman, 1986). These two disorders are different from aphasia (see Aphasia) because these people are more capable of writing and speaking than someone with aphasia (Poliva, 2014).

Nonverbal auditory agnosia is sort of the opposite of pure word deafness in the sense that people with this condition can hear and understand spoken words, but they have problems with hearing other sounds. This disorder is sometimes called *environmental sound* agnosia. These people have difficulties with nonlanguage sounds, such as cats meowing, trains whistling, and knocking on the door—experiments have shown that people with this type of brain damage have trouble identifying which object each noise belongs to (Tanaka et al., 2002). People with this disorder may not even be that inconvenienced by it, because being unable to identify sounds such as cars starting or glass breaking is a problem that affects the average person's life less than trouble with understanding speech (Yamamoto et al., 2004).

Finally, *amusia* occurs when a person has difficulties with perceiving music, which can also affect a person's ability to produce music (Clark et al., 2015). It's sort of like tone deafness, but caused by brain damage. More specifically, there may be changes to a person's perception of timbre, loudness, pitch, and other musical traits (e.g., Terao et al., 2006). They may report that singing now sounds like shouting or that all musical notes now sound the same (Piccirilli et al., 2000).

The Brain Pathology

What makes cortical deafness so rare is that it requires brain damage to large parts of both sides of the brain (Graham et al., 1980). Specifically, damage to parts of both of the *auditory cortices* located in the temporal lobes. One fun fact about the way that the brain is wired is that incoming sound wave information from both ears is shared with both auditory cortices. Therefore, a person who has damage to just one auditory cortex will not experience cortical deafness, and may not show significant impairments to hearing at all (Polster & Rose, 1998). Because the auditory cortices are located far away from one another, the typical person who develops cortical deafness first has a stroke in one auditory cortex, and then later has *another* stroke in the other one (Brody et al., 2013).

In fact, the organization of hearing in the brain has so many interconnections between the hemispheres, connections to the brain cells of other areas, and general redundancies, that even people and animals with extensive damage to these areas still show at least some abilities to respond to sound (Bamiou, 2015). For example, a woman who was seemingly "absolutely deaf" with complete destruction of both auditory cortices according to her autopsy report, was still able to react to the "loudest noises" such as a curtain rod that crashed to the floor while she was in the hospital (Mott, 1907, p. 311). The auditory system in your brain is so good at doing its job of hearing that, according to studies of brainwaves, the sense of hearing seems to be one of the last senses to fade in otherwise unresponsive people who are about to die (Blundon et al., 2020).

Instead of describing people with cortical deafness as truly deaf, it may be more accurate to describe them as unable to perceive sound, despite it entering into their brain—and experiments support this by showing that people with cortical deafness have reflexive responses to sound in places such as their *brain stem* (Bamiou, 2015). This arrangement is similar to blindsight (see Cortical Blindness). The cortically deaf person may use their sense of hearing without knowing that they are using it. For example, they may turn their head when they hear a siren or a telephone ringing, even though they don't experience "hearing" it (Tanaka et al., 1991).

What we've learned from the existence of pure word deafness, nonverbal auditory agnosia, and amusia is that speech, environmental noises, and music are processed somewhat differently in the brain, but they do depend on some of the same parts of the brain (Clark et al., 2015). All three of these disorders can occur in the same person, and then one by one be recovered independently (Mendez & Geehan, 1988). However, more needs to be learned about how these different disorders are related to one another. For example, there are areas in the human brain that are organized *tonotopically*, meaning that the brain cells at one end of the area prefer to respond to low-pitched noises while the brain cells at the other end of the area prefer to respond to high-pitched noises (Humphries et al., 2010). Is it possible that some of these disorders can be caused by damage to particular places in the tonotopic maps? Researchers aren't sure yet. It's problematic that there are a number of "anatomical constraints" that prevent easy answers to these questions, such as the fact that the auditory cortices are huge and partially buried in the folds of the brain, as well as highly distributed information processing, resulting in the fact that "functional parcellations beyond the core and their relation to anatomical landmarks are not well understood" (Hamilton et al., 2021, p. 4626). One thing that is for sure is that disorders of central hearing are complex, and often difficult to diagnose.

References

Bamiou, D. E. (2015). Hearing disorders in stroke. In G. G. Celesia & G. Hickok (Eds.), *Handbook of clinical neurology: The human auditory system* (Vol. 129, pp. 633–647). Elsevier. https://doi.org/gtm6

Blundon, E. G., Gallagher, R. E., & Ward, L. M. (2020). Electrophysiological evidence of preserved hearing at the end of life. *Scientific Reports*, *10*(1), 1–13. https://doi.org/gmb4c4

Brody, R. M., Nicholas, B. D., Wolf, M. J., Marcinkevich, P. B., & Artz, G. J. (2013). Cortical deafness: A case report and review of the literature. *Otology & Neurotology*, *34*(7), 1226–1229. https://doi.org/f5cvvx

Clark, C. N., Golden, H. L., & Warren, J. D. (2015). Acquired amusia. In G. G. Celesia & G. Hickok (Eds.), *Handbook of clinical neurology: The human auditory system* (Vol. 129, pp. 607–631). Elsevier. https://doi.org/f66q99

Graham, J., Greenwood, R., & Lecky, B. (1980). Cortical deafness: A case report and review of the literature. *Journal of the Neurological Sciences*, *48*(1), 35–49. https://doi.org/b32jg6

Hain, T. C. (2007). Cranial nerve VIII: Vestibulocochlear nerve. In C. G. Goetz (Ed.), *Textbook of clinical neurology* (3rd ed., pp. 199–215). Saunders.

Hamilton, L. S., Oganian, Y., Hall, J., & Chang, E. F. (2021). Parallel and distributed encoding of speech across human auditory cortex. *Cell, 184*(18), 4626–4639. https://doi.org/gmhtq4

Humphries, C., Liebenthal, E., & Binder, J. R. (2010). Tonotopic organization of human auditory cortex. *NeuroImage, 50*(3), 1202–1211. https://doi.org/ftkvgj

Kohn, S. E., & Friedman, R. B. (1986). Word-meaning deafness: A phonological-semantic dissociation. *Cognitive Neuropsychology, 3*(3), 291–308. https://doi.org/fkcq9s

Mendez, M. F., & Geehan, G. R. (1988). Cortical auditory disorders: Clinical and psychoacoustic features. *Journal of Neurology, Neurosurgery & Psychiatry, 51*(1), 1–9. https://doi.org/c7ktgw

Michel, F., Peronnet, F., & Schott, B. (1980). A case of cortical deafness: Clinical and electrophysiological data. *Brain and Language, 10*(2), 367–377. https://doi.org/bdbddq

Mills, C. K. (1891). On the localisation of the auditory centre. *Brain, 14*(4), 465–472. https://doi.org/bqzf8b

Mott, F. W. (1907). Bilateral lesion of the auditory cortical centre: Complete deafness and aphasia. *British Medical Journal, 2*(2432), 310–315. https://doi.org/cvnp27

Phillips, D. P., & Farmer, M. E. (1990). Acquired word deafness, and the temporal grain of sound representation in the primary auditory cortex. *Behavioural Brain Research, 40*(2), 85–94. https://doi.org/fm68kc

Piccirilli, M., Sciarma, T., & Luzzi, S. (2000). Modularity of music: Evidence from a case of pure amusia. *Journal of Neurology Neurosurgery and Psychiatry, 69*(4), 541–545. https://doi.org/dh6hqb

Pinard, M., Chertkow, H., Black, S., & Peretz, I. (2002). A case study of pure word deafness: Modularity in auditory processing? *Neurocase, 8*(1), 40–55. https://doi.org/cmmdn2

Poliva, O. (2014). *Neuroanatomical and perceptual deficits in auditory agnosia: A study of an auditory agnosia patient with inferior colliculus damage* (Doctoral dissertation, Prifysgol Bangor University).

Polster, M. R., & Rose, S. B. (1998). Disorders of auditory processing: Evidence for modularity in audition. *Cortex, 34*(1), 47–65. https://doi.org/dc5nzm

Tanaka, Y., Kamo, T., Yoshida, M., & Yamadori, A. (1991). 'So-called' cortical deafness: Clinical, neurophysiological and radiological observations. *Brain, 114*(6), 2385–2401. https://doi.org/fbv6rw

Tanaka, Y., Nakano, I., & Obayashi, T. (2002). Environmental sound recognition after unilateral subcortical lesions. *Cortex, 38*(1), 69–76. https://doi.org/bwmfvk

Terao, Y., Mizuno, T., Shindoh, M., Sakurai, Y., Ugawa, Y., Kobayashi, S., Nagai, C., Furubayashi, T., Arai, N., Okabe, S., Mochizuki, H., Hanajima, R., & Tsuji, S. (2006). Vocal amusia in a professional tango singer due to a right superior temporal cortex infarction. *Neuropsychologia, 44*(3), 479–488. https://doi.org/b4mwmq

Yamamoto, T., Kikuchi, T., Nagae, J., Ogata, K., Ogawa, M., & Kawai, M. (2004). Dysprosody associated with environmental auditory sound agnosia in right temporal lobe hypoperfusion: A case report. *Rinsho Shinkeigaku, 44*(1), 28–33.

Cotard Syndrome (Walking Corpse Syndrome)

Imagine that you believe you're no longer alive. Your feelings of attachment to the world have become muddled and dark, such that life doesn't feel "real" anymore. Not only does a gloomy mood consume you, but you feel like you no longer exist. Perhaps you can even describe which parts of your body feel like they are missing, or maybe you try to convince your doctor that there is no use treating you and they should hurry up and bury you. What has gone wrong in your brain that has convinced you that you are, in fact, dead?

The Stories

(STORY 1) A 32-year-old man with severe recurring migraine headaches developed an additional unexpected symptom. He had migraines about once per month, and his typical migraine symptoms included vomiting, sweating, and avoidance of light that lasted for around 48 hours each time. However, upon one visit to the clinic, another prominent symptom developed: Cotard syndrome. He began insisting that he was dead and had been dead for months. He claimed that what people were seeing when they looked at him was "nothing but his corpse" (p. 152). People attempted to argue with him that he was still alive, but he did not believe them. His migraine headache went away after about a day, but the delusional belief that he was dead did not disappear until about a week later. A follow-up with the patient six months later revealed that he had not experienced Cotard syndrome again after the first event. He did not appear to have any neurological lesions nor history of mental illnesses, and Cotard syndrome was not linked to any other medical anomaly, suggesting that it was due to the migraine (Bhatia et al., 1993).

(STORY 2) A 46-year-old woman with a diagnosis of bipolar disorder began having many "nihilistic delusions" (p. 197). She explained that she was "a body without content" and that she did not have an identity (p. 197). She felt as if her entire body was translucent, as if light could pass through it. She felt that her body parts were missing, especially her intestines and brain. She outright refused to shower or bathe "because she was afraid of being soluble" and washing down the drain (p. 197). Because her Cotard syndrome symptoms occurred within a depressive episode and with psychotic features, she would

DOI: 10.4324/9781003276937-22

probably be best classified as a person with *Cotard syndrome type II* (Debruyne et al., 2009, case 2).

(STORY 3) In 1989, a 28-year-old man was severely injured in a motor-cycle accident, resulting in a fluctuating coma and near-coma state for a few days. When he awoke, he couldn't remember the past three or four weeks. Scans of his brain revealed damage in multiple places, including frontal lobe atrophy, "multiple haemorrhagic contusions" in his right temporal cortex, and differences in the adjacent parietal regions (p. 800). This extensive damage was reflected in his symptoms, which included partial paralysis and partial blindness. However, the symptoms did not end there. For months after the accident, the patient believed that he was dead and had extreme feelings that events happening around him weren't real. He had trouble with recognizing previously familiar things such as places and faces, and "he described his vision as 'like listening to a foreign language'" (p. 800). When he visited a city that he knew well, he couldn't recognize the buildings, and supposed that they must have all been knocked down and replaced while he was away. When he was released from the hospital and taken on a trip to a foreign country, he was convinced that he had died and been taken to hell. At one point, there was some evidence that he was feeling depressed, but otherwise he did not seem to be suffering from any broad mental illness or "general dementing condition" (p. 803). Because the disorder was not associated with notable mental illness, this person is probably best classified as having *Cotard syndrome type I*. Later on, he showed signs of recovery from his difficulties in recognizing, and from his Cotard delusion. In the end, the "feeling of being dead resolved completely" (Young et al., 1992, p. 800).

The Features

Cotard syndrome, which occasionally goes by the name of *walking corpse syndrome*, is a disorder in which a person believes that they are dead or do not exist. When Jules Cotard described this disorder in 1882, he called it "le délire de négation"—the delusion of negation (Enoch & Ball, 2001). However, by the time the 1890s were over, the syndrome was more commonly referred to as Cotard syndrome. Of all of the disorders that one could have named after oneself, the disorder where the person believes themselves to be trapped between the worlds of the living and the dead is one of the more intriguing namesakes.

In popular media such as television shows, Cotard syndrome is usually depicted in the form of a person believing that they are dead. Sometimes this is used for comedic effect, such as in the medical comedy *Scrubs* where a patient believes that he is a ghost wandering around the hospital and narrates his thoughts out loud (Schwartz & Koch, 2005). However, the specific belief that you are *dead* is not required in order to receive a diagnosis of Cotard syndrome (Ramirez-Bermudez et al., 2010).

Many other beliefs related to death, the afterlife, non-reality, and nonexistence, have also been reported as part of Cotard syndrome. These beliefs include insistence that parts of the body are missing, that death is coming soon or will never come, or that reality isn't real. For example, Cotard himself wrote of one patient that she:

> affirms she has no brain, no nerves, no chest, no stomach, no intestines … she's nothing more than a decomposing body, and has no need to eat for living, she cannot die a natural death, she exists eternally if she's not burned, the fire will be the only solution for her.
>
> (Cotard, 1880, translated in Debruyne et al., 2011, p. 67)

Case study descriptions really went for it back then. Patients may also behave in ways that are indifferent toward life, such as practicing self-starvation in the belief that they no longer need to eat (e.g., Silva et al., 2000; Teixeira et al., 2015). Because it isn't specific to believing that you are dead, I would argue that the name "delusion of negation," as Cotard originally suggested, is a better name than both Cotard syndrome and walking corpse syndrome.

This disorder commonly occurs alongside psychiatric symptoms, such as depression, anxiety, bipolar disorder, and sometimes hallucinations. There are even cases where delusions, such as delusions of immortality, are extreme enough to merit the diagnosis of severe psychotic disorders (Berrios & Luque, 1995). When combined with psychiatric symptoms, the disorder is known as *Cotard syndrome type II*. Perhaps around 70% of reported Cotard cases occur with some type of psychosis, with schizophrenia being one example (Enoch & Ball, 2001).

However, there do appear to be cases of a *pure* disorder. That is, there are cases of Cotard syndrome *without* psychiatric symptoms. These pure cases have been referred to as *Cotard syndrome type I* (Berrios & Luque, 1995). The existence of pure cases, as well as the substantial number of times that Cotard syndrome shows up in different people, suggests that there must be underlying neurological mechanisms that lead a person to conclude that they are dead. What could those be?

The Brain Pathology

Unfortunately, the underlying neurological mechanisms leading to Cotard syndrome are far from certain. In fact, it may be the least certain of the disorders in this book. We do have theories as to why Cotard syndrome symptoms appear, but it will take more research before the cause(s) can be determined. One thing that makes pinning down the cause(s) extra tricky is that the cases of Cotard syndrome are often different from one another—both in the different symptoms that the disorder presents, and in the ways that the disorder is often combined with other disorders. This is especially true regarding the mental illnesses, such as depression, mentioned above.

One potential explanation for Cotard syndrome is that people have damaged the parts of their brains responsible for attaching emotional reactions to familiar objects or people (Wright et al., 1993). Because they have stopped feeling certain emotions that are typically attached to life experiences, they conclude that things around them are not real or that they have died, as an attempt to explain the lost feelings. As one example, they may have lost the ability to link formerly pleasurable experiences to the feeling of pleasure, leading them to lose interest in viewing art or listening to music, and instead find themselves believing that they are dead or in a dream state (Ramachandran, 2011). It is no wonder, if a person has lost "emotional contact" with the world, that they may feel depressed and zombie-like (Ramachandran & Blakeslee, 1998).

Additionally, researchers have discussed that Cotard and Capgras (see Capgras syndrome) may be closely-linked disorders (Young, 1999). In fact, Cotard syndrome and Capgras syndrome have sometimes occurred within the same patients (e.g., Butler, 2000; Wright et al., 1993). In Capgras syndrome, the person believes that people around them have been replaced by doubles, and cases of Cotard syndrome often feature people who feel disconnected from themselves when they view their own reflections. This may be due to problems with recognizing faces (Enoch & Ball, 2001). In theory, both syndromes involve patients trying to make sense of bizarre perceptual experiences, such as feeling like they are not looking at themselves when they see their reflection, by inventing an explanation that seems delusional to the rest of us (Young, 1999). Therefore, a face-processing impairment is another leading theory of the cause of Cotard syndrome (Young & Leafhead, 1996).

Cotard syndrome has resulted from various causes including migraines, epilepsy, tumors, and brain trauma. In many, but not all, cases, there is structural brain damage visible on brain scans which seems to implicate the importance of interactions between the frontal, temporal, and parietal regions of the brain in the genesis of this syndrome (e.g., Debruyne et al., 2011; Sahoo & Josephs, 2017). While structural differences such as brain damage have been detected in many people with Cotard syndrome, in many others it is unclear whether brain damage has occurred, when no structural abnormality can be discovered and blamed for the syndrome (Kudlur et al., 2007). Thus, a firm explanation for this syndrome remains elusive.

Treatment for Cotard syndrome may involve the use of prescription antidepressants and antipsychotics, although interventions such as electroconvulsive therapy have also been used (Grover et al., 2014). Patients frequently recover from Cotard syndrome, although they may still have underlying medical or neurological disorders following their improvement (Sahoo & Josephs, 2017). When people do recover, it often happens suddenly and spontaneously even in severe cases, possibly due to changes in underlying disorders such as bipolar disorder or schizophrenia (Teixeira et al., 2015). However, not all patients recover, and "prognosis can widely vary from spontaneous recovery to a very severe chronic condition" (Debruyne et al., 2011, p. 70). In any case, it's worth taking away the fact that people with this condition are just trying to make sense out of the situation that life has put them in—much like everyone has to—but the cards they have been dealt unfortunately include the lingering presence of death.

References

Berrios, G. E., & Luque, R. (1995). Cotard's syndrome: Analysis of 100 cases. *Acta Psychiatrica Scandinavica*, *91*(3), 185–188. https://doi.org/bc3tsm

Bhatia, M. S., Agrawal, P., & Malik, S. C. (1993). Cotard's syndrome in migraine (a case report). *Indian Journal of Medical Sciences*, *47*(6), 152–153.

Butler, P. V. (2000). Diurnal variation in Cotard's syndrome (copresent with Capgras delusion) following traumatic brain injury. *Australian & New Zealand Journal of Psychiatry*, *34*(4), 684–687. https://doi.org/d3nk9f

Cotard, J. (1880). Du délire hypocondriaque dans une forme grave de mélancolie anxieuse. Memoire lu à la Société médicopsychologique dans la Séance du 28 Juin 1880. *Annales Médico-Psychologiques*, *4*, 168–174.

Debruyne, H., Portzky, M., Peremans, K., & Audenaert, K. (2011). Cotard's syndrome. *Mind & Brain*, *2*(1), 67–72.

Debruyne, H., Portzky, M., Van den Eynde, F., & Audenaert, K. (2009). Cotard's syndrome: A review. *Current Psychiatry Reports*, *11*(3), 197–202. https://doi.org/ccrvbn

Enoch, D., & Ball, H. (2001). *Uncommon psychiatric syndromes* (4th ed.). Arnold.

Grover, S., Aneja, J., Mahajan, S., & Varma, S. (2014). Cotard's syndrome: Two case reports and a brief review of literature. *Journal of Neurosciences in Rural Practice*, *5*(5), S59–S62. https://doi.org/gtm8

Kudlur, S. N. C., George, S., & Jaimon, M. (2007). An overview of the neurological correlates of Cotard syndrome. *The European Journal of Psychiatry*, *21*(2), 99–116.

Ramachandran, V. S. (2011). *The tell-tale brain: A neuroscientist's quest for what makes us human.* WW Norton & Company.

Ramachandran, V. S., & Blakeslee, S. (1998). *Phantoms in the brain: Probing the mysteries of the human mind.* William Morrow.

Ramirez-Bermudez, J., Aguilar-Venegas, L. C., Crail-Melendez, D., Espinola-Nadurille, M., Nente, F., & Mendez, M. F. (2010). Cotard syndrome in neurological and psychiatric patients. *Journal of Neuropsychiatry and Clinical Neurosciences*, *22*(4), 409–416. https://doi.org/ggwh2s

Sahoo, A., & Josephs, K. A. (2017). A neuropsychiatric analysis of the cotard delusion. *The Journal of Neuropsychiatry and Clinical Neurosciences*, *30*(1), 58–65. https://doi.org/gtm9

Schwartz, M. (Writer), & Koch, C. (Director). (2005, January 25). My lucky charm (Season 4, Episode 14) [TV series episode]. In Lawrence, B. (Creator), *Scrubs.* Doozer Productions.

Silva, J. A., Leong, G. B., Weinstock, R., & Gonzales, C. L. (2000). A case of Cotard's syndrome associated with self-starvation. *Journal of Forensic Science*, *45*(1), 188–190. https://doi.org/gtnb

Teixeira, B., Araújo, A. F., & Perestrelo, J. (2015). Cotard's syndrome: Two cases of self-starvation. *Psilogos*, *13*(1), 124–132. https://doi.org/gtnc

Wright, S., Young, A. W., & Hellawell, D. J. (1993). Sequential cotard and capgras delusions. *British Journal of Clinical Psychology*, *32*(3), 345–349. https://doi.org/dvw8p9

Young, A. W. (1999). Delusions. *The Monist*, *82*(4), 571–589. https://doi.org/fz8qgm

Young A. W., & Leafhead K. M. (1996). Betwixt life and death: Case studies of the cotard delusion. In P. W. Halligan & J. C. Marshall (Eds.), *Method in madness: Case studies in cognitive neuropsychiatry* (pp. 147–171). Psychology Press.

Young, A. W., Robertson, I. H., Hellawell, D. J., De Pauw, K. W., & Pentland, B. (1992). Cotard delusion after brain injury. *Psychological Medicine, 22*(3), 799–804. https://doi .org/fkvr4r

Creutzfeldt-Jakob Disease (and Other Prion Diseases)

Imagine that you are slowly losing control of your mind and body because a 100% fatal infectious agent is marching through your brain. Your memory begins to fail, as does your very ability to think. Your muscles begin to twitch involuntarily, and you experience a loss of balance so severe that you can no longer walk. Perhaps you lose your speech, or your vision, or elements of your personality. What kind of monstrous disease is eating its way through you?

The Stories

(STORY 1) A 50-year-old man showed progressive memory loss over the course of six months leading up to his admission to a hospital. Recalling events and recognizing family members became difficult for him, and he began to lose the ability to concentrate. He had once been great with numbers, but his mathematical skills began to vanish. Over time, he began to have dizziness and jerking movements that made him unable to walk. His doctors noted a loss of appetite, loss of sleep, and how easily he became fatigued. Things worsened as he became bedridden, mute, and developed seizures. The case study about him described him as "an ill-looking gentleman lying in bed, awake but mute, and unaware of his surroundings" (p. 295). He eventually died, after about six months of symptoms. He had no known family history of such a disease, or any previous surgical interventions that could have caused it, and so he was diagnosed with *sporadic* Creutzfeldt-Jakob disease, or sCJD, meaning that there was no known cause (Haider et al., 2013).

(STORY 2) A 36-year-old man was admitted to the hospital in 2015 with a personality change. He had become easy to anger over the course of the previous nine months. He also showed signs of increasing problems with his memory, with his events from the previous day becoming more and more difficult to recall. He showed abnormalities in his eye movements and an unusual stance when balancing and walking, both of which suggested that his brain was degenerating. He died around six months after arriving at the hospital, and the cause of death was ruled to be *variant* Creutzfeldt-Jakob disease (vCJD), also known as the human version of *mad cow disease*. This patient was especially notable because his genetics were different from most other known cases of

DOI: 10.4324/9781003276937-23

vCJD, suggesting that, sometimes, eating prion-contaminated beef can lead to this deadly disease *decades* after consumption (Mok et al., 2017).

(STORY 3) Two patients developed *iatrogenic* Creutzfeldt-Jakob disease in 1976 because their physician reused silver brain electrodes that had been previously used during a brain operation on a person with Creutzfeldt-Jakob disease (CJD). Months had elapsed between the prior use of the electrodes in the CJD patient, and the electrodes had been sterilized in alcohol and formaldehyde, but this was not enough to kill the infectious prions. One of the newly infected patients was a woman who had become pregnant by the time her CJD appeared around a year after the electrode-related surgery. The surgery had helped her epilepsy, but the trade-off was rapidly worsening neurological problems including fading memory, trouble speaking, and trouble walking. The resulting brain damage from the CJD caused her to become comatose after her child was born via C-section (Bernoulli et al., 1977, case 1; Bernoulli, 1977; Rhodes, 1998, p. 138). Other iatrogenic cases of CJD stemmed from corneal transplantation (the outer layer of the eyeball) and from the injection of human growth hormone harvested from human cadavers (Rhodes, 1998, pp. 131–133 and 144–150). Since then, many more precautions have been put in place in order to avoid transmitting CJD between people.

The Features

Many human diseases and the resulting disorders are caused by "living" things like viruses, bacteria, or parasites—although the extent to which those things are alive is arguable. In contrast, many other disorders are caused by nonliving things such as poisons, or by the absence of some type of nonliving molecule from your body, like vitamins or proteins. But there's a middle ground in a category of diseases called *prion diseases*, where the disease agent is nonliving but it makes copies of itself as if it were alive.

Prion diseases cause a person's brain to slowly decay, and like other neurodegenerative diseases such as Alzheimer disease, the person gradually acts less and less like themselves. Prion diseases are caused by *misfolded proteins*—which are called prions because one guy thought that name sounded cool (Max, 2006, p. 121). Prions are not alive, they are just molecules that are bent out of shape. Despite this, they make copies of themselves just like a living thing would do. This has been compared to the way that crystals grow bigger by replicating a chemical structure (Scheckel & Aguzzi, 2018). This self-copying damages your brain as the prions accumulate.

Prion diseases are arguably the most terrifying type of brain diseases, and their formal name somehow makes them sound even scarier: *transmissible spongiform encephalopathies*. They are called transmissible because they can spread from person to person, and spongiform because they eat holes in your brain leaving behind a porous spongy consistency. If that isn't scary enough, prions are almost impossible to destroy. According to some early research on prions summarized by author Rhodes they can survive with their infectivity intact even after "thirty minutes of boiling … two months of freezing … disinfection with strong formaldehyde, carbolic acid and chloroform … [the infectious prions] 'remained viable in dried brain for at least two years, and resisted a considerable dose of ultraviolet light'" (Rhodes, 1998, p. 120). As of this writing, all prion diseases are incurable and fatal (Scheckel & Aguzzi, 2018).

This chapter focuses on prion diseases as a whole, with three exceptions that have their own chapters because of unique symptoms and stories (see Chronic Traumatic Encephalopathy; see Fatal Familial Insomnia; see Kuru). Creutzfeldt-Jakob disease is the title of this chapter because it is the most common human prion disease—but it is by no means the only one.

Creutzfeldt-Jakob (pronounced croyts'felt-yak'ob) disease, more succinctly known as CJD, was named after two people who separately worked with severely ill neurological patients. Creutzfeldt published his paper about a "peculiar" illness first, and Jakob later published several case studies of similar "peculiar" illnesses. In a twist, it was later discovered that Creutzfeldt's patient never had the disease that was later named after him—and of the five cases that Jakob reported between 1921 and 1923, only two had CJD. Some suggest a name change to Jakob-Creutzfeldt disease to more accurately reflect the researchers' contributions (Katcher, 1998). I will call it CJD because that's what pretty much everyone calls it despite the noted absurdity of the origin of the name.

What is particularly interesting about CJD and other prion diseases is that there are subtypes that a person can acquire in different ways. Prion diseases can be acquired from the environment if exposed to infectious prions, such as through ingesting brain tissue. This is *one* reason that you shouldn't eat human brains (see Kuru). Elsewise, they can appear spontaneously due to an unexpected mutation from a protein into a prion. Or, they can be obtained genetically because the body's ability to produce prions, and susceptibility to them, is passed down through family bloodlines. Respectively, these routes of getting the disease are called *acquired*, *sporadic*, and *familial*. The term *iatrogenic* is also used to describe CJD in a few cases. These people acquired the disease via medical treatment, such as by infected medical instruments, implants, transplants, or transfusions. In other words, prion diseases can hitch a ride in hospitals through infected metal, tissue, blood, etc. Are you alarmed yet?

The symptoms of CJD are irreversibly progressive, meaning that they start out small and then continue to get worse and worse until the patient dies. The symptoms typically include problems with memory and thinking, jerking contractions of muscles, difficulties with walking, and difficulties with talking. Typically, a person with CJD will live for less than a year after the onset of the symptoms, but there are some who last longer than that (Brown et al., 1986). To illustrate the symptoms for you, I have translated a portion of a case from Jakob's 1921 case series. This patient suffered a steep decline:

> letters he wrote to his wife had perfect writing … by August his writing had deteriorated … his tongue trembles … language is blurred … walking

is only possible with good support … he occasionally complains of severe pain … he is constantly anxious, confused … the patient deteriorated physically and mentally very quickly and died.

(Jakob, 1921, case 3, pp. 186–188, translated here)

In many cases, the patient declines into a semiconscious, unmoving, and unspeaking state (see Akinetic Mutism) after a few months of having the disease (Iwasaki, 2017).

There's also a type of CJD that comes from an entirely different source but causes similar symptoms, which is aptly named *variant* Creutzfeldt-Jakob disease (vCJD). vCJD is transmitted to humans through the consumption of products contaminated with *bovine spongiform encephalopathy*, which mostly includes beef products such as hamburgers. The disease is better known as *mad cow disease*. This makes vCJD a *zoonotic* disease, meaning that it can jump the species barrier to infect a different animal's brain (Comoy et al., 2015). The resulting disease does not occur immediately. Instead, the person develops vCJD years after they were exposed to the infectious prion. The amount of time that it takes to develop vCJD after being infected depends upon the person's genetics (Scheckel & Aguzzi, 2018).

When mad cow disease was first discovered, there was mass panic, and with good reason. vCJD is different from classic CJD in a few ways. It can strike younger people, the disease advances more slowly, and psychiatric disturbances are more likely (Corato et al., 2006). The psychiatric disturbances may include anxiety, aggression, insomnia, and, less commonly, hallucinations and paranoid delusions (Spencer et al., 2002). In sum, there could be a hidden disease in your food that takes years to appear, is always fatal but kills you slowly, can strike people of any age, and literally causes holes to form in your brain. And that's just one prion disease. Fortunately, food safety and prion awareness have both progressed immensely since the discovery of vCJD, and so it is very difficult to acquire this disease today. By the way, the names of prion diseases actually only get more difficult to remember from here.

Gerstmann-Sträussler-Scheinker disease (GSS) is named after researchers who studied the at-the-time unknown disease in an Austrian family (Ghetti et al., 2018). Like fatal familial insomnia (see Fatal Familial Insomnia), GSS mostly seems to run in family bloodlines, making it a familial prion disease.

Like other prion diseases, GSS is technically transmissible, but in order for someone to catch the disease, they need to somehow end up with the GSS prions in their brain. The most straightforward way of doing this is via an *injection into the brain*, which is unlikely to happen by accident. Brain injections are how scientists were able to show that other mammals can get sick from prions (Collins et al., 2001). If you want to know what some of the saddest animal research of all time was, the early studies of prion diseases involved injecting animals' brains with prions and then watching them slowly get sicker and dying over time, usually several years.

Variably protease-sensitive prionopathy (VPSPr) is another prion disease that was recently discovered (Gambetti et al., 2008). It wasn't until 2010 that it was conclusively shown to be a group of similar-but-slightly different versions of the same prion, each with differences in their sensitivity to being digested, leading to the word "variably" being used in their description (Zou et al., 2010). It has been suggested that VPSPr closely resembles GSS in some respects, and may be a sporadic variant of that generally familial prion disease (Nonno et al., 2019). In other words, anyone can get it if they are really unlucky.

The animal kingdom also has its own peculiar strains of prion diseases. The most famous of which besides mad cow disease may be *scrapie*, a prion disease found in sheep (Rhodes, 1998). Prion diseases also exist in other animals, including mink, elk, deer, cats, exotic ungulates such as kudu, and nonhuman primates (Imran & Mahmood, 2011). My point is, there are plenty of prions to go around. But how do they actually *work*?

The Brain Pathology

Prions cause damage as they tangle together and form plaques in the brain. Why do prions damage the brain, but the proteins that they are formed from don't? The protein that the prions discussed in this chapter form out of is a 253-amino-acid chain called *PrP* that serves a purpose in the cell membranes of human cells (Scheckel & Aguzzi, 2018). Usually, when those proteins are done serving their purpose, they dissolve. Prions are just PrP but twisted into a slightly different shape, often called "misfolded" because the chain of amino acids looks like it has a different fold in it (Ma & Wang, 2014). This changed shape makes them resistant to dissolving, a trait called "protease-resistant" (Scheckel & Aguzzi, 2018). Therefore, the reason that prions build up and form dangerous plaques in the brain is because they can't be dissolved and cleared away, eventually suffocating and killing brain cells (Rhodes, 1998, p. 197). That's why the spongiform holes appear in the brains of people with prion diseases, because the dead cells leave behind holes.

It is worth noting that there is still disagreement over whether the infectious agent that causes CJD and other prion diseases consists solely of a prion, or if there are other necessary components such as a virus (Botsios & Manuelidis, 2016) or lipids (Ma & Wang, 2014). In other words, prions may not be responsible for creating the diseases entirely by themselves.

Depending on the specific prion disease, there are some differences in *where* in the brain the damage is done and what the pattern of damage looks like. For example, vCJD produces unique-looking buildups of plaques in the brain, called florid plaques because they look like "chrysanthemum blooms," which distinguish that disorder from CJD where the plaques look different and are smaller (Rhodes, 1998, p. 208–209). Meanwhile, the buildup of prions inside of the brain and the damage to the brain that happens in GSS greatly resembles diseases such as Parkinson disease and Alzheimer disease (Cracco et al., 2019). Some researchers insist that common neurodegenerative diseases are also prion diseases, including CTE (see Chronic Traumatic Encephalopathy), Parkinson disease, and Alzheimer disease, but the similarities are still under investigation (Carlson & Prusiner, 2021).

It is difficult, but not impossible, to detect and diagnose prion disorders without extremely invasive brain biopsies in which a small chunk of brain tissue is examined for protease-resistant deposits—and in many cases, it is not diagnosed until the person has died and an autopsy is performed (Scheckel & Aguzzi, 2018). There is hope for the development of less invasive or deadly diagnostic procedures, however. The brainwaves of most people with CJD show what are called *periodic sharp wave complexes* which are a unique combination of brainwaves that emerge due to the deteriorating brain, and this may be useful in diagnosing the disease (e.g., Haider et al., 2013; Iwasaki, 2017). Unfortunately, even if detected early, these horrifying diseases remain fatal and transmissible, and are nightmare fuel for both patients and healthcare workers. If you're flipping through this book trying to decide which of these brain disorders you'd like to take a crack at curing someday, CJD and its ilk would be an excellent pick—the human and animal world alike would owe you an immense debt of gratitude.

References

Bernoulli, C. (1977). Danger of accidental person-to-person transmission of Creutzfeldt-Jakob disease by surgery. *Lancet*, *309*(8012), 659. https://doi.org/djb2dq

Bernoulli, C., Siegfried, J., Baumgartner, G., Regli, F., Rabinowicz, T., Gajdusek, D. C., & Gibbs Jr., C. J. (1977). Danger of accidental person-to-person transmission of Creutzfeldt-Jakob disease by surgery. *Lancet*, *309*(8009), 478–479. https://doi.org/bqgxbx

Botsios, S., & Manuelidis, L. (2016). CJD and scrapie require agent-associated nucleic acids for infection. *Journal of Cellular Biochemistry*, *117*(8), 1947–1958. https://doi.org/f8trjz

Brown, P., Cathala, F., Castaigne, P., & Gajdusek, D. C. (1986). Creutzfeldt-Jakob disease: clinical analysis of a consecutive series of 230 neuropathologically verified cases. *Annals of Neurology*, *20*(5), 597–602. https://doi.org/frqzgh

Carlson, G. A., & Prusiner, S. B. (2021). How an infection of sheep revealed prion mechanisms in Alzheimer's disease and other neurodegenerative disorders. *International Journal of Molecular Sciences*, *22*(9), Article 4861. https://doi.org/gkmwsh

Collins, S., McLean, C. A., & Masters, C. L. (2001). Gerstmann-Sträussler-Scheinker syndrome, fatal familial insomnia, and kuru: A review of these less common human transmissible spongiform encephalopathies. *Journal of Clinical Neuroscience*, *8*(5), 387–397. https://doi.org/cqdvtm

Comoy, E. E., Mikol, J., Luccantoni-Freire, S., Correia, E., Lescoutra-Etchegaray, N., Durand, V., Dehen, C., Andreoletti, O., Casalone, C., Richt, J. A., Greenlee, J. J., Baron, T., Benestad, S. L., Brown, P., & Deslys, J.-P. (2015). Transmission of scrapie prions to primate after an extended silent incubation period. *Scientific Reports*, *5*, Article 11573. https://doi.org/f7t2bk

Corato, M., Cereda, C., Cova, E., Ferrarese, C., & Ceroni, M. (2006). Young-onset CJD: Age and disease phenotype in variant and sporadic forms. *Functional Neurology*, *21*(4), 211–215.

Cracco, L., Xiao, X., Nemani, S. K., Lavrich, J., Cali, I., Ghetti, B., Notari, S., Surewicz, W. K., & Gambetti, P. (2019). Gerstmann-Sträussler-Scheinker disease revisited: Accumulation of covalently-linked multimers of internal prion protein fragments. *Acta Neuropathologica Communications, 7*(85), 1–9. https://doi.org/gtnf

Gambetti, P., Dong, Z., Yuan, J., Xiao, X., Zheng, M., Alshekhlee, A., Castellani, R., Cohen, M., Barria, M. A., Gonzalez-Romero, D., Belay, E. D., Schonberger, L. B., Marder, K., Harris, C., Burke, J. R., Montine, T., Wisniewski, T., Dickson, D. W., Soto, C., Hulette, C. M., … & Zou, W.-Q. (2008). A novel human disease with abnormal prion protein sensitive to protease. *Annals of Neurology, 63*(6), 697–708. https://doi.org/b8zd88

Ghetti, B., Piccardo, P., & Zanusso, G. (2018). Dominantly inherited prion protein cerebral amyloidoses–a modern view of Gerstmann–Sträussler–Scheinker. In M. Pocchiari & J. Manson (Eds.), *Handbook of clinical neurology: Human prion diseases* (vol. 153, pp. 243–269). Elsevier. https://doi.org/gtng

Haider, E., Wali, W., Raja, S., & Tariq, M. (2013). Creutzfeldt Jakob disease. *Journal of the College of Physicians and Surgeons Pakistan, 23*, 295–297.

Imran, M., & Mahmood, S. (2011). An overview of animal prion diseases. *Virology Journal, 8*(493). https://doi.org/bz8vcg

Iwasaki, Y. (2017). Creutzfeldt-Jakob disease. *Neuropathology, 37*(2), 174–188. https://doi.org/gmf6w3

Jakob, A. (1921). Über eigenartige Erkrankungen des Zentralnervensystems mit bemerkenswertem anatomischen Befunde. *Zeitschrift Für Die Gesamte Neurologie Und Psychiatrie, 64*, 147–228.

Katcher, F. (1998). It's Jakob's disease, not Creutzfeldt's. *Nature, 393*, 11. https://doi.org/ch424k

Ma, J., & Wang, F. (2014). Prion disease and the 'protein-only hypothesis.' *Essays in Biochemistry, 56*, 181–191. https://doi.org/f6r698

Max, D. T. (2006). *The family that couldn't sleep: A medical mystery.* Random House.

Mok, T., Jaunmuktane, Z., Joiner, S., Campbell, T., Morgan, C., Wakerley, B., Golestani, F., Rudge, P., Mead, S., Jäger, H., Wadsworth, J. D., Brandner, S., & Collinge, J. (2017). Variant Creutzfeldt–Jakob disease in a patient with heterozygosity at PRNP codon 129. *New England Journal of Medicine, 376*(3), 292–294. https://doi.org/bxk3

Nonno, R., Notari, S., Di Bari, M. A., Cali, I., Pirisinu, L., d'Agostino, C., Cracco, L., Kofskey, D., Vanni, I., Lavrich, J., Parchi, P., Agrimi, U., & Gambetti, P. (2019). Variable protease-sensitive prionopathy transmission to bank voles. *Emerging Infectious Diseases, 25*(1), 73–81. https://doi.org/gtnh

Rhodes, R. (1998). *Deadly feasts: Tracking the secrets of a terrifying new plague.* Simon and Schuster.

Scheckel, C., & Aguzzi, A. (2018). Prions, prionoids and protein misfolding disorders. *Nature Reviews Genetics, 19*(7), 405–418. https://doi.org/gdrp6w

Spencer, M. D., Knight, R. S., & Will, R. G. (2002). First hundred cases of variant Creutzfeldt-Jakob disease: Retrospective case note review of early psychiatric and neurological features. *British Medical Journal, 324*(7352), 1479–1482. https://doi.org/dp73kt

Zou, W. Q., Puoti, G., Xiao, X., Yuan, J., Qing, L., Cali, I., Shimoji, M., Langeveld, J. P. M., Castellani, R., Notari, S., Crain, B., Schmidt, R. E., Geschwind, M., DeArmond, S. J., Cairns, N. J., Dickson, D., Honig, L., Torres, J. M., Mastrianni, J., … & Gambetti, P. (2010). Variably protease-sensitive prionopathy: A new sporadic disease of the prion protein. *Annals of Neurology, 68*(2), 162–172. https://doi.org/dvfgns

Diminished Decision–Making Capacity

Imagine that you can't make decisions. Even if you carefully consider the options and consequences of a choice, you simply can't bring yourself to choose. Pretend that you are attempting to pick a movie to see at the local cinema. You could see an action movie, or a scary movie, or perhaps a romantic comedy. You know that you have preferences for types of movies, and you know that because you came all this way to the movie theater, you should probably see a movie or else it would be a waste of a trip. Despite this, you cannot make a decision. Instead, you ask the movie attendant which movie you should see. "I don't know," they say, "they're all good, why don't you pick?" How can you explain that you can't?

The Stories

(STORY 1) A man with a "cerebral defect" involving both frontal lobes was the subject of an extensive case study (p. 479). He had either been born with brain damage or it came to him in early childhood. Psychologists studied him for decades, taking note of his behavioral differences. While the authors do not specifically note decision-making impairments in the case history, they do describe many instances of what I would call *inhibition inhibition*. For example, he stole the cars of his relatives and neighbors on multiple occasions to go on poorly planned cross-country road trips. He also had a habit—beginning when he was less than 3 years old—of wandering off without any fear of becoming lost. As a child, he walked for blocks beyond a mile, and as an adult would wander for *thousands* of miles. He ascribed his wandering behavior to "impulse" (p. 485). When he was young he was unable to make friends, had anger problems, and was caught stealing and participating in other reckless activities. As he grew up, he showed poor planning abilities for the future, was unable to keep jobs, and spent money compulsively. When discussing right and wrong actions with a counselor, he could identify behaviors that a person *ought* to do in particular situations—but when it came time for him to make decisions in his own life, he consistently made impulsive choices that led to disaster (Ackerly & Benton, 1948).

DOI: 10.4324/9781003276937-24

(STORY 2) After a severe concussion, a professor wrote a book about the aftermath of the brain damage and his road to recovery. Among his many symptoms was an interesting case of what I refer to as *acquired decision paralysis*. He wrote in his book, *The Ghost in My Brain*, that "it is the troubling loss of the *innate ability* to pull the trigger on a decision" (p. 64). He vividly described one situation where he could not seem to make a decision about what to eat even though he was very hungry. He was feeling mentally drained, and when it came time to decide what to eat, he found himself staring at two options laid out on his cutting board: an apple and a salami. He simply had to decide which to prepare so that he could eat. But he found himself utterly paralyzed, and unable to decide. He eventually gave up, and tried again later. When he returned to the cutting board, now even hungrier, he was still unable to decide. After his "forced fasting" had lasted two days, he called his friend to ask for help, at which point his friend gave him instructions on what to eat (p. 66). He was able to follow that plan easily in order to eat, demonstrating the contrast between the difficulty of generating decisions in his own brain versus easily following commands coming from outside of his own brain (Elliott, 2016, pp. 64–66).

(STORY 3) At the age of 35, a man experienced vision problems and changes to his personality, leading to the revelation that he had a tumor pressing on the frontal lobes of his brain. Following the removal of the tumor, many pronounced behavioral symptoms appeared, including diminished decision-making capacity. He suffered severe *acquired decision paralysis* when deciding which restaurant to visit, such that "deciding where to dine might take hours, as he discussed each restaurant's seating plan, particulars of menu, atmosphere, and management" (p. 1732). He would even "drive to each restaurant to see how busy it was" but still could not choose (p. 1732). Similarly, shopping decisions took a long time because he would consider all of the information that he had access to, such as price, brand, and purchase method, even for small items. He also seemed to experience *inhibition inhibition*. He went bankrupt after he invested his life savings in a business partnership that his friends and family had warned him against. Due to regularly arriving late to work as well as disorganization, he was fired from several jobs. For similar reasons, he was divorced by his wife. He then remarried against the advice of his relatives, and was divorced again. During clinical tests, he could logically reason through questions about morality and social problems. This showed that he still had the *knowledge* required for typical decision-making behaviors. However, when actually making similar decisions in real life, he took poor actions, "often with disastrous consequences" (Eslinger & Damasio, 1985, p. 1737).

The Features

The frontal lobe of the brain, located behind your forehead, is arguably the most human part of your body. Not only does it contribute to consciousness, but it also plays a major role in *executive functions*. Executive functions are processes that your brain does that assist you in controlling your own behavior, such as planning ahead and switching between tasks. There are general terms that apply to many kinds of damage to these executive functions, such as *dysexecutive syndrome* or *frontal lobe syndrome*, but those terms are not very useful for describing a person's specific problems, because the frontal lobe contributes to many different behaviors (Schneider & Koenigs, 2017). So, let's look a little closer.

It is debated what the different executive functions have in common with one another, but they often have to do with the *inhibition* of behavior and *reasoning* abilities (Ardila, 2013). Inhibition simply means preventing yourself from doing something, like stopping yourself from drinking an alcoholic beverage even if part of your brain wants to drink it. Reasoning is a bit more difficult to define, but it is essentially following a series of mental steps to a logical conclusion. An example of this is determining that bear tracks in the mud mean that a bear has been in the area recently, and because bears are dangerous, you should leave the area. Damage to the executive functions of the brain may therefore result in disorders where a person has trouble with inhibiting behaviors and completing logical reasoning—which are both important for *decision-making* (Wood & Worthington, 2017). Other types of frontal lobe damage may result in symptoms that are subtle or difficult to describe, but problems with decision-making tend to be noticeably impactful on a person's life, which is why decision-making has a chapter in this book.

People with diminished decision-making capacity seem to be unusually insensitive to future consequences. In other words, they may be guided only by what is currently happening as opposed to the positive or negative events that may occur in the future because of the decision (Bechara et al., 1998). They often fail to learn from repeated mistakes and do not correctly anticipate the outcomes of their actions (Wood & Worthington, 2017).

However, there is more than one way in which decision-making can break down. For example, a person may find themselves repeatedly making *poor* decisions, or they may find themselves unable to efficiently *make* decisions. Decision-making capacity as it refers to making poor decisions is connected to a person's ability to *prevent* impulsive behaviors. I will call this *inhibition inhibition*. In contrast, inefficient decision-making is connected moreso to the brain's ability to *compare* choices. I will call this *acquired decision paralysis*. Neither of those terms is commonly used in the literature, but they are useful for illustration.

Inhibition inhibition reduces a person's ability to say no to the impulsive thoughts that pop into their head—you know, the things that you *think* but decide not to *do* because they are bad ideas? Imagine unleashing those because you are unable to stop them. Inhibition inhibition occurs in different forms, ranging from an increase in making poor choices such as gambling or using drugs dangerously, to a person becoming more easily persuaded to carry out dangerous behaviors.

Acquired decision paralysis can be a more visible symptom than inhibition inhibition. Being unable to complete decisions, even trivial ones, or taking much longer than expected to carry out decisions, is a noticeable symptom. Inhibition inhibition and acquired decision paralysis may sound like opposites—the former may lead a person to take *more* actions wherein the latter may lead them to take *fewer* actions—but they are both coping strategies for brain damage to the parts of the brain that typically evaluate and make decisions.

The Brain Pathology

The brain location in question for diminished decision-making capacity is often the ventromedial prefrontal cortex (vmPFC) which is located near the front of your skull (Schneider & Koenigs, 2017). The vmPFC isn't really one specific place in the brain, but more of a highly complex and interconnected brain region that is involved in a lot of different brain disorders (Hiser & Koenigs, 2018). This complexity is an important point. When comparing the symptoms of people with damage in this region to people with brain damage located somewhere other than prefrontal regions, the people with the vmPFC damage showed more "blunted emotional experience, apathy, low emotional expressiveness, inappropriate affect, poor frustration tolerance, irritability, lability, indecisiveness, poor judgment, social inappropriateness, lack of planning, lack of initiation and persistence, and lack of insight" (Barrash et al., 2000, p. 355). Each symptom from this wide variety may be involved in diminished decision-making capacity. Evidence from a variety of studies suggests that people with damage to the vmPFC have trouble "both generating feasible options and choosing the best decision" (Schneider & Koenigs, 2017, p. 86). This may appear as symptoms of inhibition inhibition, acquired decision paralysis, or both.

In terms of inhibition inhibition, people with vmPFC damage may gamble more, and some people with drug addictions have been shown to also have vmPFC abnormalities (Bechara, 2005). People with vmPFC damage seem more likely to make decisions that are "against their best interests" and lead to several kinds of losses: financially, in general social standing, and in terms of the support of family and friends (Bechara & Van der Linden, 2005, p. 735). In some cases, those impulsive behaviors such as gambling and dangerous drug use may not seem like symptoms of brain damage unless you compare the person's current behavior to their past behavior. That is, brain damage to a person's ability to inhibit behavior may appear to be a change in *personality*.

One theory as to how acquired decision paralysis arises is that the brain has difficulty *making mental comparisons* due to damage to the brain's working memory, attentional, and task-switching processes. To compare two options, a brain must hold both options in memory, gather information about those options using the ability to pay attention, and switch between paying attention to those different options. But if one or more of those processes is interrupted, as they may be in acquired decision paralysis, then seemingly simple decisions can become unsolvable burdens.

For example, vmPFC damage may cause a person to lose the ability to represent the *value* of things, to lose the ability to generate alternative options, and/or to lose the ability to choose which option is the best one (Schneider & Koenigs, 2017). Those value-related abilities are not entirely located in the vmPFC, but the frontal lobe is an important component, as indicated by studies in rats and monkeys which featured damaging selective parts of the animals' brains to see how it impacted the way that the animals made value-based decisions about food (Hiser & Koenigs, 2018). As a result of being unable to correctly represent value, people with acquired decision paralysis may spend more time considering the aspects of one potential decision than they do in comparing the decisions (Fellows, 2006). Thus, the person may get stuck considering and reconsidering options, spending more time thinking over the task instead of making the decision.

Interestingly, because the prefrontal cortex develops until a person is in their twenties, we can consider teenagers to have a form of inhibition inhibition. Not due to brain damage, but due to incomplete development. The average teenager brain is different from the brains of younger children and the brains of adults (Luna et al., 2010). Brain scans that reveal the communication abilities of the prefrontal cortex show that adolescents are poorer than adults at integrating information, which leads to worse impulse control, planning, and decision-making (Davis, 2017). This may explain the riskier behaviors of children when compared to adults: their brains haven't finished developing decision-making capacity (Levin et al., 2007). Of course, adults wrote those studies, so maybe they're just being buzzkills that hate dangerous fun. Another important piece of the puzzle is that cognitive control in adolescent brains is more sensitive to emotions—and if your decision-making is overly controlled by emotions, you might make worse decisions (Cohen et al., 2016). Perhaps this helps to explain the questionable dating decisions that some of us make as teenagers.

Decision-making capacity is important for determining whether a person can safely control their medical decisions. Due to this, there are tests for determining decision-making capacity (Dunn et al., 2006). However, those types of tests do not always detect the sort of decision-making impairments that people with vmPFC damage have (Schneider & Koenigs, 2017). Plus, mild impairments are notoriously difficult to detect. A study that carefully looked at decision-making in people receiving medical care found much cognitive impairment including low scores on decision-making tests (Burton et al., 2012). Elderly people may show good intelligence and memory but have poor decision-making due to subtle changes in the brain's cognitive functions (Bechara & Van der Linden, 2005). The real-world implication here is that decisions made by sick or dying people, including important end-of-life arrangements, may be more impacted by diminished decision-making capacity than is realized.

References

Ackerly, S. S., & Benton, A. L. (1948). Report of case of bilateral frontal lobe defect. *Research Publications-Association for Research in Nervous and Mental Disease, 27*, 479–504.

Ardila, A. (2013). There are two different dysexecutive syndromes. *Journal of Neurological Disorders, 1*(1), 1–4. https://doi.org/gtrw

Barrash, J., Tranel, D., & Anderson, S. W. (2000). Acquired personality disturbances associated with bilateral damage to the ventromedial prefrontal region. *Developmental Neuropsychology, 18*(3), 355–381. https://doi.org/dxj6wn

Bechara, A. (2005). Decision making, impulse control and loss of willpower to resist drugs: A neurocognitive perspective. *Nature Neuroscience, 8*(11), 1458–1463. https://doi.org/b5qmjh

Bechara, A., Damasio, H., Tranel, D., & Anderson, S. W. (1998). Dissociation of working memory from decision making within the human prefrontal cortex. *Journal of Neuroscience, 18*(1), 428–437. https://doi.org/gtrx

Bechara, A., & Van der Linden, M. (2005). Decision-making and impulse control after frontal lobe injuries. *Current Opinion in Neurology, 18*(6), 734–739. https://doi.org/b3b5jm

Burton, C. Z., Twamley, E. W., Lee, L. C., Palmer, B. W., Jeste, D. V., Dunn, L. B., & Irwin, S. A. (2012). Undetected cognitive impairment and decision-making capacity in patients receiving hospice care. *The American Journal of Geriatric Psychiatry, 20*(4), 306–316. https://doi.org/gtrz

Cohen, A. O., Breiner, K., Steinberg, L., Bonnie, R. J., Scott, E. S., Taylor-Thompson, K. A., Rudolf, M. D., Chein, J., Richeson, J. A., Heller, A. S., Silverman, M. R., Dellarco, D. V., Fair, D. A., Galván, A. & Casey, B. J. (2016). When is an adolescent an adult? Assessing cognitive control in emotional and nonemotional contexts. *Psychological Science, 27*(4), 549–562. https://doi.org/d5gc

Davis, K. A. (2017). *The brain defense: Murder in Manhattan and the dawn of neuroscience in America's courtrooms*. Penguin.

Dunn, L. B., Nowrangi, M. A., Palmer, B. W., Jeste, D. V., & Saks, E. R. (2006). Assessing decisional capacity for clinical research or treatment: A review of instruments. *American Journal of Psychiatry, 163*(8), 1323–1334. https://doi.org/cpw9

Elliott, C. (2016). *The ghost in my brain: How a concussion stole my life and how the new science of brain plasticity helped me get it back*. Penguin.

Eslinger, P. J., & Damasio, A. R. (1985). Severe disturbance of higher cognition after bilateral frontal lobe ablation patient EVR. *Neurology, 35*(12), 1731–1741. https://doi.org/gg5vpr

Fellows, L. K. (2006). Deciding how to decide: Ventromedial frontal lobe damage affects information acquisition in multi-attribute decision making. *Brain, 129*(4), 944–952. https://doi.org/fk7bzd

Hiser, J., & Koenigs, M. (2018). The multifaceted role of the ventromedial prefrontal cortex in emotion, decision making, social cognition, and psychopathology. *Biological Psychiatry, 83*(8), 638–647. https://doi.org/gc9h6j

Levin, I., Weller, J., Pederson, A., & Harshman, L. (2007). Age-related differences in adaptive decision making: Sensitivity to expected value in risky choice. *Judgment and Decision Making, 2*(4), 225–233.

Luna, B., Padmanabhan, A., & O'Hearn, K. (2010). What has fMRI told us about the development of cognitive control through adolescence? *Brain and Cognition, 72*(1), 101–113. https://doi.org/b9psrx

Schneider, B., & Koenigs, M. (2017). Human lesion studies of ventromedial prefrontal cortex. *Neuropsychologia, 107,* 84–93. https://doi.org/gcs93m

Wood, R. L., & Worthington, A. (2017). Neurobehavioral abnormalities associated with executive dysfunction after traumatic brain injury. *Frontiers in Behavioral Neuroscience, 11,* Article 195. https://doi.org/gch6pg

Echophenomena and Coprophenomena

Imagine that you are saying things that you don't intend to say, and making movements that you don't intend to make. Perhaps you hear someone say something, and this sets off a reaction in your brain that causes you to say that same thing in response, like an echo. Perhaps you've just said something and now find yourself stuck in a loop, saying the same thing over and over again. The same types of things can happen with movements as well, where you can find yourself making inappropriate gestures or mimicking the movements of others when you don't want to do so. What has grabbed control of your voice and muscles?

The Stories

(STORY 1) In the case of an 11-year-old girl, both *echolalia* and *echopraxia* were displayed. She would echo words addressed to her as well as other words said by people in the room around her. The child mimicked both the "tones and inflections of the examiner's voice" automatically (p. 215). Some of the movements that she echoed included the medical examiner drawing shapes on paper, which the patient would try to imitate, although the result was often not identical to the original drawing. Besides her repetition of speaking and moving, no true responses could be elicited, such as original thoughts or opinions. The physician described her as lacking the ability to behave independently (Hollingworth, 1917, case II).

(STORY 2) A 15-year-old was described in a case report after he developed *coprolalia* and *copropraxia*. At first, his verbal tic took the form of shouting the first word or two of a sentence before returning to his normal speaking volume. He then began to occasionally "emit an explosive utterance" during conversations (p. 522). At first, these explosive utterances were formless and inarticulate, but eventually developed into coprolalia such that he was shouting obscenities and vulgarities "of a sexual nature" (p. 522). When confronted about this behavior by his parents, he said "I don't mean them towards you, it just flashes through my mind" (p. 522). Some echolalia was also noted such that he repeated things that he heard, and he also developed copropraxia in the form of spitting at inappropriate times (Mazur, 1953).

DOI: 10.4324/9781003276937-25

(STORY 3) A woman who had previously suffered from encephalitis lethargica began experiencing *palilalia* following her treatment with L-DOPA. She developed an uncontrollable tendency to repeat the things that she was saying. Her voice would rise from its normal soft and low-pitched state to one that was shrill and piercing as she shouted the same phrase over and over, such as "my arms, my arms, my arms, my arms, please move my arms, my arms, move my arms" (p. 52). During these attacks she felt "anguish and terror and shame" and tried to express that she was not controlling her voice during these attacks: "oh, oh, oh, oh … please don't … I'm not myself, not myself … It's not me, not me, not me at all" (Sacks, 1999, case FD, p. 52).

(STORY 4) A 12-year-old boy developed *coprolalia* and *echolalia* around 1886. He would yell obscenities during quiet moments, especially if surprised. He withdrew from his schooling because his coprolalia was disturbing to others, and he reportedly also disturbed his neighbors in the early mornings when the coprolalia was at its worst. In his echolalic moments, he would imitate the last parts of sentences that he heard, including the tone and accent of the person speaking. Being physically punished by his parents seemed to do little to diminish his outbursts. As part of his treatment, the physician prescribed arsenic, which would certainly not be prescribed for a case like this if it occurred today (Dana & Wilkin, 1886, case I).

The Features

Mimicking others can be useful. For example, imitating the things that other people say and do is a necessary part of learning as a child grows up. Especially when young humans and other animals mimic the actions of others that they are observing, and much of this imitation seems automatic (Ganos et al., 2012). Mimicry is useful not only for acquiring language, but also for skills that use particular muscle movements. However, those automatic mimicking behaviors can sometimes persist after childhood, or they may disappear but then re-emerge later in life. At that point, when the mimicry is no longer useful for learning, automatic mimicking behaviors may be considered symptoms of *echophenomena*.

The prefix "echo-" refers to *repetition*. Echophenomena are behaviors that a person does that are repetitions of other behaviors. The person's repetitions may be repeats of the actions of others or repeats of their own actions. Two commonly discussed "echo-" symptoms are *echolalia* and *echopraxia*.

The suffix "-lalia" refers to *speech*. Echolalia occurs when a person *involuntarily* repeats sounds, words, or entire phrases. The word involuntary is important here, because these are automatic responses, and not something that the person chooses to do. In many cases, the speech repetition is of things that they hear, such as words that the people around them say. Some people with echolalia repeat only sounds that are directed toward them, or only the words of certain people, but others with this symptom repeat anything that they hear around them (Schuler, 1979). Words may be more likely to be repeated if they draw the attention of the person in some way, such as if the words are unfamiliar (Mazur, 1953). Oftentimes, the person seems not to have understood the words that they are echoing, and some researchers have even suggested that "the language which is least understood is best echoed" (Brown, 1972, p. 75).

In contrast, sometimes the repetitions may be of the person's own speech. They may appear to get stuck repeating themselves over and over. This form of echophenomena has a special name of *palilalia* (Sacks, 1999). Echolalia and palilalia can occur together, such that a person first hears something from the environment around them, repeats it, and then hears themselves saying it, and then they repeat themselves (Linetsky et al., 2000).

The suffix "-praxia" refers to *action*. Echopraxia occurs when a person involuntarily mimics and repeats an action. If you want an example, try yawning while someone is looking at you—if they yawn back, you've got your example. Although the contagiousness of yawning is not acquired echopraxia because most people experience it. A better clinical example of echopraxia is contagiousness of other actions like waving your hand or touching your nose. A person may also repeat gestures that they themselves just made, which is called *palipraxia* (Kurvits et al., 2020).

There are other echophenomena as well, although less commonly described. Echomimia refers to mimicking facial expressions, echographia is the repetition of writing, and echoplasia refers to the copying of contours, such as by repeatedly tracing shapes (Ganos et al., 2012).

Related to echophenomena are *coprophenomena*. The prefix "copro-" refers to feces. Therefore, coprophenomena are vile or rude behaviors. When attached to the suffixes "-lalia" and "-praxia," we get terms for involuntarily using rude speech and using rude gestures.

Coprolalia is when a person says something rude without willing themselves to do so. The most common examples are curse words, often with sexual connotations. When a person with coprolalia speaks, they may involuntarily add obscenities into pauses between their sentences, sometimes in a louder voice than the voice otherwise used for the conversation (Lees et al., 1984). Mental coprolalia—thinking but not saying something obscene—may sometimes be more common than verbally expressing coprolalia (Enoch & Ball, 2001).

Copropraxia is the act of making vulgar gestures when not intending to do so. Which gestures this consists of varies by culture, depending on which gestures are rude and forbidden. Many of these rude gestures involve hand signs, but other vulgar displays such as hip thrusting at inappropriate times are also reported (Lees et al., 1984). Spitting at rude times is also a behavior associated with copropraxia (Mazur, 1953). Remember, these gestures are involuntary: these people may find themselves interrupting an otherwise pleasant conversation by showing off their middle fingers.

These various symptoms tend to be at least somewhat related to one another. For example, if someone has copropraxia, they probably also have coprolalia (Kurvits et al., 2020). What can account for this wide variety of echophenomena and coprophenomena?

The Brain Pathology

Echophenomena and coprophenomena can be thought of as *tics*, which are compulsive and difficult-to-control behaviors. Echophenomena and coprophenomena may occur in tic disorders, especially Tourette syndrome. The disorder got its name from the French researcher who described many symptoms of various echophenomena and coprophenomena in patients in the 1880s. For example, he laid out the symptoms of a 15-year-old boy with "convulsive movements of his head and waist. After all of these movements, he almost always screams *merde* (shit) … if one talks in front of him, the boy carefully repeats the two or three words that ended the sentence just said" (Gilles de la Tourette, 1884, translated in Lajonchere et al., 1996, p. 572).

People with Tourette syndrome often describe their tics as similar to the urge to sneeze, with the urge vanishing temporarily after completing the tic (Finkelstein, 2018). Even though coprophenomena, such as shouting swear words, are closely associated with Tourette syndrome, fewer than half of people with that disorder exhibit coprophenomena behaviors, and the symptoms may vary widely between two people (Freeman et al., 2009). Other than Tourette syndrome, echophenomena may occur with epilepsy (see Seizures), dementia, autoimmune disorders, aphasia (see Aphasia), and schizophrenia (Ganos et al., 2012). Similarly, coprophenomena may occur in epilepsy, dementia, and after strokes (Kobierska et al., 2014). But what is actually happening in the brain when a person experiences these symptoms?

The pathophysiology of tic disorders is extremely complex, and there isn't just one part of the brain that can be pointed to as the source of the symptoms. Instead, symptoms such as echophenomena and coprophenoma are related to "multiple brain areas and complex pathways" (Yael et al., 2015, p. 1171). More specifically, research has indicated the importance of cortico-striatal-thalamo-cortical circuits of brain cells, as well as other circuits such as frontoparietal connections, to the features of tic disorders (Naro et al., 2020). Essentially, the symptoms arise because of functional abnormalities in the ways that these various regions of the brain communicate with one another. However, this still isn't a very satisfying answer as to what is occurring in the brain that causes the symptoms.

At the risk of oversimplifying these complex brain communications, one explanation for the phenomena is that the person's brain is failing to stop itself from acting out impulsive actions. In Tourette syndrome research, this is known as the *disinhibition* hypothesis. It is based on the theory that the brain has "either insufficient inhibitory motor control … or imbalance in the selection and suppression of competing motor programs" (Hashemiyoon et al., 2017, p. 9). Essentially, this hypothesis puts the blame on the parts of the brain that are supposed to prevent unwanted behaviors (see Diminished Decision-Making Capacity). Those parts of the brain are located in the *frontal* areas, where processes of planning and decision-making take place. In theory, echophenomena and coprophenomena occur because the frontal areas of the brain are not strong enough to inhibit or suppress the tics that are being generated in the motor areas of the brain (Yael et al., 2015). Research has successfully identified abnormalities in brain cell communication patterns that support this theory (Naro et al., 2020).

Problematically, the disinhibition explanation must be incomplete because one of the hallmark signs of Tourette syndrome is the ability for the person to temporarily suppress tics by concentrating—this is one of the features that differentiates jerking movements due to Tourette syndrome from other disorders that cause jerking movements, such as CJD (see Creutzfeldt-Jakob Disease) or other severe neurodegenerative diseases (Ganos et al., 2018). Meanwhile, some of these phenomena, especially echophenomena, occur outside of Tourette syndrome and may have entirely different explanations in the brain for their occurrence, but they are not as well studied (Kurvits et al., 2020). For these reasons, echophenomena and coprophenomena are still not yet well understood.

References

Brown, J. W. (1972). *Aphasia, apraxia, and agnosia: Clinical and theoretical aspects*. CC Thomas.

Dana, C. L., & Wilkin, W. P. (1886). On convulsive tic with explosive disturbances of speech (so-called Gilles de la Tourette's Disease). *The Journal of Nervous and Mental Disease, 13*(7), 407–412.

Enoch, D., & Ball, H. (2001). *Uncommon psychiatric syndromes* (4th ed.). Arnold.

Finkelstein, S. R. (2018). Swearing and the brain. In K. Allan (Ed.), *The oxford handbook of taboo words and language* (pp. 107–139). Oxford University Press. https://doi.org/gtr3

Freeman, R. D., Zinner, S. H., Müller-Vahl, K. R., Fast, D. K., Burd, L. J., Kano, Y., Rothenberger, A., Roessner, V., Kerbeshian, J., & Stern, J. S. (2009). Coprophenomena in Tourette syndrome. *Developmental Medicine & Child Neurology, 51*(3), 218–227. https://doi.org/dpsbvs

Ganos, C., Ograzal, T., Schnitzler, A., & Münchau, A. (2012). The pathophysiology of echopraxia/echolalia: Relevance to Gilles de la Tourette syndrome. *Movement Disorders, 27*(10), 1222–1229. https://doi.org/f363qw

Ganos, C., Rothwell, J., & Haggard, P. (2018). Voluntary inhibitory motor control over involuntary tic movements. *Movement Disorders, 33*(6), 937–946. https://doi.org/gtr4

Gilles de la Tourette, G. (1884). Jumping, latah, myriachit. *Archives de Neurologie, 8*, 68–74.

Hashemiyoon, R., Kuhn, J., & Visser-Vandewalle, V. (2017). Putting the pieces together in Gilles de la Tourette syndrome: Exploring the link between clinical observations and the biological basis of dysfunction. *Brain Topography, 30*(1), 3–29. https://doi.org/f9nbk7

Hollingworth, L. S. (1917). Echolalia in idiots: its meaning for modern theories of imitation. *Journal of Educational Psychology, 8*(4), 212–219. https://doi.org/bspkvn

Kobierska, M., Sitek, M., Gocyła, K., & Janik, P. (2014). Coprolalia and copropraxia in patients with Gilles de la Tourette syndrome. *Neurologia i Neurochirurgia Polska, 48*(1), 1–7. https://doi.org/f5zxsb

Kurvits, L., Martino, D., & Ganos, C. (2020). Clinical features that evoke the concept of disinhibition in Tourette Syndrome. *Frontiers in Psychiatry, 11*, Article 21. https://doi.org/gtr5

Lajonchere, C., Nortz, M., & Finger, S. (1996). Gilles de la Tourette and the discovery of Tourette syndrome: Includes a translation of his 1884 article. *Archives of Neurology*, *53*(6), 567–574. https://doi.org/dz6br6

Lees, A. J., Robertson, M., Trimble, M. R., & Murray, N. M. (1984). A clinical study of Gilles de la Tourette syndrome in the United Kingdom. *Journal of Neurology, Neurosurgery & Psychiatry*, *47*(1), 1–8.

Linetsky, E., Planer, D., & Ben-Hur, T. (2000). Echolalia–palilalia as the sole manifestation of nonconvulsive status epilepticus. *Neurology*, *55*(5), 733–734. https://doi.org/gtr6

Mazur, W. P. (1953). Gilles de la Tourette's syndrome. *Canadian Medical Association Journal*, *69*(5), 520–522.

Naro, A., Billeri, L., Colucci, V. P., Le Cause, M., De Domenico, C., Ciatto, L., Bramanti, P., Bramanti, A., & Calabrò, R. S. (2020). Brain functional connectivity in chronic tic disorders and Gilles de la Tourette syndrome. *Progress in Neurobiology*, *194*, Article 101884. https://doi.org/hh6t

Sacks, O. (1999). *Awakenings*. Vintage Books.

Schuler, A. L. (1979). Echolalia: Issues and clinical applications. *Journal of Speech and Hearing Disorders*, *44*(4), 411–434. https://doi.org/gtr7

Yael, D., Vinner, E., & Bar-Gad, I. (2015). Pathophysiology of tic disorders. *Movement Disorders*, *30*(9), 1171–1178. https://doi.org/f7p554

Environmental Tilt (Visual Allesthesia)

Imagine that you can't keep the world from flipping around. Sometimes, while going about your day, everything that you are looking at suddenly shifts. Perhaps what was up now looks like down, or what was above you now looks straight ahead. Your visual field, including everything you can see, may suddenly begin to rotate. What has changed in your brain to make it so that the world around you seems to literally turn upside down?

The Stories

(STORY 1) In the case of a 30-year-old woman, episodes of strange visual phenomena became daily occurrences. Besides visual blurring and changes to the way she experienced color, she also began to experience tilting of her visual field in a clockwise direction. The rotations were variable in their degrees of tilt, sometimes almost reaching 90°. She reported that on two occasions, she was driving her car when the symptoms of environmental tilt hit, and she swerved her car onto the shoulder of the road as a result. Her episodes of environmental tilt lasted only a matter of seconds each, and the researcher suspected migraines as the culprit despite a lack of pain in this case (Ropper, 1983, case 4).

(STORY 2) A 70-year-old man developed environmental tilt symptoms after having a shunt inserted into his brain to manage excess cerebrospinal fluid. After the insertion of the shunt, he had periods of ten to 20 minutes where his environment would appear tilted. Strangely, the rotation of the environment was 90° in the coronal axis, meaning that when he looked forwards, he felt that he was looking toward the ceiling. The illusions occurred several times each day until the patient had another surgery, and then never occurred again (Girkin et al., 1999).

(STORY 3) A 12-year-old boy had some brain damage in the form of lesions in his brain, but he didn't seem to have many resulting symptoms. However, on some tests that required him to draw, he would unintentionally draw the pictures in a rotated way. He described his most notable experience of allesthesia to medical workers. He was working on his homework when he got up from the table to make some tea, and when he returned and sat back down, he felt that

DOI: 10.4324/9781003276937-26

what he had written was upside down. When he looked up from his homework, he saw that the entire kitchen seemed to have flipped upside down. With some effort, he made his way to the door and opened it, to see that the world outside had also flipped upside down. He closed his eyes and rubbed them, and when he reopened them his vision was back to normal. The next day, while looking at a tree, his vision appeared to slowly rotate until it was upside down again. He experienced problems with his vision like this at least a few more times, but later on he told doctors that it had stopped happening to him (Solms et al., 1988).

The Features

Usually, our brains are pretty good at figuring out which way is up. There are environmental situations that can cause disorientation in space, such as being buried in an avalanche or trapped underwater—but it's also possible for the problem to come from inside your brain as well. One way that the brain can disorient a person is through environmental tilt.

Environmental tilt is the experience of seeing your environment tilted on its side or upside down, as if your brain has rotated everything that you can see. This symptom has been known about for a long time, such as demonstrated by this case study from 1805 wherein a woman, who was probably experiencing a seizure,

> could not resist the impulse she felt to place the chairs in the room hori-zontally, lest they should fall, finding they would not stand on the other end. She expressed her surprise, and laughed heartily, on seeing the attend-ants all standing, as she thought, upon their heads.
>
> (Bishopp, 1805, pp. 117–118)

After about an hour, her vision returned to its correct orientation, but the at-the-time unnamed symptom repeatedly recurred.

We've learned a lot about environmental tilt since then. Another name for this symptom is *room tilt illusion* because it really can look like the room has been tilted. An alternate name that never really caught on was "tortopia," which is what this chapter was almost called (Ropper, 1983). If we want to be extra scientific, *visual allesthesia* is a term that refers to rotation of the visual field, or the transposition of points in the visual field, and it includes the phe-nomenon of environmental tilt (Girkin et al., 1999).

Perhaps the most common form of environmental tilt is a complete 180° rotation of the visual field, such that things that are in the top right of your vision now appear in the bottom left (Solms et al., 1988). This 180° rotation goes by many names, such as upside-down reversal of seeing, the floor-on-ceiling phenomena, or reversal of vision metamorphopsia (e.g., Blom, 2014; River et al., 1998).

However, rotations other than 180° are also possible. Rotations of 90° appear to be the second-most-common form of environmental tilt, but other rotations such as 45° or 150° have also been reported (Sierra-Hidalgo et al., 2012). The transformations can occur suddenly, or the person may experience the feeling of their visual field actively rotating. When the direction of the rotation can be observed as it is happening, it may be in a clockwise or counterclockwise direction (Ropper, 1983).

The duration of the feeling of rotation can be variable, but most cases last only seconds or minutes (Sierra-Hidalgo et al., 2012). In most, and possibly all, cases, the person's vision eventually returns to normal (Solms et al., 1988). Some people who experience environmental tilt find that the best way to treat it is to close their eyes for several seconds and hope that the world is back to normal when they reopen them. Others have found success in ending the environmental tilt by moving their hands in front of themselves or repositioning their bodies (River et al., 1998).

The Brain Pathology

How is environmental tilt possible? We have a number of systems in our brain that work together to figure out what our position in the environment is, and where the things around us are located. One such system is vision, but there are at least two other important systems: the *vestibular sense* and the *proprioceptive sense*.

The vestibular sense is your sense of balance, and it is primarily sensed by structures in your inner ear. Some of these structures are sensitive to the rotation of your head because they are full of fluid that sloshes around, and others are sensitive to gravity because they contain calcium crystals that you can sense being pulled in various directions (Hain, 2007). When your sense of balance goes wrong, the consequences are unsettling (see Vertigo).

Proprioception, on the other hand, is the feeling of knowing where parts of your body are located. Proprioception is similar to the sense of touch: it uses receptors all over the body in the muscles, tendons, joints, and skin, in order to gather information about the position of the body (Morgan, 2003). It tells you, for example, whether you are stretching or relaxing a particular muscle (Sierra-Hidalgo et al., 2012). When this sense of body part location goes wrong, the results can be quite remarkable (see Somatoparaphrenia).

When your brain tries to build a map of the surrounding space, it uses these different senses in order to figure out where the real positions of objects are (Arntzen & Alstadhaug, 2020). In a case of environmental tilt, something goes wrong and the positioning of things relative to the head becomes confused, even though the objects' colors, shapes, and sizes are all correctly seen (Girkin & Miller, 2001). This *multisensory* theory can help explain why people who stare at objects with known orientations such that the right way up is unchanging, or grasp unmoving objects, can sometimes forcibly correct the environmental tilt (Arjona & Fernández-Romero, 2002). Their vision returns to normal because they are using one sense (vision or proprioception) to correct another sense (vestibular) that has made a mistake.

Environmental tilt has been associated with causes including strokes, brain tumors, head injury, migraine, and multiple sclerosis (Gondim et al., 2014). Many cases involve damage to the brain stem and/or cerebellum, which both work with the vestibular system (River et al., 1998). However, damage to other areas has also been reported, including the inner ear, the parieto-occipital lobe, and more (Sierra-Hidalgo et al., 2012). Damage in different places may cause the illusory tilt through different mechanisms (Deniz et al., 2012). Cases which involve interruption of blood supply to the brain, such as in strokes, may be more commonly associated with 180° rotations, while cases involving more direct vestibular damage may produce variable angles of rotation, such as 90° or less (Arjona & Fernández-Romero, 2002).

It may take some work to figure out the specific cause for each person. A doctor should be consulted though, because this symptom can indicate severe underlying conditions in the brain (Arntzen & Alstadhaug, 2020). Overall, losing your sense of up and down is unpleasant, and a case of tortopia can be quite shocking to suddenly experience. You know what, the word tortopia is growing on me. Is it too late to change the name of this chapter?

References

Arjona, A., & Fernández-Romero, E. (2002). Room tilt illusion: Report of two cases and terminological review. *Neurologia (Barcelona, Spain)*, *17*(6), 338–341.

Arntzen, K., & Alstadhaug, K. B. (2020). Room tilt illusion and subclavian steal - A case report. *BMC Neurology*, *20*(1), 2–6. https://doi.org/gtr8

Bishopp, M. T. (1805). Case of optical illusion from hysteria. *The Medical and Physical Journal*, *14*(78), 117–118.

Blom, J. D. (2014). *A dictionary of hallucinations*. Springer.

Deniz, O., Keklikoglu, H. D., Vural, G., Temel, S., & Dilbaz, F. A. (2012). Acute "upside-down" visual inversion in a patient with multiple sclerosis. *Neurological Sciences*, *33*(3), 635–637. https://doi.org/ff6fqb

Girkin, C. A., & Miller, N. R. (2001). Central disorders of vision in humans. *Survey of Ophthalmology*, *45*(5), 379–405. https://doi.org/d5q2cf

Girkin, C. A., Perry, J. D., & Miller, N. R. (1999). Visual environmental rotation: A novel disorder of visiospatial integration. *Journal of Neuro-Ophthalmology*, *19*(1), 13–16.

Gondim, F. D. A. A., De Araújo, D. F., & Sales, P. M. G. (2014). Acute reversal of vision metamorphopsia: Report of two cases. *Journal of Health & Biological Sciences*, *2*(4), 224–226. https://doi.org/gtr9

Hain, T. C. (2007). Cranial nerve VIII: Vestibulocochlear nerve. In C. G. Goetz (Ed.), *Textbook of clinical neurology* (3rd ed., pp. 199–215). Saunders.

Morgan, G. W. (2003). Proprioception, touch, and vibratory sensation. In C. G. Goetz (Ed.), *Textbook of clinical neurology* (2nd ed., pp. 333–350). Saunders.

River, Y., Hur, T. B., & Steiner, I. (1998). Reversal of vision metamorphopsia: Clinical and anatomical characteristics. *Archives of Neurology*, *55*(10), 1362–1368. https://doi.org/d8nhq9

Ropper, A. H. (1983). Illusion of tilting of the visual environment. Report of five cases. *Journal of Clinical Neuro-Ophthalmology*, *3*(2), 147–151.

Sierra-Hidalgo, F., De Pablo-Fernández, E., Martín, A. H. S., Correas-Callero, E., Herreros-Rodríguez, J., Romero-Muñoz, J. P., & Martín-Gil, L. (2012). Clinical and imaging features of the room tilt illusion. *Journal of Neurology*, *259*(12), 2555–2564. https://doi.org/f4f9t3

Solms, M., Kaplan-Solms, K., Saling, M., & Miller, P. (1988). Inverted vision after frontal lobe disease. *Cortex*, *24*(4), 499–509. https://doi.org/gtsb

Exploding Head Syndrome

Imagine that you can't fall asleep easily because whenever you try to do so, there's a chance that you will be woken up by an exploding sound. The sound startles you, causing your heart to race, and you become wide awake from the shock. While the noises are not painful, they are both alarming and disturbing, sometimes occurring in the middle of the night while you are already asleep. Is this something that you should be worried about?

The Stories

(STORY 1) A 43-year-old woman developed exploding head syndrome. Suddenly, she began having nearly nightly episodes in which, just before falling asleep, she heard a loud noise lasting roughly one second. This noise was described by the patient as "electrical current running" (p. 602). Like other EHS (exploding head syndrome) cases, it was occasionally accompanied by other symptoms such as bodily convulsions or flashes of light. Occasionally, it would happen twice in a row, but afterward she could successfully fall asleep (Evans & Pearce, 2001).

(STORY 2) A 57-year-old man had irregular experiences with exploding head syndrome. He described four instances over a period of two years in which he was suddenly awakened by an explosion sound on the right side of his head. The sound was described as an electrical jolt-like sound. The four instances all occurred during the early portion of his sleep, near bedtime. He did not have any pain or experience a headache, but the symptom was disturbing enough that he visited the doctor and received an MRI and EEG, which did not reveal any underlying issues with his brain (Ganguly et al., 2013).

(STORY 3) A woman began having episodes of exploding head syndrome at the age of 67. She reported periods of attacks in which she had two or three per week, as well as remission periods in which she had no attacks for up to three weeks. She described the experience as "bursting with a flash of light over both fields of vision, after which I would be dazed for a split second and would come round, terrified, my heart thumping. There was no pain, just a frightening sense of explosion" (Pearce, 1988, p. 270). These attacks continued

DOI: 10.4324/9781003276937-27

for many years, but she otherwise seemed to be healthy (Pearce, 1988, case 1; Pearce, 1989).

The Features

Exploding head syndrome is a humorous name for a problem that is not very humorous. Don't be too concerned though, because this disorder is not at all dangerous, although it can be quite disruptive to a good night's sleep.

The primary symptom of exploding head syndrome is hearing a loud noise just as you are falling asleep or, less commonly, upon waking up (Sharpless, 2018). People with this condition report that it feels like the noise is deep inside of their heads (Pearce, 1988). The startling noise typically lasts for only a fraction of a second and may be accompanied by a flash of light or sudden jerking of the limbs (Evans & Pearce, 2001). Most people do not experience flashing lights as part of exploding head syndrome, but they do occur in about a third of people (Sharpless, 2018). This condition is usually not painful, but it is "unpleasant and sometimes terrifying" (Queiroz, 2013, p. 13).

A variety of different sounds have been reported. These include explosions, high-pitched noises, doors slamming, gunshots, a scream, breaking glass, and "dropping an object from a height" (Sharpless, 2018, p. 596). Some reports are quite dramatic, including people who described the incidents as "noise as if head will burst open," "fierce explosions as if house crashed," and an "enormous roar so loud it could kill me" (Pearce, 1989, p. 908). In 1897, one researcher wrote that the typical noises were "like that of a pistolshot or of the crash of broken glass, or as of a bell, or a wire sharply twanged … even those who are used to them greatly dread their return" (Mitchell, 1897, pp. 80–81). Understandably, a person's heart is usually beating very fast and they feel afraid following the noise (Sharpless, 2018).

Exploding head syndrome is surprisingly common. One study that asked over 1600 adults about exploding head syndrome found that around 30% had experienced it at least once (Denis et al., 2019). Some people experience symptoms rarely, perhaps having only a single episode of exploding head syndrome in their lives (Sharpless, 2015). However, a few people report that it occurs reliably, such as *every day* for a period of years (Weiler et al., 2019). These people presumably explain to those around them that they haven't been sleeping much lately because "my head keeps exploding."

People who experience the symptoms of exploding head syndrome also frequently experience other sleep-related phenomena. These may include difficulties in falling asleep or staying asleep, unpleasant dreams around the times of falling asleep or waking up, and "dissociative experiences" such as "finding yourself in a place and having no idea how you got there" (Denis et al., 2019, pp. 5–7). Other dissociative experiences that people with this condition sometimes report include out-of-body sensations and feeling like their body is floating (Sharpless, 2018). Exploding head syndrome is also associated with sleep paralysis (see Narcolepsy) and lucid dreaming in some cases

(Denis et al., 2019). Essentially, the more difficult and strange your typical night of sleep, the more likely you are to have symptoms of exploding head syndrome.

The Brain Pathology

It has been theorized that the cause of exploding head syndrome is a problem with *attentional processing*, leading the person to amplify the sensations that they are sensing with their ears and/or eyes (Sakellariou et al., 2020). In other words, the noise and lights may be real sensations coming from the environment outside of the person's head, but those sensations become *distorted* once they enter the almost-sleeping person's brain. The reason that the person's brain may be distorting light and sound could be due to an incomplete shutdown of the sensory parts of the brain as the person sleeps—a job that is normally done by the *reticular formation* in the brain stem (Evans & Pearce, 2001). In other words, because the brain didn't completely shut down for sleep, the person can hear or see strange things. It has also been theorized that exploding head syndrome can result from movement in the middle ear, seizures (see Seizures), withdrawal from certain medications, and problems with the flow of calcium ions in the brain (Ganguly et al., 2013).

There is not yet a consistent treatment for exploding head syndrome, but that is probably fine because the condition is considered benign—that is, it's not dangerous (Sakellariou et al., 2020). At least one team of physicians concluded that the syndrome is not usually disruptive enough to a person's life to warrant treatment beyond reassurance to the patient that they are healthy (Ganguly et al., 2013). However, people who are deeply disturbed by the symptoms do sometimes seek medical help, and some reported that they feared they were having a stroke (Sachs & Svanborg, 1991). In some cases, treatment with drugs has been successful—but this has only occurred in a "small subgroup of patients" (Ganguly et al., 2013, p. 16).

While there are not yet any universally agreed-upon interventions for eliminating symptoms of exploding head syndrome, one study asked thousands of adults about what they do to relieve their symptoms and found some possible prevention strategies. Strategies included changing their intake of alcohol, changing sleep positions (especially avoiding lying on the back), adjusting sleep patterns, meditation and relaxation, and getting out of bed for a while if it happens before trying to sleep again (Sharpless et al., 2020). Overall, it can be a tough condition to grapple with but, fortunately, the bang is usually louder than the bite.

References

Denis, D., Poerio, G. L., Derveeuw, S., Badini, I., & Gregory, A. M. (2019). Associations between exploding head syndrome and measures of sleep quality and experiences, dissociation, and well-being. *Sleep*, *42*(2), 1–11. https://doi.org/gtsc

Evans, R. W., & Pearce, J. M. S. (2001). Exploding head syndrome. *Headache, 41*(6), 602–603. https://doi.org/dx4mq9

Ganguly, G., Mridha, B., Khan, A., & Rison, R. A. (2013). Exploding head syndrome: A case report. *Case Reports in Neurology, 5*(1), 14–17. https://doi.org/gtsd

Mitchell, S. W. (1897). *Clinical lessons on nervous diseases.* Lea Brothers & Co.

Pearce, J. M. S. (1988). Exploding head syndrome. *The Lancet, 332*(8605), 270–271. https://doi.org/d9gdjf

Pearce, J. M. (1989). Clinical features of the exploding head syndrome. *Journal of Neurology, Neurosurgery & Psychiatry, 52*(7), 907–910. https://doi.org/cs8xfj

Queiroz, L. P. (2013). Unusual headache syndromes. *Headache, 53*(1), 12–22. https://doi.org/f4hg8k

Sachs, C., & Svanborg, E. (1991). The exploding head syndrome: Polysomnographic recordings and therapeutic suggestions. *Sleep, 14*(3), 263–266. https://doi.org/gtsf

Sakellariou, D. F., Nesbitt, A. D., Higgins, S., Beniczky, S., Rosenzweig, J., Drakatos, P., Gildeh, N., Murphy, P. B., Kent, B., Williams, A. J., Kryger, M., Goadsby, P. j., Leschziner, G. D., & Rosenzweig, I. (2020). Co-activation of rhythms during alpha band oscillations as an interictal biomarker of exploding head syndrome. *Cephalalgia, 40*(9), 1–10. https://doi.org/gtsg

Sharpless, B. A. (2015). Exploding head syndrome is common in college students. *Journal of Sleep Research, 24*(4), 447–449. https://doi.org/f7mjph

Sharpless, B. A. (2018). Characteristic symptoms and associated features of exploding head syndrome in undergraduates. *Cephalalgia, 38*(3), 595–599. https://doi.org/f9zpkt

Sharpless, B. A., Denis, D., Perach, R., French, C. C., & Gregory, A. M. (2020). Exploding Head Syndrome: Clinical features, theories about etiology, and prevention strategies in a large international sample. *Sleep Medicine, 75*, 251–255. https://doi.org/gtsh

Weiler, E., Wiegand, R., Brill, K., & Schneider, D. (2019). Quantitative electroencephalography and exploding head syndrome: A case study. *Neuropsychiatry, 9*(1), 2131–2135. https://doi.org/gtsj

Fatal Familial Insomnia

Imagine that you are incapable of falling asleep. You may think such a fate would allow you to get more work done because you no longer have to lie down and take a break for many hours each night. However, sleep is incredibly important, and without it you will eventually die. Plus, this insomnia has more symptoms on top of the maddening wakefulness: uncontrollable body temperature, wild bouts of sweating, frantic involuntary muscle jerking, and demented delirium lasting for months. What has gone wrong in your brain to wake you up for the rest of your life?

The Stories

(STORY 1) A 48-year-old woman began having troubling symptoms, beginning with a bout of dizziness one day in 1973. She began feeling as if she were always tired and that sleep was no longer restful. When doctors began treating her with sleeping pills, they made her problems worse by triggering agitation and nightmares. Combined with sweating and tremors, her symptoms continued to worsen, while doctors incorrectly diagnosed her with conditions such as alcoholism. In the end, she lost her abilities to walk and to swallow, but retained a remarkable awareness of herself and the people around her, holding conversations up until the day that she passed away (Max, 2006, chapter 7).

(STORY 2) A woman began losing sleep for multiple days at a time, leading to her receiving prescriptions for sleep aid medications. Unfortunately, they didn't work, and she continued to get worse. She had memory disturbances, as well. Over time, she lost the ability to walk and could no longer sit still—she had a tremor in her body as if she was shivering. At one point, physicians were unable to take measurements of her brain activity because she was involuntarily moving so much. Eventually she found herself confined to bed but unable to sleep. After around two years of symptoms, she passed away. Following her death, she was diagnosed with sporadic fatal insomnia, which was not considered while she was alive because of her lack of familial history of fatal insomnia (Moody et al., 2011).

(STORY 3) A 53-year-old man with progressive insomnia was described in a case study from 1986, which also investigated his family history. Insomnia

DOI: 10.4324/9781003276937-28

began by reducing his hours slept each night to around two or three. After a couple of months, he would only sleep about one hour per night. Eventually, he lost the ability to sleep altogether. Instead, he would occasionally enter dreamlike trances that included stupor as if asleep but included complex gestures, and from which he could be awakened easily. He began to have memory disturbances, constant fevers, and was overall losing control of his body. He died after around nine months of symptoms. Investigations of his brain and those of his family members were extremely informative to researchers, helping to move investigations of fatal insomnia forwards (Lugaresi et al., 1986).

The Features

Fatal familial insomnia (FFI) is a disorder that is pretty much exactly what its name makes it sound like. It's a disease that is fatal, runs in families, and involves severe insomnia, eventually including the complete loss of the ability to sleep (Schenkein & Montagna, 2006). In regular insomnia, a person cannot fall asleep or stay asleep, perhaps because they are running through a mental list of every mistake that they have ever made. In FFI, people cannot sleep because the brain literally forgets how. And that's just the beginning.

The loss of the ability to sleep happens gradually. First, the person begins to sleep less and has trouble falling asleep. When they do sleep, they often report vivid and disturbing dreams, and throughout the day they may have severe daytime sleepiness and lapse randomly into dreamlike states (Polnitsky, 2005). Then, usually over the course of several months, they lose the ability to sleep entirely. For the final three months or so of their life they are awake and suffering as the other symptoms catch up to the severity of the insomnia (Lindsley, 2017).

There are several other symptoms that make the experience even more awful. Two big ones are motor dysfunction such as tremors or thrashing limbs and irregular breathing (Wu et al., 2018). Others include the loss of the abilities to walk and swallow, and *sympathetic hyperactivity* (Lindsley, 2017). Sympathetic hyperactivity refers to the sympathetic nervous system becoming out of control—leading to symptoms such as excess sweating and tearing up of the eyes (Wu et al., 2018). Temperatures of patients may gyrate wildly, including severe fevers (Max, 2006).

Additional symptoms are those of *progressive cognitive dysfunction* and depression (Gistau et al., 2006). Progressive cognitive dysfunction means that the person slowly gets worse at remembering and thinking, much like a person with dementia. Depression is common in FFI (Harder et al., 1999). Have you ever lost so much sleep that you felt your ability to think was worse, and that your mood was terrible? Now imagine that, except you literally can't sleep. The cognitive and mood symptoms of FFI are already understandable considering all of that lost sleep, even before we discuss the spreading brain damage.

Eventually, the people may fall into akinetic mutism (see Akinetic Mutism) and remain bedridden and unable to speak, although some patients die before reaching this point (Montagna, 2005). Symptoms can vary quite a lot between patients—believe it or not, there have been some cases of FFI where insomnia was not a symptom (e.g., Bär et al., 2002; Wu et al., 2018). However, the disorder is always fatal. Death itself generally occurs because of pneumonia, specifically aspiration pneumonia, which occurs after fluid or food enters the lungs due to the patients' loss of controlled swallowing (e.g., Fukuoka et al., 2018; Harder et al., 1999). The symptoms last an average of 18 months before death occurs (Schenkein & Montagna, 2006). However, the time that it takes the disease to progress to death depends upon the person's specific genetics, with some people lasting less than a year and others lasting multiple years (Montagna et al., 1998).

One of the many unusual things about FFI is that it is an inherited *prion* disease. Prion diseases are thought to be caused by misfolded proteins that replicate and cause damage in the brain over time (see Creutzfeldt-Jakob Disease). FFI follows family bloodlines over generations in what's called an *autosomal dominant pattern*, meaning that one mutated gene is enough to develop the disease and risk passing it along to your children (Wu et al., 2018). If one parent has FFI, you have a 50% chance of having it too (Lindsley, 2017).

The average age at which people begin to show FFI signs is 50 years old; however this can vary, with some people developing it decades earlier (Schenkein & Montagna, 2006). It may even appear past the age of 70 (Harder et al., 1999). Most people have children in the first few decades of life, so they may pass on the disease before finding out that they have it.

However, it is possible to develop this kind of insomnia without belonging to a specific family line. Mutations in the brain can lead to prions as well. These cases are exceptionally rare, and are referred to as just plain old *fatal insomnia*—because it's no longer familial—or as *sporadic fatal insomnia*. The symptoms resemble FFI, except the person does not have the genetic mutation that causes the disease (Montagna, 2005). Sporadic fatal insomnia is so rare that it sometimes isn't even considered as a diagnosis until it is already too late (e.g., Moody et al., 2011).

The Brain Pathology

Technically, fatal insomnia can infect others, but it requires getting the prions from inside of one person's brain into the brain of someone else. You could do this by eating human brains (see Kuru) or by transplanting infected tissues. As far as I know, fatal insomnia has never been transmitted like that. However, fatal insomnia has been transmitted to animals by intentionally infecting them with human prions (Montagna et al., 2003).

As discussed in the chapter about more general prion disorders (see Creutzfeldt-Jakob Disease), it is the accumulation of the prions into plaques in the brain that seems to cause the actual brain damage in prion disorders such as FFI. However, there is an additional risk associated with FFI specifically. Namely, the loss of the ability to sleep probably makes the brain damage even worse than in other similar disorders in which the ability to sleep is not lost. This is because the brain creates waste products as it functions, and clearing those waste products away especially takes place while the person sleeps. This "clearance" process is a leading theory for why humans need to sleep: to allow their brains to be more effectively cleaned (Xie et al., 2013). In theory, during FFI, the brain is dealing with prion plaques as well as the loss of sleep and therefore a loss of clearance, and so the brain damage compounds over time.

Scientists have found that the part of the brain most affected by the disease is the *thalamus*, although other brain regions are also affected (Bär et al., 2002). FFI seems to destroy specific parts of the thalamus while keeping other parts more intact (Lugaresi et al., 1986). The thalamus is a complicated part of the brain, but one thing that it does is monitor and control signals going from the brain to the body. Some of those signals include things like the temperature of the body, sweating, production of tears, dilation of the pupils, and so on. Sometimes 50% or more of the cells are missing from those thalamus regions by the time the person dies, leading to the aforementioned symptoms of fatal insomnia (Montagna et al., 2003).

The specific genetic mutations of FFI have been identified, and some options for disease management have been investigated (e.g., Schenkein & Montagna, 2006). However, there is currently no cure or standard treatment, and attempting to treat insomnia with sleep-inducing drugs seems to worsen the symptoms (Lindsley, 2017). Yes, that's right, sleeping pills actually make the problem worse for these poor people. Fortunately, FFI is rare, but it has been found in families across the world (Montagna et al., 2003). It affects only about one out of every 30 million people (Lindsley, 2017). So, statistically speaking, you probably won't develop it. Sleep tight?

References

Bär, K. J., Häger, F., Nenadic, I., Opfermann, T., Brodhun, M., Tauber, R. F., Patt, S., Schulz-Schaeffer, W., Gottschild, D., & Sauer, H. (2002). Serial positron emission tomographic findings in an atypical presentation of fatal familial insomnia. *Archives of Neurology*, *59*(11), 1815–1818. https://doi.org/cdxkfp

Fukuoka, T., Nakazato, Y., Yamamoto, M., Miyake, A., Mitsufuji, T., & Yamamoto, T. (2018). Fatal familial insomnia initially developing parkinsonism mimicking dementia with Lewy bodies. *Internal Medicine*, *57*(18), 2719–2722. https://doi.org/gtsk

Gistau, V. S., Pintor, L., Matrai, S., & Saiz, A. (2006). Fatal familial insomnia. *Psychosomatics*, *47*(6), 527–528. https://doi.org/fdz2kg

Harder, A., Jendroska, K., Kreuz, F., Wirth, T., Schafranka, C., Karnatz, N., Théallier-Janko, A., Dreier, J., Lohan, K., Emmerich, D., Cervós-Navarro, J., Windl, O., Kretzschmar, H. A., Nürnberg, P., & Witkowski, R. (1999). Novel twelve-generation kindred of fatal familial insomnia from Germany representing the entire spectrum of disease expression. *American Journal of Medical Genetics*, *87*(4), 311–316. https://doi.org/fvfqnn

Lindsley, C. W. (2017). Genetic and rare disease of the CNS. Part I: Fatal familial insomnia (FFI). *ACS Chemical Neuroscience*, *8*(12), 2570–2572. https://doi.org/gtsm

Lugaresi, E., Medori, R., Montagna, P., Baruzzi, A., Cortelli, P., Lugaresi, A., Tinuper, P., Zucconi, M., & Gambetti, P. (1986). Fatal familial insomnia and dysautonomia with selective degeneration of thalamic nuclei. *New England Journal of Medicine, 315*(16), 997–1003. https://doi.org/b63kqp

Max, D. T. (2006). *The family that couldn't sleep: A medical mystery.* Random House.

Montagna, P. (2005). Fatal familial insomnia: A model disease in sleep physiopathology. *Sleep Medicine Reviews, 9*(5), 339–353. https://doi.org/dpqvqc

Montagna, P., Cortelli, P., Avoni, P., Tinuper, P., Plazzi, G., Gallassi, R., Portaluppi, F., Julien, J., Vital, C., Delisle, M. B., Gambetti, P., & Lugaresi, E. (1998). Clinical features of fatal familial insomnia: Phenotypic variability in relation to a polymorphism at codon 129 of the prion protein gene. *Brain Pathology, 8*(3), 515–520. https://doi.org/c9pbt2

Montagna, P., Gambetti, P., Cortelli, P., & Lugaresi, E. (2003). Familial and sporadic fatal insomnia. *Lancet Neurology, 2*(3), 167–176. https://doi.org/fgc9tw

Moody, K. M., Schonberger, L. B., Maddox, R. A., Zou, W. Q., Cracco, L., & Cali, I. (2011). Sporadic fatal insomnia in a young woman: A diagnostic challenge: Case Report. *BMC Neurology, 11*(136), 1–8. https://doi.org/dc3ssp

Polnitsky, C. A. (2005). Fatal familial insomnia. In T. L. Lee-Chiong (Ed.), *Sleep: A comprehensive handbook* (pp. 111–115). John Wiley & Sons. https://doi.org/fwmksm

Schenkein, J., & Montagna, P. (2006). Self management of fatal familial insomnia. Part 1: What is FFI? *Medscape General Medicine, 8*(3), Article 65.

Wu, L.-Y., Zhan, S.-Q., Huang, Z.-Y., Zhang, B., Wang, T., Liu, C.-F., Lu, H., Dong, X.-P., Wu, Z.-Y., Zhang, J.-W., Zhang, J.-H., Han, F., Huang, Y., Lu, J., Gauthier, S., Jia, J.-P., Wang, Y.-P. (2018). Expert consensus on clinical diagnostic criteria for Fatal Familial Insomnia. *Chinese Medical Journal, 131*(13), 1613–1617. https://doi.org/gkxtnv

Xie, L., Kang, H., Xu, Q., Chen, M. J., Liao, Y., Thiyagarajan, M., O'Donnell, J., Christensen, D. J., Nicholson, C., Iliff, J. J., Takano, T., Deane, R., & Nedergaard, M. (2013). Sleep drives metabolite clearance from the adult brain. *Science, 342*(6156), 373–377. https://doi.org/pb7

Gerstmann Syndrome (Dysgraphia, Dyscalculia, Finger Agnosia, and Left-Right Disorientation)

Imagine that you've developed a collection of difficulties. Your writing ability has vanished. You now mix up your spelling, and the former fluidity of your writing motions is gone, replaced with slow, inconsistent lettering. Your ability to do math has evaporated, leading to confusion with even simple addition. You can't quite understand fingers. When you are asked to move your pinky, you flex the wrong digit. When asked to point to the ring finger on a drawing of a hand, you choose wrong. Telling the right apart from the left has become challenging. What has caused this array of difficulties?

The Stories

(STORY 1) A 52-year-old woman showed the classic tetrad of symptoms for Gerstmann syndrome in 1960. She was admitted to hospital with writing difficulties, showing *dysgraphia*, such that she could not form letters correctly with a pen. She also placed letters out of their correct order such that words were often severely misspelled. She could read, however, and could do so in a mostly unimpaired fashion. One of her main complaints was that she couldn't work out the correct change to give customers at her job as a cashier. Even simple tasks of addition and subtraction were difficult, and she "invariably failed if numbers had to be carried from one column to the next" (p. 57). She also showed somewhat severe left-right disorientation such that telling left and right apart was challenging, and she showed general clumsiness. She was part of a study that showed that people with Gerstmann syndrome treated their fingers "as if they were an undifferentiated mass" (p. 56). When asked to point to specific fingers, she could not, although she correctly pointed to and named other body parts (Kinsbourne & Warrington, 1962, case 2).

(STORY 2) A 55-year-old woman resigned from her position as a second-grade teacher when she discovered that she was losing the ability to write and do math. She was described as alert, cooperative, and pleasant and was able to do most of her daily activities by herself. However, she was unable to do a few things. The researcher noted that her "calculations were severely impaired," showing prominent *dyscalculia* or *acalculia* (p. 129). Two example math problems that she did not solve correctly were 8 + 4 and 4 + 2. She could not recite

DOI: 10.4324/9781003276937-29

the months in order, and she had severe spelling difficulties, even for simple words. She also showed some problems with telling the different fingers on a hand apart from one another and showed mild signs of left-right disorientation. She could, however, read and draw certain pictures. She was classified as having Gerstmann syndrome, and her brain scans showed some evidence of changes in the frontoparietal regions of her brain, especially on the left side (Gitelman, 2003).

(STORY 3) A 59-year-old man suddenly lost the ability to calculate, write, and dial phone numbers in 1994. A brain scan revealed that he had suffered a small stroke on the left side of his brain, and he stayed in the hospital for ten days. While there, he was examined for the classic Gerstmann syndrome symptoms. He was tested for *digit agnosia* (fingers as well as toes) in many different ways. He could correctly complete some tasks regarding fingers. For example, when asked which finger was used to hitchhike, he correctly indicated the thumb. When asked which finger a wedding ring is placed on, he was also correct. However, when his fingers were touched while he couldn't see them, he made several errors when asked to name which finger had been touched. When asked to judge left from right, he tended to show *left-right disorientation* as he generally "hesitated, looked at his hands or feet, turned them, etc., before giving his response" (p. 1113). This, combined with his very slow responses, showed how impaired he was at distinguishing left from right. They also thoroughly tested his writing and calculating abilities, and found that "every task requiring numbers was severely impaired" (p. 1115). For example, he was asked to count out the numbers from 1 to 20. Counting on his fingers for this task, he took over 5 seconds to name some of the numbers and accidentally skipped over three of the numbers. The researchers found this particular case study to be theoretically interesting because the region of brain damage in this case was very small, but the person showed all four of the classic Gerstmann syndrome symptoms without showing many other symptoms, suggesting that this was a relatively "pure" case (Mayer et al., 1999).

The Features

According to the traditional view, Gerstmann syndrome is a collection of four symptoms that frequently, but not always, occur together. This grouping of symptoms is named after Josef Gerstmann, not to be confused with the other brain disorder named after him (see Gerstmann-Sträussler-Scheinker disease in the Creutzfeldt-Jakob Disease chapter). The modern view, on the other hand, is that this group of four symptoms may not be some special category—but we will get to that later on. Together, the four symptoms are known as a *tetrad*, which is the raddest-known way to refer to a group of four.

The first symptom is *dysgraphia*, also called *agraphia* when severe. Mild dysgraphia may involve a decrease in the legibility of handwriting and an increase in spelling errors, while severe agraphia may result in the loss of the ability to write even single letters.

Many people spend a great deal of time during their childhood training their brains to trace loops and arrange shapes into legible letters that face in the correct directions. That practice helps to make writing an almost automatic process once you are an adult. But, behind the scenes, the brain is constantly following electrochemical recipes to produce those detailed strings of symbols. Agraphia may result from damage to these recipes or, more specifically, damage to the processes in the brain that contribute to selecting words, arranging letters, spelling, and a number of other complex calculations that the brain usually performs relatively effortlessly (Anderson et al., 2009).

The second symptom is *dyscalculia*, which is called *acalculia* when severe. This is trouble with, or the complete loss of, the ability to do mathematical operations such as addition and subtraction. If a person has some mathematical computations memorized, such as times tables (4 × 5) or simple single-digit addition (2 + 2), those may also be harder to remember (Willmes, 2008). It can also involve trouble with numerical concepts in general, such as counting (Pyrtek et al., 2020). In severe cases, the knowledge of numbers is so eroded that telephone numbers or the numbers in the time of day become incomprehensible (Willmes, 2008).

The third symptom is called *finger agnosia*. Here's how Gerstmann described this symptom: "it manifests itself as an isolated disturbance in the recognition, naming, choosing, and differential exhibition of the various fingers of both hands—one's own fingers as well as those of another person" (Gerstmann, 1930, translated by Wilkins & Brody, 1971, p. 476). What Gerstmann missed back then is that the symptom would be better called *digit agnosia* because the toes can also be involved (Tucha et al., 1997). Specifically, a person with digit agnosia has trouble pointing to and naming individual fingers or toes when they are touched or pointed at, especially the middle three fingers (Pyrtek et al., 2020). For example, the doctor may point to the person's middle finger and ask them to bend it, but they may move their ring finger instead. Or, the doctor may point to their middle finger and ask them which finger is being pointed at, but the person might incorrectly say, "that's my pointer finger." Digit agnosia should be specifically tested for in cases of brain damage due to how easy it is to overlook in some cases, because it doesn't cause many problems in day-to-day life (Della Sala & Spinnler, 1994).

The fourth and final symptom of the classic tetrad is *left-right disorientation*, in which a person has trouble telling their left from their right. They often don't know where the directions of "left" and "right" are relative to their own body, and they also have trouble figuring out left from right on the body of a person who is facing them. This symptom can be tested by asking the person to follow directions such as "place left hand to right ear" and noting how many times their motions are incorrect (Heimburger et al., 1964, p. 52). People with this symptom may adapt, perhaps learning to rely on an external cue, such as which of their wrists has a watch (Miller & Hynd, 2004).

The Brain Pathology

Damage to a part of the brain called the angular gyrus, located near where the parietal and temporal lobes meet, appears to be enough to produce this syndrome. However, there are reports of people developing some of the symptoms even with brain damage in different areas (Bhattacharyya et al., 2014). For example, dyscalculia can be a symptom of damage to many different brain locations, including frontal, temporal, parietal, and subcortical structures, although the angular gyrus is probably the most frequently implicated (e.g., Grafman et al., 1982; Willmes, 2008). Importantly, Gerstmann syndrome is commonly associated with damage to the *dominant* hemisphere of a person's brain (Tucha et al., 1997). In right-handed people, the left side of the brain is usually dominant, and because most people are right-handed, Gerstmann syndrome is usually associated with damage to the left half of the brain. Therefore, Gerstmann syndrome is most frequently associated with left-sided damage of the angular gyrus... but there are exceptions to all of this (Lebrun, 2005). In fact, there are a *lot* of exceptions to the guidelines of this syndrome, which brings us to an important question.

We need to ask: does Gerstmann syndrome exist? I sure hope so, because I just made you read a whole chapter about it. Researchers have evaluated for many decades whether Gerstmann syndrome should be considered a discrete diagnosis, or if it's just made up of smaller types of brain damage (e.g., Benton, 1961; Pyrtek et al., 2020). When electrostimulation is applied to the angular gyrus during open brain surgery, the four individual symptoms of the syndrome can be turned on and off somewhat individually, although they are located close together (Rusconi & Kleinschmidt, 2011). In other words, the syndrome may not be caused by damage to one specific region in the brain, but by damage across small regions that are located right next to one another. Because the brain's cells and blood supplies are so interconnected, like the roots of two plants growing together in the same pot, the regions probably don't have clean boundaries between them. This is why you don't automatically have all four of the symptoms, but you often have more than one, because damaging the roots of one plant probably damages the other.

And there's no guarantee that the symptoms will stay within the confines of those four, either. Gerstmann syndrome often occurs with other brain damage symptoms such as language difficulties (see Aphasia), reading difficulties (see Alexia), and others (Pyrtek et al., 2020). As you might expect, when a person has more Gerstmann syndrome symptoms, such as the entire tetrad, they usually have a bigger area of brain damage, and are therefore more likely to have other additional brain damage symptoms (Heimburger et al., 1964). For example, it's possible to produce agraphia by widely damaging a person's language processing centers in the brain, which may also harm their abilities to speak and read, but that's not necessarily the same type of agraphia that a person with Gerstmann syndrome develops. That is, in some cases of Gerstmann syndrome, the person struggles with writing but can successfully speak and read, possibly due to damage to the nonlinguistic components of writing ability in the brain while keeping the more linguistic regions intact (Pyrtek et al., 2020). Therefore, lots of possibilities exist.

In other words, the brain is complex enough that there are multiple ways to cause many symptoms and you could probably find a way to selectively damage areas in order to produce just one symptom, but the brain is also interconnected enough that causing one symptom may cause others. This makes it difficult to argue that there is anything special about the classic tetrad. However, the name Gerstmann syndrome may still be useful in describing how common it is for these symptoms to go hand in hand, which may tell a doctor which other possible symptoms should be examined. Each of the components of the tetrad should be measured and diagnosed individually. Sorry Gerstmann, but your syndrome was really just four smaller symptoms standing on top of each other's shoulders while wearing a trench coat so that they only needed to purchase a single ticket to the movie theater.

References

Anderson, S. W., Tranel, D., & Denburg, N. L. (2009). Agraphia. In L. R. Squire (Ed.), *Encyclopedia of neuroscience* (pp. 227–229). Academic Press (Elsevier).

Benton, A. L. (1961). The fiction of the Gerstmann syndrome. *Journal of Neurology, Neurosurgery, and Psychiatry, 24*, 176–181. https://doi.org/d2nx8c

Bhattacharyya, S., Cai, X., & Klein, J. P. (2014). Dyscalculia, dysgraphia, and left-right confusion from a left posterior peri-insular infarct. *Behavioural Neurology, 2014*. Article 823591. https://doi.org/gb5d88

Della Sala, S., & Spinnler, H. (1994). Finger agnosia: Fiction or reality? *Archives of Neurology, 51*(5), 448–450. https://doi.org/d2ztmz

Gerstmann, J. (1930). Zur Symptomatologie der Hirnläsionen im Übergangsgebiet der unteren Parietal-und mittleren Occipitalwindung. (Das Syndrom: Fingeragnosie, Rechts-Links-Störung, Agraphie, Akalkulie). *Nervenarzt, 3*, 691–695.

Gitelman, D. R. (2003). Acalculia: A disorder of numerical cognition. In M. D'Esposito (Ed.), *Neurological foundations of cognitive neuroscience* (pp. 129–163). MIT Press.

Grafman, J., Passafiume, D., Faglioni, P., & Boller, F. (1982). Calculation disturbances in adults with focal hemispheric damage. *Cortex, 18*(1), 37–49. https://doi.org/gtsn

Heimburger, R. F., Demyer, W., & Reitan, R. M. (1964). Implications of Gerstmann's syndrome. *Journal of Neurology, Neurosurgery, and Psychiatry, 27*(1), 52–57. https://doi.org/btv7qq

Kinsbourne, M., & Warrington, E. K. (1962). A study of finger agnosia. *Brain, 85*(1), 47–66. https://doi.org/cb6czx

Lebrun, Y. (2005). Gerstmann's syndrome. *Journal of Neurolinguistics, 18*(4), 317–326. https://doi.org/dmw8sz

Mayer, E., Martory, M. D., Pegna, A. J., Landis, T., Delavelle, J., & Annoni, J. M. (1999). A pure case of Gerstmann syndrome with a subangular lesion. *Brain, 122*(6), 1107–1120. https://doi.org/bph

Miller, C. J., & Hynd, G. W. (2004). What ever happened to developmental Gerstmann's syndrome? Links to other pediatric, genetic, and neurodevelopmental syndromes. *Journal of Child Neurology, 19*(4), 282–289. https://doi.org/dpxhdz

Pyrtek, S., Badziński, A., Adamczyk-Sowa, M., & Pąchalska, M. (2020). Does Gerstmann syndrome exist? *Acta Neuropsychologica, 18*(2), 259–284.

Rusconi, E., & Kleinschmidt, A. (2011). Gerstmann's syndrome: Where does it come from and what does that tell us? *Future Neurology, 6*(1), 23–32. https://doi.org/bs2n4k

Tucha, O., Steup, A., Smely, C., & Lange, K. W. (1997). Toe agnosia in Gerstmann syndrome. *Journal of Neurology, Neurosurgery & Psychiatry, 63*(3), 399–403. https://doi.org/brhv2p

Wilkins, R. H., & Brody, I. A. (1971). Gerstmann's syndrome. *Archives of Neurology, 24*(5), 475–476. https://doi.org/c3x3zq

Willmes, K. (2008). Acalculia. In G. Goldenberg & B. L. Miller (Eds.), *Handbook of clinical neurology* (pp 339–358). Elsevier. https://doi.org/bsp25k

Hemianopsia (and Scotoma)

Imagine that you can't see part of the world in front of you. In the case of hemianopsia, a dark void eats up one entire half of your visual field, such that there is a middle line beyond which you cannot see anything. In the case of a scotoma, you have a missing part of your vision in any variety of shape with hard or soft edges that eats away at the environment around you. In order to be able to see things, you have to look at them in a certain way such that your blind areas do not cover the objects up. What has gone wrong in your brain such that there are suddenly places that you can't see?

The Stories

(STORY 1) A 32-year-old woman had migraine headaches since about the age of 12, and each time that she had one, she would temporarily gain a blind spot in the upper-right part of her central vision. If drawn on a clock, she was blinded from 12 o'clock to 3 o'clock, but only in the middle part where the hands of the clock are located, not on the outer edge where the clock numbers are located. This transient *scotoma* would appear along with the headache, slowly as if shading itself in from the top toward the middle. However, the "haze" in her eyes had recently become perpetually present for unknown reasons and was always there regardless of whether she had a headache or not. In essence, her temporary partial blindness had become permanent (Rich, 1948, p. 592).

(STORY 2) A 60-year-old schoolteacher was hit in the head by a basketball, which triggered a series of events that led to seeing "kaleidoscopic spots before her eyes" and a surgery (p. 959). She complained of bad headaches and that she felt like she was looking through a cloud. Even as her vision began to return to normal, it was discovered that she was suffering from a *homonymous* paracentral scotoma on the right side of her visual field. She could still see if she looked straight ahead, and the far edges of her vision were okay, but between the center and edges there was a big missing chunk from about 1 o'clock to 5 o'clock on a clock's face. With this hole in her visual field, she found it difficult to locate lines of words when attempting to read, and it was also difficult to find objects in general, such as a thimble or needle while she was sewing. Over

DOI: 10.4324/9781003276937-30

time, her visual field slowly improved and her ability to read became better (Barkan & Boyle, 1935).

(STORY 3) As part of a 1960 study into migrainous scotomas of hundreds of people, Walter Alvarez shared his experience over the course of dozens of his own recurring migrainous scotomas. He wrote that the scotoma would begin in the form of his vision becoming a bit fuzzy as if he could not focus his eyes, then a bright dot would appear. That bright dot would then change shape as he watched, becoming "a luminous zigzag line which runs almost always vertically … the line pulsates rapidly as if it were a tiny rubber tube through which some fluid was being pumped with rapid impulses" (pp. 490–491) From there, he reported that the line would bow outwards until it went "beyond the edge of the field of vision" (p. 491). These transformations of his scotoma took place over the course of about 20 minutes, after which his vision returned to normal (Alvarez, 1960, p. 491).

(STORY 4) A 36-year-old woman lost consciousness and was taken to a hospital. Six months before that, she had major cranial surgery to remove a large tumor. At the hospital, it was discovered that she had developed a right-sided *homonymous hemianopsia* such that she was blind in most of her right field of vision. Interestingly, however, she retained the ability to detect movement on the right side of her visual field, even though she could not see color or form. She could detect movement even in the most extreme periphery of her visual field, despite it appearing completely dark and empty. The researchers noted in the case study that "we lack an explanation for this observation even though there may be many hypotheses" (p. 410). Since then, scientists have discovered many more examples of what is now called "blindsight" (see Cortical Blindness) and have begun to piece together how such a symptom is possible. This patient displayed both homonymous hemianopsia and blindsight at the same time (Bender & Kanzer, 1939, case 5).

The Features

Huge swaths of your brain contribute to processing the visual information that your eyes collect. Usually, your brain does this automatically behind the scenes. However, when the brain is damaged, your visual centers may no longer receive all of the visual information from your eyes. You may lose the ability to see a chunk of the space in front of you. This leaves behind an inky void of partial blindness like someone has drawn with a black permanent marker on the inside of your eye.

Hemianopsia (also spelled hemianopia) is a type of partial blindness that affects *half* of a person's vision. This partial blindness can be annoying, such as when this affects a person's ability to read, and it can be dangerous, when affecting a person's ability to navigate around objects or avoid falling over (Goodwin, 2014). There are several types of hemianopsia, and they all have long names that can take some getting used to.

Homonymous hemianopsia is the type that neurologists are usually referring to when they say "hemianopsia." Homonymous hemianopsia is a visual defect where you can't see out of one half of each eye—the *same* half on each side. Pretend that for each of your eyeballs, there is a black line running from the top to the bottom right down the middle. Now, pretend that you have a marker with black ink and shade in everything on one side—left or right—of that line, turning your eyes into half-moons. Now, you are effectively blind to one side of your nose. This is similar to what homonymous hemianopsia is like.

Homonymous means "on the same side." However, in rare cases, the halves of your eyes that are not working properly do not need to be on the same side. If the halves are on opposite sides, it is called *heteronymous hemianopsia*. There are two subtypes of this heteronymous type: *binasal* and *bitemporal*. Binasal is when the two halves that are blind are the inside halves by your nose, and it is extremely rare (Tsokolas et al., 2020). Bitemporal is when the blind halves are the outside halves by the temples, and it can be caused, for example, by a rare type of tumor in the pituitary gland (Azmeh, 2018).

There is also a less severe version of hemianopsia called *quadrantanopsia*, which affects only a quarter of a person's visual field instead of half of their visual field. For example, you could have an upper-left quadrantanopsia or a lower-right quadrantanopsia, and so on.

Now we get into the really rare stuff: it is possible to experience something called *crossed-quadrant homonymous hemianopsia*, which is also called a "checker-board visual field defect" if you're low on syllables (Cross & Smith, 1982). This visual defect involves what is essentially two quadrantanopsias at the same time, although they may not originally appear at the same time (Dyer et al., 1990). A person with this condition might be blind, for example, in the lower-left quadrant and the upper-right quadrant of their vision.

Another type of partial vision loss that can be due to brain damage is the *scotoma*. Scotomas are "blind spots" in a person's vision, often with irregularly shaped borders that make them resemble blobs. You know those "floater" shapes that you sometimes notice floating around inside of your eye, especially in bright places? Scotomas can be kind of like those, except fixed in place and, generally, larger.

There are different types of scotomas. The kind that completely removes a person's ability to see in a part of their eye is called an *absolute scotoma*, which resembles a black shape drawn inside of the eyeball. But some scotomas are partially transparent, allowing some vision, called a *relative scotoma*. People may have a part of their visual field where they cannot perceive color, or perhaps have distorted color, in a *color scotoma*. Additionally, people may experience *metamorphosias* which distort space "like a bubble in a pane of glass" (New & Scholl, 2018, p. 6).

People who have scotomas that are far away from the center of their eyes or have certain mild types, especially metamorphosias, may not even be aware that they have a scotoma. But if the scotoma gets worse and begins to include central vision, the person will probably begin to notice the problem (Midena & Vujosevic, 2016).

People can get along without noticing scotomas because their brain fills in missing information as part of its ordinary process of creating vision. The brain does this in at least two ways. The first is through *nystagmus*, which are tiny automatic eye movements, which allow your eyes to gather information from around the scotoma, letting you fill in some missing information (Valmaggia & Gottlob, 2002). The second is through *filling in*, or *perceptual completion*, wherein your brain basically makes an educated guess about what things are *supposed* to look like (New & Scholl, 2018). Don't believe me? Your brain is doing this *right now* because you have a minimum of one scotoma in each of your eyes.

The scotoma that everyone has is called the *blind spot*, which occurs in the location at which your optic nerve fibers exit the back of your eye in order to carry information from your light-sensitive *retina* to your brain. But the optic nerve fibers themselves cannot see; they are blind and, therefore, you are blind in that spot in each of your eyes. However, your brain does a great job of filling the blind spot in, making you forget that it's there. We're so good at forgetting about it, that it wasn't officially discovered until the 1600s even though it's *right there* (Finger, 1994). The discovery of the blind spot was so important that it was demonstrated before King Charles II of England (Faraday's Eyesight and the Blind Spot, 1935). Similarly, people with additional scotomas often get used to having them and adapt their viewing habits, especially reading, to compensate for missing information.

The Brain Pathology

The causes of these symptoms of vision loss are, in most cases, relatively well understood. Hemianopsia and scotomas can be caused by many things such as vascular diseases in the eyes, nutritional deficiency, and diseases that affect the myelin sheaths of nerve cells (Gillig & Sanders, 2009). Hemianopsia and scotomas can also be caused by direct damage to the brain, such as area V1 in the occipital lobe (Corballis, 1994). Because that part of the brain is *topographically organized*, like a map of your visual field, you can actually predict which part of a person's vision a scotoma will appear in based on where their brain is damaged, and vice versa (Kosslyn et al., 2006).

Hemianopsia and scotomas can be permanent, such as in cases where brain matter is actually destroyed, for example in strokes, traumatic brain injuries, and tumors. Or they may be temporary, especially in cases of migraine (see Migraine Headaches), seizures (see Seizures), and sometimes with variation in blood sugar (Goodwin, 2014). One such case was described in 1825: "I have known an instance of obfuscation of sight of many hours duration in a patient after an epileptic fit … in this case the patient could see only a perpendicular half of any object at which he looked" (Parry, 1825, p. 559). As you might imagine, temporary blindness can be very disturbing for a person when they open their eyes to see that they are now partially unable to see.

Improving your vision after hemianopsia or a scotoma is a tricky subject. On the one hand, there is very little evidence that interventions, in order to force a person's visual deficit to improve, actually work (Pollock et al., 2019; Riggs et al., 2007). In other words, researchers have been unable to definitively show that a person with one of these disorders can intentionally train themselves to see better following the brain damage. But, on the other hand, someone who has developed a visual deficit such as a homonymous hemianopsia may see some improvement in their ability to use visual information as their brain recovers. At the very least, people with partial vision loss tend to do an amazing job of adapting, and over time their brain helps them to gather what information it can and then tries to fill in the rest.

References

Alvarez, W. C. (1960). The migrainous scotoma as studied in 618 persons. *American Journal of Ophthalmology, 49*(3), 489–504. https://doi.org/gtsp

Azmeh, A. (2018). Neuro-ophthalmology findings in pituitary disease (review of literature). In F. Assaad, H. Wassmann, & M. Khodor (Eds.), *Pituitary diseases*. IntechOpen. https://doi.org/gtsq

Barkan, O., & Boyle, S. F. (1935). Paracentral homonymous hemianopic scotoma. *Archives of Ophthalmology, 14*(6), 957–959. https://doi.org/fxgntr

Bender, M. B., & Kanzer, M. G. (1939). Dynamics of homonymous hemianopias and preservation of central vision. *Brain, 62*(4), 404–421. https://doi.org/ccd4j7

Corballis, M. C. (1994). Neuropsychology of perceptual functions. In D. W. Zaidel (Ed.), *Neuropsychology* (2nd ed., pp. 83–104). Academic Press. https://doi.org/gtsr

Cross, S. A., & Smith, J. L. (1982). Crossed-quadrant homonymous hemianopsia. The "checkerboard" field defect. *Journal of Clinical Neuro-Ophthalmology, 2*(3), 149–158.

Dyer, J. A., Hirst, L. W., Vandeleur, K., Carey, T., & Mann, P. R. (1990). Crossed-quadrant homonymous hemianopsia. *Journal of Clinical Neuro-Ophthalmology, 10*(3), 219–222.

Faraday's Eyesight and the Blind Spot (1935). *Nature, 136*, 542. https://doi.org/cd942m

Finger, S. (1994). *Origins of neuroscience: A history of explorations into brain function*. Oxford University Press.

Gillig, P. M., & Sanders, R. D. (2009). Cranial nerve II: Vision. *Psychiatry (Edgemont), 6*(9), 32–37.

Goodwin, D. (2014). Homonymous hemianopia: Challenges and solutions. *Clinical Ophthalmology, 2014*(8), 1919–1927. https://doi.org/gtss

Kosslyn, S. M., Thompson, W. L., & Ganis, G. (2006). *The case for mental imagery*. Oxford University Press. https://doi.org/ct8kh5

Midena, E., & Vujosevic, S. (2016). Metamorphopsia: An overlooked visual symptom. *Ophthalmic Research, 55*(1), 26–36. https://doi.org/gtst

New, J. J., & Scholl, B. J. (2018). Motion-induced blindness for dynamic targets: Further explorations of the perceptual scotoma hypothesis. *Journal of Vision, 18*(9), Article 24. https://doi.org/gtsv

Parry, C. H. (1825). *Collections from the unpublished medical writings of the late Caleb Hillier Parry* (Vol. 1). Underwoods.

Pollock, A., Hazelton, C., Rowe, F. J., Jonuscheit, S., Kernohan, A., Angilley, J., Henderson, C. A., Langhorne, P., & Campbell, P. (2019). Interventions for visual field defects in people with stroke. *Cochrane Database of Systematic Reviews*, *5*, Article CD008388. https://doi.org/gg66d9

Rich, W. M. (1948). Permanent homonymous quadrantanopia after migraine. *British Medical Journal*, *1*(4551), 592–594. https://doi.org/cr6h35

Riggs, R. V., Andrews, K., Roberts, P., & Gilewski, M. (2007). Visual deficit interventions in adult stroke and brain injury: A systematic review. *American Journal of Physical Medicine & Rehabilitation*, *86*(10), 853–860. https://doi.org/ff2p8c

Tsokolas, G., Khan, H., Tyradellis, S., George, J. & Lawden, M. (2020). Binasal congruous hemianopia secondary to functional visual loss: A case report. *Medicine*, *99*(27), Article e20754. https://doi.org/gtsw

Valmaggia, C., & Gottlob, I. (2002). Optokinetic nystagmus elicited by filling-in in adults with central scotoma. *Investigative Ophthalmology and Visual Science*, *43*(6), 1804–1808.

Hemispatial Neglect (and Autosomatagnosia)

Imagine that you can't remember that "left" exists. Yes, the entire spatial direction of left. You cannot recall that you have a left side of your body, and neglect to groom your hair and face on that side. You cannot perceive the left side of space, such that when you look at a room you will only see objects located to your right. You may even see only the right side of objects and neglect their other half. Whenever you must turn your body, you only turn it to the right. After all, what other direction is there?

The Stories

(STORY 1) In the case of an 81-year-old woman, a hemorrhagic stroke produced brain damage resulting in neglect. While hospitalized, the clinicians made careful observations of her behavior. She would run into objects on her left side without realizing that they were there, and she would drop objects from her left hand without realizing that it was happening. She could pay attention to things on her left if she was directly instructed to do so but otherwise seemed to forget about them. She would sometimes stop what she was doing when she reached the midline of her visual field, where the left meets right, such that she would not draw the left side of drawings or complete the left side of writings. When she was asked to draw a clock, she neglected the numbers located on the left side of the clockface and struggled repeatedly to decide where to draw. When medical workers entered her room from the left side of her bed, she experienced "distress," probably because they surprised her when they appeared—she wasn't able to realize that they were entering the room due to her neglect on that side. To fix this, she was moved to a room with a right-sided entrance so that she could more easily realize when people were approaching (DeVore et al., 2017).

(STORY 2) A 51-year-old woman experienced a sudden temporary *autosomatagnosia* in her left hand. That is, she experienced a period during which she could no longer sense or move that hand. She could see her left arm only above her elbow and felt as if there was only empty table space where her hand was resting on the table. As she sat and waited, she slowly began to be able to perceive her hand again, beginning with the pinky and moving toward her

DOI: 10.4324/9781003276937-31

thumb but leaving what seemed like holes in the middle of her hand. Her lost hand re-emerged completely after a few minutes, and she regained the ability to sense it and move it as before. When examined several days after this incident, it was discovered that she had experienced a blood clot in the right side of her brain, leading to two small lesions in the motor and premotor cortex on that side (Arzy et al., 2006).

(STORY 3) A stroke resulted in left-sided neglect in a 65-year-old woman. Brain scans revealed that her right middle cerebral artery in her brain had become blocked, leading to a stroke in her posterior inferior parietal lobe and the resulting neglect symptoms. While hospitalized, she tended to lie in bed at an angle that was "oriented to her right" while ignoring the left side of her body (p. 1). She had *somatoparaphrenia* for her left arm, such that when she was shown her own arm by a medical examiner holding it in front of her, she claimed that the arm belonged to the examiner, and not to herself. She would turn to look to the right even when someone spoke to her from her left side. Additionally, at mealtimes she would ignore the food on the left half of her meal tray and eat only the right-handed portion, and the food she ate would occasionally collect in the left side of her mouth where she neglected it. At first, she denied that anything was wrong with her, other than feeling a bit weak, but eventually improved enough to realize the severe extent of her left-sided weakness. She eventually regained some feelings for her left side, and the obvious signs of neglect faded away (Chatterjee, 2003).

The Features

If there's a disorder in this book that is most difficult to wrap your head around, it just might be neglect. Neglect refers to the tendency of a person to *ignore parts of space* around them or to *ignore parts of themselves*. In plain but vague terms, the person acts as if parts of the world do not exist when those parts are in specific locations.

Unfortunately for science communication books, experts disagree on the different types of neglect (Marsh & Hillis, 2008). The categories of neglect disorders "overlap and shift" (Brock & Merwarth, 1957, p. 366). Thus, the shades and tints of this disorder are a bit muddy, so hold my hand tightly as we explore.

Let's begin with people who lose perception of part of *space*. Commonly, a single "half" of space is affected, usually the left half. For example, one early description described this as a condition in which a person "never attended to his left body half, apparently never missed it, and seemed to have completely forgotten about it" and "appeared grossly perplexed when one started to talk about his left body side" (Zingerle, 1913, translated in Benke et al., 2004, p. 268). Because this type of neglect tends to affect halves—that is, it encompasses half of space in one direction—it is often called *hemispatial neglect* or unilateral neglect. Think about where you are sitting right now, whether it is in a room or outside. Take note of everything that is located to your left: your left arm, that stack of books, that cloud. Now, imagine if you had no idea that those things existed. Not because you can't see them, but because your brain isn't paying *attention* to them. They *do not enter your conscious awareness*.

Hemispatial neglect sparked much philosophical debate regarding the nature of consciousness. Many people with hemispatial neglect are *unaware* that they are neglecting part of space, which can make this disorder a type of anosognosia (see Anosognosia). If you want a book that deals with the philosophy of not knowing that a direction in space exists, I highly recommend *Flatland* by Abbott (1884), although it is surprisingly sexist for a book about geometry. However, some people with neglect are actually aware of their problem with remembering that left exists, so we can't generalize too far (McGlynn & Schacter, 1989).

Hemispatial neglect can be broken down further into *personal* and *extrapersonal* neglect. Personal neglect refers to the person's own body, such that everything on the left side of their body does not exist as far as they are concerned. Instead, they neglect those body parts. They may forget to lace up their left shoe, incorrectly position their glasses on their left ear, and otherwise forget their left half (Baas et al., 2011). Some people may rarely or never use the arm or leg on their neglected side—although they may still use those limbs when pressured to do so (Sampanis & Riddoch, 2013). One way that personal neglect is tested for is by using a *comb and razor test* to see how the person grooms themselves—specifically, whether they ignore one side of their face and only comb and shave the other side (Beschin & Robertson, 1997). Personal neglect is closely related to the disorders of body imperception that are discussed a bit further on in this chapter.

Now let's get *extra*personal. That's the type of neglect where a person neglects objects that are out in the space around them. A person may forget to look to the left, for example, when searching a room for an object, concluding that it is not there when it would be in plain sight for someone without a neglect disorder. Or, if you hand them a crossword puzzle, they may only fill in the squares on the right side of the puzzle (Vallar & Bolognini, 2014). To make things more complicated, there are two subtypes of extrapersonal neglect that concern the position of the center of the neglected space.

Subject-centered neglect (also called egocentric neglect) is neglect from the point of view of the person with the neglect disorder. One way of testing for this type is with a *cancellation task*, in which the person is given a sheet of paper with many "targets" such as little lines or shapes. They are then asked to cross out all of a specific type of target. A person with typical subject-centered neglect is able to search for, find, and cross out all of the targets on the right-hand side of the piece of paper but is unable to complete the task for the targets on the left-hand side of the paper (Chatterjee, 2003).

Object-centered neglect (also called allocentric neglect) is neglect from the center of an object, such that it is the left side of the object that is not perceived by the neglect patient. Common examples of this include being unable to see food on the left side of a plate or being unable to see the left side of a clock's face. A common way of testing object-centered neglect is with *drawing* tasks, where the person is asked to copy a drawing of an image. A person with object-centered neglect draws an incomplete left side of the image or mistakenly draws features from the left side on the right side of the drawing (Chatterjee, 2003).

Subject-centered and object-centered neglect often occur in the same person, and some researchers have argued that object-centered neglect may only occur if subject-centered neglect is also present (Rorden et al., 2012). Whether or not object-centered and subject-centered neglect are actually separable disorders is still debated, with some evidence suggesting that the symptoms depend on the situation (Leyland et al., 2017). Subtypes of neglect can be even further specified with regard to distance from the body and sense used (seeing, touching, etc.), but those matters are even less clear-cut (Marsh & Hillis, 2008). Like I said, neglect is a muddy diagnosis.

Then there are the disorders of *body imperception*. The names given to disorders of body imperception are complex. Be careful not to mispronounce these words because your phone might start levitating while a dove shoots out of your shirtsleeve.

As a start, *asomatognosia* is the general feeling of nothingness surrounding physical parts, in other words, a lack of awareness of one's own body. If you've ever had the feeling that a part of your body has stopped existing—maybe you laid on top of your arm for too long and no longer know where it is located thanks to a complete feeling of numbness—you've had temporary asomatognosia. Asomatognosia and neglect often happen in the same person at the same time, but this is not always true—either one is possible without the occurrence of the other (Jenkinson et al., 2018). It gets even more complicated, because there are at least two subtypes of asomatognosia.

One subtype of asomatognosia is called *autosomatagnosia*, where a person experiences the feeling of nothingness *and* has a lack of conscious recognition for part of their body (Gerstmann, 1942). If a person has autosomatagnosia, they will not consciously experience a neglected body part as belonging to them even if you show them that body part; instead, they may experience nonexistence as if the body part was not physically present (Vallar & Ronchi, 2009).

There is also a subtype of asomatognosia called *somatoparaphrenia* that has its own chapter. It is a delusion of ownership related to a body part affected by asomatognosia, such as believing that your leg belongs to someone else (see Somatoparaphrenia).

Interestingly, during the phase of sleep called *rapid eye movement*, some people with neglect have shown evidence that their eye movements avoid their neglected area—this may mean that the direction of left doesn't exist in their *dreams*, either (Doricchi et al., 1993). And, if you ask a person with neglect to imagine a scene, such as standing in the center of a town, they may be unable to *imagine* parts of the scene located in their neglected space (Bisiach & Luzzatti, 1978). Imagination blindness is further discussed elsewhere in this book (see Aphantasia).

Now that we've discussed neglect, let's explore how it's possible for a person to forget that an entire direction of space exists. Especially: how is it possible that a person can have a limb attached to them without knowing about it?

The Brain Pathology

Neglect is a common disorder. It has a variety of possible causes including neurodegenerative diseases and trauma, but it is especially well known as a symptom following a stroke (Li & Malhotra, 2015). It has long been debated exactly where brain damage needs to occur in order to cause symptoms of hemispatial neglect, but it turns out that "exactly where" may have been too specific a question.

Some candidates for brain damage that may cause neglect are the "middle and superior temporal gyrus, inferior parietal lobule, intraparietal sulcus, precuneus, middle occipital gyrus, caudate nucleus, and posterior insula, as well as in the white matter pathway corresponding to the posterior part of the superior longitudinal fasciculus" (Molenberghs et al., 2012). Thus, neglect seems to be a possible symptom of brain damage in a variety of places including the frontal, temporal, and parietal lobes, as well as subcortical structures underneath (Li & Malhotra, 2015). If you flipped open a brain atlas to a random page and pointed at an illustration of a brain structure, there is a decent chance for that structure to be involved in neglect. My point is that the calculations that the brain uses to understand space are intricate (see Topographical Disorientation). This is why researchers have switched "from trying to identify a single brain area to investigations of brain areas that are involved as sub-components of a more complex network, responsible for space attention and representation" (Gammeri et al., 2020).

Something that we do know is that damage to the *right* side of the brain is more likely to produce symptoms of neglect than damage to the left side. This explains why *left* is the direction that is most likely to be forgotten—because the right side of the brain is responsible for sensing the left side of the body. But what makes right-sided damage especially likely to cause this disorder? One possible answer is that the right side of the brain is more likely to pay attention to both sides of space, while the left side of the brain often prefers to pay attention only to the right side of space (Heilman & Van Den Abell, 1980). In other words, the right brain tends to pay attention to more space than the left brain. To oversimplify, imagine that your right brain has security cameras that monitor both your right side and your left side, while your left brain only has security cameras for your right side. Therefore, when the right brain is damaged the left brain neglects part of space as a result of the missing camera feed. In contrast, when the left brain is damaged, the right brain typically *does* continue to pay attention to both sides.

Similarly, there is a theory that neglect arises because the two halves of the brain actively *inhibit* the attention being paid by the other half of the brain—that is, the hemispheres of the brain compete with each other to pay attention to their respective regions of space by slowing each other down (Kinsbourne, 1977). Trust no one, not even your own brain. Thus, when one half is damaged, the remaining half suppresses attention to that side of space, essentially "forgetting" that it is there in favor of paying attention to its preferred side of space. Because the left brain tends to have a strong preference for the right side of space, when the right side of the brain is damaged and stops inhibiting the left brain, the left brain takes over a bunch of attentional resources that used to be shared more equally, and instead dedicates them to monitoring the right side of space.

Oftentimes, neglect symptoms go away on their own over time as the person recovers. However, sometimes they continue to linger for months or longer following the brain injury (Gammeri et al., 2020). There are a few things that doctors can do to try and help neglect patients recover. While some drugs have been tried, most neglect treatments are not based on medication (Chatterjee, 2003). One of the first methods that was used successfully to temporarily treat neglect was called "caloric stimulation" which involved pouring cold water into the left ear (Rubens, 1985). But because of the "general impracticality of ear irrigation"—or earigation, as it is called by no one—other methods such as galvanic stimulation are used (Wilkinson et al., 2014). That involves sending tiny electric shocks into the bones just behind the ears in order to remind the brain that there are two different sides of the body. Another approach to treating neglect is prismatic adaptation, in which a person wears special reality-warping glasses or goggles that bend light in a way that allows them to interact with and understand more of their environment, and sometimes this prism training takes place in virtual environments designed to retrain the person's brain (Gammeri et al., 2020). As more is learned about the different subtypes of neglect, it will become easier to treat people with specific issues, as we begin to determine exactly why their left was left behind.

References

Abbott, E. A. (1884). *Flatland: A romance of many dimensions.* Seeley & Co.

Arzy, S., Overney, L. S., Landis, T., & Blanke, O. (2006). Neural mechanisms of embodiment: Asomatognosia due to premotor cortex damage. *Archives of Neurology, 63*(7), 1022–1025. https://doi.org/cdrrzt

Baas, U., de Haan, B., Grässli, T., Karnath, H. O., Mueri, R., Perrig, W. J., Wurtz, P., & Gutbrod, K. (2011). Personal neglect–A disorder of body representation? *Neuropsychologia, 49*(5), 898–905. https://doi.org/fsfm2s

Benke, T., Luzzatti, C., & Vallar, G. (2004). Hermann Zingerle's "Impaired perception of the own body due to organic brain disorders" An introductory comment, and an abridged translation. *Cortex, 40*(2), 265–274. https://doi.org/fqx3nr

Beschin, N., & Robertson, I. H. (1997). Personal versus extrapersonal neglect: A group study of their dissociation using a reliable clinical test. *Cortex, 33*(2), 379–384. https://doi.org/csks24

Bisiach, E., & Luzzatti, C. (1978). Unilateral neglect of representational space. *Cortex, 14*(1), 129–133. https://doi.org/ggbwbw

Brock, S., & Merwarth, H. R. (1957). The illusory awareness of body parts in cerebral disease. *Archives of Neurology & Psychiatry*, 77(4), 366–375. https://doi.org/gtsx

Chatterjee, A. (2003). Neglect: A disorder of spatial attention. In M. D'Esposito (Ed.), *Neurological foundations of cognitive neuroscience* (pp. 1–26). MIT Press.

DeVore, B. B., Campbell, R. W., Harrison, P. K., & Harrison, D. W. (2017). Left gaze bias with left sensory hemineglect syndrome: Hallucinations and hemispatial neglect following right middle cerebral artery cerebrovascular accident. *BAOJ Neurology*, 3(4), Article 44.

Doricchi, F., Guariglia, C., Paolucci, S., & Pizzamiglio, L. (1993). Disturbances of the rapid eye movements (REMs) of REM sleep in patients with unilateral attentional neglect: Clue for the understanding of the functional meaning of REMs. *Electroencephalography and Clinical Neurophysiology*, 87(3), 105–116. https://doi.org/fbfxj2

Gammeri, R., Iacono, C., Ricci, R., & Salatino, A. (2020). Unilateral spatial neglect after stroke: Current insights. *Neuropsychiatric Disease and Treatment*, 16, 131–152. https://doi.org/gtsz

Gerstmann, J. (1942). Problem of imperception of disease and of impaired body territories with organic lesions. *Archives of Neurology and Psychiatry* 48(6), 890–913. https://doi.org/gts2

Heilman, K. M., & Van Den Abell, T. (1980). Right hemisphere dominance for attention: The mechanism underlying hemispheric asymmetries of inattention (neglect). *Neurology*, 30(3), 327–327. https://doi.org/gts3

Jenkinson, P. M., Moro, V., & Fotopoulou, A. (2018). Definition: Asomatognosia. *Cortex*, 101, 300–301. https://doi.org/gc8zbv

Kinsbourne, M. (1977). Hemi-neglect and hemisphere rivalry. *Advances in Neurology*, 18, 41–49.

Leyland, L. A., Godwin, H. J., Benson, V., & Liversedge, S. P. (2017). Neglect patients exhibit egocentric or allocentric neglect for the same stimulus contingent upon task demands. *Scientific Reports*, 7(1941), 1–9. https://doi.org/f99c7h

Li, K., & Malhotra, P. A. (2015). Spatial neglect. *Practical Neurology*, 15(5), 333–339. https://doi.org/f8rcrp

Marsh, E. B., & Hillis, A. E. (2008). Dissociation between egocentric and allocentric visuospatial and tactile neglect in acute stroke. *Cortex*, 44(9), 1215–1220. https://doi.org/bcstxz

McGlynn, S. M., & Schacter, D. L. (1989). Unawareness of deficits in neuropsychological syndromes. *Journal of Clinical and Experimental Neuropsychology*, 11(2), 143–205. https://doi.org/fvzpkj

Molenberghs, P., Sale, M. V., & Mattingley, J. B. (2012). Is there a critical lesion site for unilateral spatial neglect? A meta-analysis using activation likelihood estimation. *Frontiers in Human Neuroscience*, 6, Article 78. https://doi.org/ggcpfr

Rorden, C., Hjaltason, H., Fillmore, P., Fridriksson, J., Kjartansson, O., Magnusdottir, S., & Karnath, H. O. (2012). Allocentric neglect strongly associated with egocentric neglect. *Neuropsychologia*, 50(6), 1151–1157. https://doi.org/f3x64q

Rubens, A. B. (1985). Caloric stimulation and unilateral visual neglect. *Neurology*, 35(7), 1019–1024. https://doi.org/gts4

Sampanis, D. S., & Riddoch, J. (2013). Motor neglect and future directions for research. *Frontiers in Human Neuroscience*, 7, Article 110. https://doi.org/gts5

Vallar, G., & Bolognini, N. (2014). Unilateral spatial neglect. In A. C. Nobre & S. Kastner (Eds.), *The Oxford handbook of attention* (pp. 972–1027). Oxford University Press. https://doi.org/hqnx

Vallar, G., & Ronchi, R. (2009). Somatoparaphrenia: A body delusion. A review of the neuropsychological literature. *Experimental Brain Research*, *192*(3), 533–551. https://doi .org/cw8spn

Wilkinson, D., Zubko, O., Sakel, M., Coulton, S., Higgins, T., & Pullicino, P. (2014). Galvanic vestibular stimulation in hemi-spatial neglect. *Frontiers in Integrative Neuroscience*, *8*, Article 4. https://doi.org/gts6

Zingerle, H. (1913). Über Störungen der Wahrnehmung des eigenen Körpers bei organischen Gehirnerkrankungen. *Monatsschrift für Psychiatrie und Neurologie*, *34*, 13–36.

Klüver–Bucy Syndrome

Imagine that your behavior was completely impulsive. Specifically, you found yourself full of uncontrollable impulses to look at objects, grab them, and to try and put them in your mouth. Hunger never goes away, even after you have eaten, and you find yourself drawn to eat things that aren't even food. Extreme sexual impulses cause you to touch yourself and others in inappropriate places at extremely inappropriate times. You no longer respond to events that should make you angry. The parts of yourself that previously managed your behavior vanish, leaving behind a version of yourself that behaves on impulse, without considering consequences. Was this version of you always hiding somewhere in your brain?

The Stories

(STORY 1) In the case of a 14-year-old boy, Klüver–Bucy syndrome (KBS) developed following an attack of mycoplasmal bronchitis that caused a fever, sore throat, cough, and unusual drowsiness. His fever broke and he became fully awake again on the tenth day of his illness, but his behavior had completely changed. He had become entirely sexually uninhibited, exposing himself in public and grabbing people in inappropriate places as a result of this new *hypersexuality*. He began to use his mouth to explore objects, a classic *hyperorality* behavior associated with KBS. He lost some memories, and he also lost the ability to "recognize some possessions and some people, such as his school friends" (p. 321). A brain scan revealed abnormalities in the temporal lobes of his brain, and he was treated with medication. The behavioral symptoms of KBS stopped a few days later and did not return over the course of six months, indicating successful treatment (Auvichayapat et al., 2006).

(STORY 2) A 12-year-old girl collapsed and had a 20-minute seizure following the running of a two-mile race during which "no fluids were available" (p. 73). As a result, she acquired brain damage as a complication of heatstroke. She "did not seem to recognize family members," her ability to use language disappeared, and she showed a lack of emotional responses to the world around her (p. 73). When objects were placed in her hand, she "immediately brought them to her mouth to examine orally and attempt to eat" (p. 73). She showed

DOI: 10.4324/9781003276937-32

hypermetamorphosis, with an increased interest in exploring objects visually, and especially liked to look at the reflection of her own face in the mirror while she wiggled her facial features such as her eyebrows and tongue. She showed some clear evidence of hypersexuality, as well, including attempts to kiss people. During her rehabilitation at a facility for brain injury recovery, she began to show the return of some language abilities, such as singing, and completing sentences or nursery rhymes that other people started for her. However, in this unfortunate case, the patient did not fully recover and continued to be dependent on caregivers for her basic needs (Pitt et al., 1995).

(STORY 3) A 14-year-old boy developed several symptoms over the course of a few days including drooping eyelids, crossed eyes, and difficulties with walking. After being hospitalized, he began to show new symptoms including excessive sleepiness and problems with his speech—such as speaking incoherently. Over the course of the next three weeks in the hospital, his condition worsened and new signs began to appear, including classic KBS signs. Hyperorality led him to impulsively nibble on many things including bedsheets and "everything on which he could lay hands" (p. 105). He self-inflicted "deep bite marks" on both of his arms (p. 105). In addition, hypersexuality, explosive anger, and short-term memory loss developed. The symptom of hypermetamorphosis developed, and he increased the attention he paid to "everything around him," becoming hypervigilant (p. 105). An autoimmune disorder was suspected, and he began to be treated with various medicines. Eventually, the hyperorality, drooping eyelids, short-term memory problems, hypersexuality, and other problems went away. However, some behavioral problems lingered, including a diagnosis of oppositional defiant disorder, which is defined by uncooperativeness toward other people (Juliá-Palacios et al., 2017, case 1).

The Features

In 1939, a research team including two men named Heinrich Klüver and Paul Bucy published research about what happened when they removed large sections of the brains of macaque monkeys (Klüver & Bucy, 1939). Specifically, they removed both of the temporal lobes—the large peninsula-like area of the cerebral cortex located above and behind your ear. I want to make a joke here about "monkeying around inside of their brains" but frankly the results were just too sad to joke about. The monkeys developed a collection of unfortunate symptoms that were detailed in the published research. Following the monkey studies, these symptoms appeared in some humans that also had parts of both of their temporal lobes removed—the notable difference was that the human surgeries were for the treatment of epilepsy and not just removing brain parts for the sake of seeing what would happen (Terzian & Ore, 1955). At that point, the syndrome was named after them—Klüver-Bucy syndrome (KBS) was born.

KBS symptoms may include difficulties in recognizing objects (see Visual Form Agnosia), short-term memory loss (see Amnesia), increased attentiveness to visual stimuli, oral tendencies and changes in dietary habits, loss of fear and/ or anger responses, and hypersexuality. Let's examine those symptoms that don't have their own chapters more closely.

Increased attentiveness to visual stimuli is referred to as *hypermetamorphosis*, which is defined as the "tendency to attend to and manipulate objects in the visual field" (Clay et al., 2019, p. 7). Essentially, the person will become interested in every object that they can see and will often reach out and play with that object. In its mild form, the person may merely touch items within reach, but in a more severe form, the person may snatch the items and try to stuff them into their mouth. This severe type overlaps with the next symptom of *hyperorality*.

The symptom of hyperorality can be summarized as changes to dietary habits and the tendency to put objects into the mouth whether or not they are food. A person with this symptom will eat more food, may eat things that are *not* food (such as toilet paper, tea bags, and shoe polish), and may put inedible objects into their mouths to feel them—this can lead to the person gaining a considerable amount of weight (Lilly et al., 1983). Hyperorality is the most commonly reported symptom of KBS when the disorder occurs in children (Juliá-Palacios et al., 2017).

The loss of fear and anger responses is called *placidity* in KBS cases and refers to a *blunting* of displayed emotion. Sufferers may not show warmth toward relatives or react emotionally to situations that would typically alarm or anger them. In severe cases, people with KBS may be "absolutely resistant to any attempt to arouse aggressiveness and violent reactions" such that they may not defend themselves when it is called for (Terzian & Ore, 1955, p. 376). In other cases, the placidity may come and go with time and be intermixed with states of agitation or aggression (Clay et al., 2019).

Hypersexuality as a symptom includes a sudden increase of highly sexual behaviors such as making indiscriminate sexual advances, attempts at the inappropriate sexual touching of others, and general sexual disinhibition. All of these behaviors tend to be "exhibitionistic" such that the person performs these actions and makes these comments in the presence of others instead of hiding them (Terzian & Ore, 1955). Many cases describe medical staff needing to be careful around such patients to ensure that they avoid the act of groping during medical examinations. Hypersexuality is frequently reported in KBS cases, with one review finding nearly 96% of cases in adolescents and adults included this symptom (Clay et al., 2019).

The Brain Pathology

At first glance, the brain pathology of KBS seems simple to explain: KBS occurs because of damage to the temporal lobes. That is the literal definition of the disorder, after all. But to investigate deeper, I should note that there are a few different ways to acquire the temporal lobe damage that leads to this constellation of symptoms.

KBS can exist from birth due to genetic disorders and grow worse with age (Hu et al., 2017). It can also occur suddenly due to traumatic brain injury, and many people with KBS acquire the injury from road traffic accidents (Clay et al., 2019). It sometimes also develops over time due to neurodegenerative diseases such as Alzheimer disease (Auvichayapat et al., 2006). Other possibilities of damaging events also exist, but what these causes have in common is relatively *extensive* damage leading to extremely reduced functioning of the temporal lobes of the brain, especially two parts called the hippocampus and the amygdala (Caro & Jimenez, 2016). Because the hippocampus plays a role in memory, and the amygdala plays a role in a person's emotional responses such as fear and anger, damage to these areas make intuitive sense for explaining the symptoms of KBS as discussed in this chapter. However, because the temporal lobes are such large parts of the brain, and there are two of them, the condition really ought to be thought of more complexly than simply "damage to those areas." Unfortunately, because this condition is uncommon and symptoms vary between people, much more work is needed in order to understand the nuances of how temporal lobe damage leads to KBS.

Interestingly, some people do recover from KBS, either partially or completely (Clay et al., 2019). Medication can help somewhat, but disruptive behaviors may continue. Klüver and Bucy discovered that their monkey … participants … were very resilient to developing the full disorder and showed that when only one temporal lobe was removed, or only certain connections were cut, the full constellation of symptoms did not appear (Klüver & Bucy, 1939). This, in combination with the fact that humans often partially recover, shows just how extreme the brain damage needs to be in order for KBS to take over completely. It appears that deep inside all of our brains are wild impulses that are kept in check by our temporal lobes.

References

Auvichayapat, N., Auvichayapat, P., Watanatorn, J., Thamaroj, J., & Jitpimolmard, S. (2006). Kluver–Bucy syndrome after mycoplasmal bronchitis. Epilepsy & Behavior, 8(1), 320–322. https://doi.org/bvxjk4

Caro, M. A., & Jimenez, X. F. (2016). Mesiotemporal disconnection and hypoactivity in Klüver-Bucy syndrome. The Journal of Clinical Psychiatry, 77(8), e982–e988. https://doi.org/gts7

Clay, F. J., Kuriakose, A., Lesche, D., Hicks, A. J., Zaman, H., Azizi, E., Ponsford, J. L., Jayaram, M., & Hopwood, M. (2019). Klüver-Bucy syndrome following traumatic brain injury: A systematic synthesis and review of pharmacological treatment from cases in adolescents and adults. The Journal of Neuropsychiatry and Clinical Neurosciences, 31(1), 6–16. https://doi.org/gts8

Hu, H., Hübner, C., Lukacs, Z., Musante, L., Gill, E., Wienker, T. F., Ropers, H.-H., Knierim, E., & Schuelke, M. (2017). Klüver–Bucy syndrome associated with a recessive variant in HGSNAT in two siblings with Mucopolysaccharidosis type IIIC (Sanfilippo C). European Journal of Human Genetics, 25(2), 253–256. https://doi.org/f9kxq5

Juliá-Palacios, N., Boronat, S., Delgado, I., Felipe, A., & Macaya, A. (2017). Pediatric Klüver–Bucy syndrome: Report of two cases and review of the literature. Neuropediatrics, 49(2), 104–111. https://doi.org/gc998t

Klüver, H., & Bucy, P. C. (1939). Preliminary analysis of functions of the temporal lobes in monkeys. Archives of Neurology & Psychiatry, 42(6), 979–1000. https://doi.org/gts9

Lilly, R., Cummings, J. L., Benson, D. F., & Frankel, M. (1983). The human Klüver-Bucy syndrome. Neurology, 33(9), 1141–1145. https://doi.org/gh5v2s

Pitt, D. C., Kriel, R. L., Wagner, N. C., & Krach, L. E. (1995). Kluver-Bucy syndrome following heat stroke in a 12-year-old girl. Pediatric Neurology, 13(1), 73–76. https://doi.org/c7z7gr

Terzian, H., & Ore, G. (1955). Syndrome of Klüver and Bucy: Reproduced in man by bilateral removal of the temporal lobes. Neurology, 5(6), 373–380. https://doi.org/gttc

Korsakoff Syndrome

Imagine that you can't form proper memories and instead invent your own. Whenever you need to fill in something that you don't remember, you just start talking. You make up lies about what happened to you in the past because you can't remember the truth. However, you yourself are unaware that the things that you are making up are not true. Where have your memories gone, and why have all of these untruths taken their place?

The Stories

(STORY 1) A woman over the age of 40 developed a severe memory disturbance diagnosed as Korsakoff syndrome. She believed that she was living in Ireland, despite having left that country long ago, when she was 19 years old. She had no memory of her subsequent marriage or the raising of her four children and *confabulated* untrue events to make sense of her world. Interestingly, she did retain small "islands" of memories from her adult years that she would haphazardly connect to other memories without realizing that the sequence of time was illogical. These fabricated sequences of events sometimes contained errors on the scale of years, such that events that had happened long ago were remembered as recent, and recent events were sometimes remembered as having happened long ago. She had been in hospital for over six years but, at one point, was confused about that time period, believing that the hospitalization had only lasted for a few days (Victor et al., 1971, pp. 53–54).

(STORY 2) A man who "remembered nothing for more than a few seconds" freely confabulated unending improvised truths about everything that he saw around him as a replacement for his ability to understand what was actually happening (p. 109). It seemed that he didn't know where he was, and misidentified the people that he interacted with, but he would speak in a rapid-fire way "without any appearance of uncertainty" continuously guessing and re-guessing what was going on around him (p. 109). He used to work as a grocer, and sometimes when people would greet him he would try to sell them delicatessen meats—or he would answer the phone in the hospital ward with a traditional delicatessen's greeting. When he was around people he never seemed to stop talking, and he immersed himself in a funny-but-tragic string of

DOI: 10.4324/9781003276937-33

narratives containing little, if any, truth. His Korsakoff syndrome allowed him to "literally make himself (and his world) up every moment" (p. 110). He once took a taxi and told the taxi driver amazing stories for the duration of the trip, which the driver could scarcely believe. Later, the doctor explained the situation to the taxi driver, which cleared things up (Sacks, 1998, pp. 108–115).

(STORY 3) A 67-year-old woman had begun drinking heavily following the death of her husband a few years prior. She was sometimes described as "confused" by her relatives (p. 526). She continued her work at a grocery store until her symptoms extended into muscle weakness and a more permanent confused state. During her hospitalization, it was discovered that she had severe problems with memory. Not only was she unable to recognize her hospital room and the medical staff, but she also had no idea what year or day it was. She also showed severe problems with her muscular system, including difficulty walking due to weakness and an absence of some reflexes. She was diagnosed with Wernicke-Korsakoff syndrome due to a lack of nutrients in her diet, partially stemming from alcoholism, but also a lack of nutritious food. She would confabulate freely about where she thought she was, and frequently claimed to be at home despite being in the hospital. When asked about why she was wearing a nightgown, she would sometimes claim that she was "in a hurry and had no time to change [into] … more appropriate clothing" (p. 527). Or she would claim that the reason she was in the hospital was to visit a friend. She would also confabulate past events, such as the reason why she couldn't walk. The real reason was nerve damage, but she claimed that burning coals had fallen on her toes (Dalla Barba et al., 1990).

(STORY 4) A 48-year-old woman with a history of excessive intake of alcohol was hospitalized with extreme symptoms of confabulation and received a diagnosis of Korsakoff syndrome. Her memory of recent events was very poor, and she often did not know where she was. She was given a series of tests where she was asked to name and draw images after looking at them. The images were presented at various levels of illumination and sometimes were presented with so little lighting that they could not be seen. However, these invisible pictures did not bother the patient; she confabulated a made-up image whenever she couldn't actually see it and seemed to actually believe that she had seen the things that she was confabulating and drawing. Sometimes, "the patient reported seeing material bearing no relation whatsoever to the visual stimuli presented, and made ready answers without regard to reality" (p. 332). When the pictures could be seen, she completed the tasks successfully. It seemed that whenever she was missing a detail in her mind, she would make something up and just go with it as if it were true (Wyke & Warrington, 1960).

The Features

Drinking excessive alcohol causes lots of problems for the brain. You might feel like you already know that much, but trust me, the problems that we are about to talk about are more troubling than you may be expecting. Not only does alcohol cause short-term changes that wear off when you sober up, but it also causes long-term damage if you drink enough of it. People who drink a lot of alcohol end up with smaller brains overall, whether you measure by reductions in brain volume, weight, or number of brain cells (Shahani et al., 2015). For alcoholics, even if they stop drinking, there may be permanent damage to the way that they think. One function that can become especially damaged is that of memory.

One memory-related disorder that can develop from alcohol abuse is called Korsakoff syndrome. It's named after the Russian neuropsychiatrist who discovered it. He preferred to call it "psychosis associated with polyneuritis," or rather, the Russian equivalent of that, so you can see why Korsakoff syndrome, or KS, sticks a bit better as a name (Victor & Yakovlev, 1955, p. 395). This syndrome includes amnesia (see Amnesia), as well as other characteristics.

The major component of KS is called *confabulation*. Confabulation is a type of amnesia that occurs when a person makes up a lie in order to fill in a gap in their memory (Wyke & Warrington, 1960). Korsakoff described this particular kind of forgetting back in the 1800s: "after a long conversation with the patient, one may note that at times he utterly confuses events and that he remembers absolutely nothing of what goes on around him … on occasion, such patients invent some fiction and constantly repeat it" (Korsakoff, 1889, as translated by Victor & Yakovlev, 1955, pp. 394–406). As the quote notes, it can take an entire conversation with the person with KS before you begin to sense that anything is off with their memory, but eventually their stories can no longer hold the weight of the falsehoods.

What makes confabulation different from lying is that the person is *unaware* that they are telling a lie (see Anosognosia). For example, if you ask a person with KS what they were doing last night, and they don't have any memory of that night, instead of saying that they don't know, they may misremember by accidentally generating an incorrect answer. They may tell you that they were playing video games with their brother at a local hotel, when they were really in the hospital at that time—and they often truly believe their mis-memory. Confabulation is sometimes called "honest lying" for this reason (Arts et al., 2017, p. 2883). Sometimes the confabulations are based on real memories that have been jumbled up and "recalled out of temporal sequence" (Kopelman et al., 2009, p. 149). In extreme cases called "fantastic" confabulations, the confabulations may be wild, quite grandiose, and may even include impossible events (Arts et al., 2017, p. 2883). For example, perhaps their brother is currently in a different country and the local hotel *burned down years ago*.

Besides confabulation, KS also includes several other cognitive and behavioral symptoms. One common symptom is retrograde amnesia, wherein the person might be unable to recall the last few decades of their life (Kopelman et al., 2009). Symptoms may also include lowered ability to form new memories, generally impaired executive functioning such as lowered ability to plan ahead, and lowered responsiveness and lack of self-initiated actions (Arts et al., 2017). These symptoms are not as attention-grabbing as confabulation and so are less often written about, but they are also important.

The Brain Pathology

Even though KS is often closely associated with excessive use of alcohol—which is indeed commonly the culprit—alcoholism is not strictly required in order to develop this disorder. What actually seems to cause KS is a nutritional deficiency, which will take some further explaining.

Korsakoff syndrome is often preceded by a condition called *Wernicke enceph-alopathy*, or WE (Kopelman et al., 2009). How often? Often enough that WE and KS were once considered by some physicians to be the same disease (Victor et al., 1971). It has been argued that WE *always* precedes KS, but because WE is difficult to diagnose, it is missed in some cases before it evolves into KS (Arts et al., 2017).

Wernicke encephalopathy is a condition that is "short-lived and severe" that includes mental confusion, difficulties in coordinating the movements of the lower limbs (see Ataxia), and difficulties in moving the eyes—these people may be so confused that they cannot figure out how to leave a room, and may even be unable to walk (Martin et al., 2003, p. 135). WE is a medical emergency that is frequently deadly, so treatment should begin as soon as it is discovered (Kopelman et al., 2009).

Wernicke encephalopathy is caused by a lack of the vitamin thiamine, also called vitamin B1, which is one of the vitamins that the human body does not make and therefore must be obtained through the diet (Martin et al., 2003). The two main ways to develop a deficiency of thiamine are via excessive alcohol intake or via malnourishment, and these often overlap, with alcoholics often lacking proper nourishment. There are, however, other ways to get it, such as when a person receives weight loss surgery that makes it difficult for them to intake and absorb thiamine (Shahani et al., 2015).

Thiamine is a "helper molecule" that allows the brain to function, assisting in the transformation of sugar into other useful molecules (Martin et al., 2003, p. 134). Treating a thiamine deficiency is as simple as adding thiamine back into the person, often with intravenous doses, but the treatment should be completed quickly (Shahani et al., 2015). Korsakoff syndrome is more likely to develop in people who had Wernicke encephalopathy and were not treated quickly or effectively enough for the vitamin deficiency (Arts et al., 2017). Fortunately, fast treatment of WE may prevent the development of KS (Shahani et al., 2015).

When KS does develop following WE, it is sometimes permanent. Many people with KS end up in long-term care facilities, where their confabulations may continue across years (Oudman et al., 2021). The lesson here is to keep an eye on your nutrition, as it really can make or break your brain.

References

Arts, N. J., Walvoort, S. J., & Kessels, R. P. (2017). Korsakoff's syndrome: A critical review. *Neuropsychiatric Disease and Treatment, 13*, 2875–2890. https://doi.org/gcnkcp

Dalla Barba, G., Cipolotti, L., & Denes, G. (1990). Autobiographical memory loss and confabulation in Korsakoff's syndrome: A case report. *Cortex, 26*(4), 525–534. https://doi.org/gttd

Корсаков, С.С. [Korsakoff, S. S.] (1889). Психическое расстройство в сочетании с множественным невритом. [Psychic disorder in conjunction with multiple neuritis]. Мед обзор [*Medizinskoje Obozrenije*], *32*(13), 3–18.

Kopelman, M. D., Thomson, A. D., Guerrini, I., & Marshall, E. J. (2009). The Korsakoff syndrome: Clinical aspects, psychology and treatment. *Alcohol and Alcoholism, 44*(2), 148–154. https://doi.org/cxjzmv

Martin, P. R., Singleton, C. K., & Hiller-Sturmhofel, S. (2003). The role of thiamine deficiency in alcoholic brain disease. *Alcohol Research & Health, 27*(2), 134–143.

Oudman, E., Rensen, Y., & Kessels, R. P. C. (2021). Confabulations in post-acute and chronic alcoholic Korsakoff's syndrome: a cross-sectional study conducted in two centres. *International Journal of Psychiatry in Clinical Practice.* https://doi.org/gj98pw

Sacks, O. (1998). *The man who mistook his wife for a hat and other clinical tales.* Touchstone.

Shahani, L., Noggle, C. A., & Thompson, J. C. (2015). Neuropsychological disturbance and alcoholism: Korsakoff's and beyond. In C. A. Noggle, R. S. Dean, S. S. Bush, & S. W. Anderson (Eds.), *The neuropsychology of cortical dementias* (pp. 199–220). Springer. https://doi.org/gttf

Victor, M., Adams, R. D., and Collins, G. H. (1971). *The Wernicke–Korsakoff syndrome.* F. A. Davis Company.

Victor, M., & Yakovlev, P. I. (1955). S. S. Korsakoff's psychic disorder in conjunction with peripheral neuritis to clinical medicine: A translation of Korsakoff's original article with brief comments on the author and his contribution to clinical medicine. *Neurology, 5*(6), 394–406. https://doi.org/gttg

Wyke, M., & Warrington, E. (1960). An experimental analysis of confabulation in a case of Korsakoff's syndrome using a tachistoscopic method. *Journal of Neurology, Neurosurgery, and Psychiatry, 23*(4), 327–333. https://doi.org/dhvhmw

Kuru

Imagine that you can't stop trembling and laughing. Formerly known as the laughing disease, kuru is no joke, because it is always deadly. Once you catch kuru, it is only a matter of time before you lose the ability to walk and instead lay in a shaky pile all day. But at the same time, you find yourself bursting into fits of inappropriate laughter. What is happening to your brain? What could you have done to acquire this disease? Maybe you should take a closer look at your diet.

The Stories

(STORY 1) In 1957, the first scientific report of kuru was published. The report discussed "a disease syndrome new to western medicine" that was ravaging the native people in "the Eastern Highlands of New Guinea" (p. 745). The stages of the disease were described as "uniform" in that specific symptoms appeared in a specific order (p. 746). In this report, the authors noted that the disease was primarily affecting women and that many of the older people in the villages claimed that the disease was not around when they were younger, indicating that the disease had shown up only within the past few decades. The kuru epidemic was ravaging the villages of the native people at this time, and in some communities "50% of all deaths … over the past five years have been from kuru" (p. 750). Interestingly, even though kuru is always fatal, the authors discussed a few reports of people seemingly recovering from kuru—but these cases turned out to be mimicry, such that they never really had the disease (Zigas & Gajdusek, 1957).

(STORY 2) In the case of a 42-year-old man who contracted kuru, he spent the last seven months of his life in a hospital, which allowed doctors to observe the progression of his disease. Physicians offered to return him to his home in Papua New Guinea, "but he refused and said he preferred to remain [at the hospital] in New Britain" (p. 266). He revealed to the medical workers that his father had died of kuru and that he had participated in some cannibalistic rituals when he was younger, including as a teenager. The doctors took careful notes on the progression of his disease, giving him many neurological tests at several points throughout the months that he was cared for at the hospital. In total,

DOI: 10.4324/9781003276937-34

his illness lasted for around one year, and he spent the last few of those months unable to sit up or speak. After his death, some of his brain tissue was injected into the brains of monkeys. Those monkeys later contracted kuru themselves, years later, which demonstrated that the disease could take a very long time to emerge after exposure (Scrimgeour et al., 1983).

(STORY 3) An 11-year-old boy was examined in 1957, after he had already been ill with kuru for around four months. His speech was described as "blurred," and he could not stand up without help (p. 16). His muscles were vibrating with an uncontrolled tremor. He had trouble when he was asked to touch his nose or bring his feet up to run along his shins in classic tests of coordination. A few months later, he spent his time curled up in bed, with his eyes reacting "poorly to light" and his face occasionally seized by attacks of smiling—he was described as looking "demented" (p. 16). However, even in the final month of his life, he demonstrated that he could still hear the doctors and follow simple commands. In all, he survived for ten months after the first signs of kuru. A brain autopsy revealed the extensive damage to his brain cells, which helped give new clues to the researchers about what was causing such a vicious disease (Fowler & Robertson, 1959, case 1).

The Features

Unlike all of the other conditions listed in this book, you will not find a single person on the face of the planet that has the disease known as kuru. It is, as far as anyone can tell, completely extinct. And that is a very good thing, as you will learn momentarily.

According to the oral history of the indigenous people from what is now called Papua New Guinea in the English language, the first cases of kuru appeared around the year 1910 (Alpers, 2007). Cases of kuru began to be discovered by people from the world outside of Papua New Guinea in the 1940s and 1950s, where the disease was seen to mostly affect a group of indigenous people called the Fore (Anderson, 2008). According to researchers at the time, "both the disease and descriptions of its phases have become part of the traditional magic lore of the Fore people" (Gajdusek & Zigas, 1959, p. 446). The word *kuru* in the Fore language loosely means "to tremble from fever," and the disease was also sometimes called *negi nagi*, which means "a silly or foolish person" (Liberski et al., 2019, pp. 2–4). These names were derived from symptoms of kuru: trembling uncontrollably as if shivering and wild laughing.

The shivering tremor was due to a loss of muscle coordination (see Ataxia), and became progressively worse over time. Sufferers slowly lost the ability to walk, then the ability to sit up, then the ability to leave bed at all, and then eventually the ability to swallow, which sometimes led to death by starvation. Other victims of kuru died from infected bedsores that came from lying still in bed for many days in a row. When one researcher tried to prolong their lives by treating the bedsores, he discovered that the dying people did not want to be treated and preferred to die as quickly as possible (Rhodes, 1998, p. 40).

Compulsive laughter was another sign of kuru. The laughter was such a striking symptom that kuru was sometimes called *laughing disease*, especially by journalists at the time (Liberski et al., 2019). Researchers noted that the Fore people with the disease were more likely to have a "sustained over-demonstrative smile" and/or laugh when compared to those without the disease (Simpson et al., 1959, p. 12). However, the medical workers who were studying the disease were appalled when newspapers at the time sensationalized kuru as the "laughing death" and "laughing sickness" because those accounts were played up and highly distorted from the reality of the disease (Anderson, 2008, p. 82). In truth, the emotional changes in kuru victims could include not only laughter, but also inappropriate euphoria, aggression, or deep depression (Gajdusek & Zigas, 1959). Although it is true that wild laughter is a much more noticeable sign than deep depression, so no wonder that's what made it into the newspapers.

The most famous researcher associated with kuru is Carlton Gajdusek, who began his work on the disease in 1956, and eventually won a Nobel Prize for that work. Many unusual things about the disease stuck out to Gajdusek and his colleagues. For example, the affected people were mainly women and children, with adult men rarely developing the disease (Alpers, 2007). The disease had the signs of neurodegenerative diseases such as dementia but seemed to spread as an epidemic. Additionally, the infected people showed no signs of inflammation, which was baffling, because that suggested that no foreign substance had entered the body to trigger the immune system, such as what happens in the course of an infection (Rhodes, 1998, pp. 33–37). What could explain all of this?

The Brain Pathology

There were suspicions from the beginning that kuru was being spread by an unusual behavior in which the Fore people engaged. Specifically, they were ritualistic cannibals that would sometimes eat their dead relatives. The other leading theory at the time was that kuru was a genetic disease, but it was later confirmed that *eating the brains* of other humans led to kuru due to the spread of *prions*. Yes, kuru turned out to be a prion disease, similar to other conditions discussed in this book (see Creutzfeldt-Jakob Disease; see Fatal Familial Insomnia).

This explained why people didn't have immune responses to kuru. It was because the infectious prions were essentially just slightly misshapen human proteins and therefore weren't flagged by the body as foreign agents requiring an immune response of inflammation (Rhodes, 1998, p. 166). Because the immune system did not fight the prions, they were free to make holes in many places in the person's brain, causing symptoms depending on the locations of the holes (Liberski et al., 2019). Because women and children were most likely to eat the brains of deceased relatives, this also explained the pattern in which women were much more affected than men (Alpers, 2007). The first person to die from kuru may have had a sporadic mutation in the brain that led to kuru prions, and then the prions were passed on to others who ate that person's brain, and so on, creating the kuru epidemic (Liberski et al., 2019). According to at least one account, the prions continued to spread because kuru victims— unable to walk for long periods before their death—built up fatty tissues and were especially "tender and appetizing" (Anderson, 2008, p. 168).

Eating the dead was practiced by the Fore until around the years of 1957–1962 in various villages, after which both cannibalism and kuru disappeared. However, kuru did not die out immediately because it had an incredibly long incubation period. In other words, the symptoms of the disease often did not appear until long after the person ate brains. The incubation period of kuru depended on the amount of infected tissue that the person ate, and the incubation period could last for more than 20 years (Scrimgeour et al., 1983). Incubation perhaps lasted for more than *50 years* in a few cases (Alpers, 2007).

Once the symptoms of kuru itself began to emerge, death typically followed within a year or so, sometimes in just a few months (Gajdusek, 1977). Like the other prion diseases in this book there was no known cure and kuru was always fatal. The discovery of prions and research into how they work eventually led to two more Nobel Prize winners (Prusiner and Wüthrich), meaning that studying kuru directly or indirectly led to at least three Nobel Prizes. At least humans ended up gaining a lot of knowledge from this terrifying epidemic.

References

Alpers, M. P. (2007). A history of kuru. *Papua New Guinea Medical Journal, 50*(1–2), 10–19.

Anderson, W. (2008). *The collectors of lost souls: Turning kuru scientists into whitemen.* Johns Hopkins University Press.

Fowler, M., & Robertson, E. G. (1959). Observations on kuru. III: Pathological features in five cases. *Australasian Annals of Medicine, 8*(1), 16–26. https://doi.org/gtth

Gajdusek, D. C. (1977). Unconventional viruses and the origin and disappearance of kuru. *Science, 197*(4307), 943–960. https://doi.org/dp2c4v

Gajdusek, D. C., & Zigas, V. (1959). Kuru: clinical, pathological and epidemiological study of an acute progressive degenerative disease of the central nervous system among natives of the Eastern Highlands of New Guinea. *The American Journal of Medicine, 26*(3), 442–469. https://doi.org/cp5gw6

Liberski, P. P., Gajos, A., Sikorska, B., & Lindenbaum, S. (2019). Kuru, the first human prion disease. *Viruses, 11*(3), Article 232. https://doi.org/gttj

Rhodes, R. (1998). *Deadly feasts: Tracking the secrets of a terrifying new plague.* Simon and Schuster.

Scrimgeour, E. M., Masters, C. L., Alpers, M. P., Kaven, J., & Gajdusek, D. C. (1983). A clinico-pathological study of a case of kuru. *Journal of the Neurological Sciences, 59,* 265–275. https://doi.org/c8bgcc

Simpson, D. A., Lander, H., & Robson, H. N. (1959). Observations on kuru: II. Clinical features. *Australasian Annals of Medicine, 8*(1), 8–15. https://doi.org/gttk

Zigas, V., & Gajdusek, D. C. (1957). Kuru: Clinical study of a new syndrome resembling paralysis agitans in natives of the Eastern Highlands of Australian New Guinea. *Medical Journal of Australia, 2*(21), 745–754. https://doi.org/gttm

Locked-In Syndrome

Imagine that, because you can't move the muscles of your body, everyone thinks that you are unconscious. But you are not in a coma. You are very much awake and aware of what is going on around you. You want to use your voice to tell everyone that you are trapped inside of your body, but despite your attempts to do so, your body won't listen. Will you ever be able to tell those around you that you are still in here?

The Stories

(STORY 1) Jean-Dominique Bauby wrote a book called *The Diving Bell and the Butterfly* following a major stroke that caused locked-in syndrome. The book speaks of his everyday life with locked-in syndrome as well as his memories and hopes. He could only blink his left eyelid, and he also had severe hearing problems that made interacting with the outside world extremely difficult. In one chapter, he details how infuriating it was when someone would leave the door to his hospital room open, because the noises were endless and he could not get up to close it. Bauby wrote about the alphabet system that he used to dictate his memoir to his transcriber—who read the letters in a row until Bauby blinked—and how some of his visitors such as fans of crossword puzzles and scrabble players did much better at communicating with the code than others. He wrote about his children and how much he missed physically eating food. His friends told him that they had overheard people at a cafe discussing how he had become a "vegetable," which motivated him to do more writing because he "wanted to prove that [his] IQ was still higher than a turnip's" (p. 82). He finished dictating his book via blinking and then died suddenly just two days after its original publication (Bauby, 1997).

(STORY 2) Martin Pistorius wrote in *Ghost Boy* about his experiences with a mysterious ailment. First, around the age of 12, he gradually lost the ability to move and then fell into unresponsive wakefulness. He spent the next few years unaware of what was happening to him, but around the age of 16, his consciousness began to return. By the age of 19, he was fully conscious again, but mostly unable to voluntarily move due to a partial locked-in syndrome. He wasn't paralyzed, but he said that it was as if his body moved

DOI: 10.4324/9781003276937-35

"independently of me ... If I ever walked, it was to take just a few shuffling steps with someone holding me up because otherwise I would crumple to the floor" (pp. 13–14). He eventually developed a few movements that he could reliably make—"jerking my head down to the right and smiling" (p. 21). He tried to respond to questions using smiles and moving his head slightly, but it wasn't enough for most people to notice that he was conscious. Eventually, around the age of 25, a massage therapist that worked with him noticed that he seemed to be responsive to her words and recommended that he be brought to a facility to test his communication abilities. He was then able to learn how to use a computer to communicate with his family for the first time since he was a child. He continued to recover the use of his body and went on to marry and start a business (Pistorius & Davies, 2011).

(STORY 3) A 17-year-old boy was hit by a car and ended up in hospital where he appeared to be "totally unresponsive" and "exhibited no evidence of any spontaneous movement" (p. 63). A number of tests suggested that he was in a coma. For example, they squirted cold water into his ear canals to judge his reaction, which was described as "unpredictable movements" (p. 63). However, there were some movements around his eyelids and eyes that led his examiner to consider locked-in syndrome as a possibility. It's a good thing that they did. When they began asking him questions, he was able to respond with small eye movements. He was taught to blink once for "yes" and blink twice for "no." Using this system, he was able to communicate and stay "intellectually stimulated" during his time at the hospital (p. 64). Unfortunately, he did not regain control of any muscles beyond those around his eyes. The researchers specify in his case study the importance of medical workers quickly identifying that patients with locked-in syndrome are conscious. They argue that such consciousness demands additional care when compared to patients that are unconscious. For example, they suggest that "appropriate ongoing vocal interaction with the patient (care to mind and body)" should begin immediately in order "to enrich their environment. Otherwise they may truly remain locked-in" (Shivji et al., 2003, p. 66).

The Features

If you're like most people, you probably spend very little time thinking about your brain stem. That part of your body usually does its job quietly, automatically, and without complaint. But it deserves more recognition, because the brain stem is absolutely essential. It contains neural wiring that allows your body to send signals to the motor and sensory areas in your upper brain, and vice versa. This allows you to move your muscles, as well as sense information from the outside world such as through the sense of touch. It is also your brain stem that is responsible for many functions that keep you alive, such as your breathing, heartbeat, and ability to wake up from sleep. Perhaps I should have mentioned those crucial functions first—they are very important. In rare cases, it is possible to damage that first part of the brain stem that relays signals between the brain and the body while keeping that second part that keeps you alive and awake more intact. This can result in a condition known as locked-in syndrome, which may look a lot like a coma from the outside (see Coma). But from the inside—through the eyes of the one experiencing it—locked-in syndrome is far more terrifying than any coma.

Almost all movement becomes impossible in locked-in syndrome. That's because most of your motor nerves that travel through your brain stem are cut off from sending signals to your muscles. *Quadriplegia*—the complete inability to move the trunk and all four limbs—is just the beginning. The person also experiences *swallowing palsy*, meaning that they cannot use the muscles involved in eating, and *aphonia*, meaning that they cannot use the muscles involved in speaking. Their facial muscles are also typically paralyzed, including some of their eye movements. Specifically, a person with locked-in syndrome typically cannot look from side to side due to *horizontal gaze palsy*.

However, some movements and sensations may still be possible. Most notably, blinking of their eyes and the ability to move their eyes up and down is still possible for many people with locked-in syndrome. This is because the neural wires that allow some eye movements, such as the supranuclear oculomotor pathways, are located higher up in the brain than the bundle of nerves typically damaged in locked-in syndrome (Khanna et al., 2011; Shivji et al., 2003). Because speaking and all other facial movement is lost, people with locked-in syndrome use eye movements in order to communicate what they are thinking. In addition to eye movements, the person is often still able to see and smell because the nerves feeding those senses—the optic nerve and the olfactory nerve, respectively—are also located higher up in the brain than the typical damage that causes locked-in syndrome. Sight and breathing are also generally affected, leading to blurry vision and sub-optimal breathing patterns (Halan et al., 2021).

If you're wondering about the sensations of touch and hearing, well, those are a bit more complicated. The neural pathways for those senses also run through the brain stem, but in a *slightly* different location—further back in the brain stem than the motor nerves (Bleck, 2003). In most people who have locked-in syndrome, they can still experience at least some touch and hearing because those nerve fibers were just slightly out of the range of the brain damage. This may lead to cases where the person can feel the prick of a pin, but can't move any muscles to indicate that they can feel it, leading the medical workers to conclude that they are deeply unconscious due to the lack of a response—a terrifying situation to be in.

The pattern of symptoms described above is considered *classical locked-in syndrome*. However, there are also cases where touch and hearing sensations are partially or completely lost, and cases in which movement of the eyes is completely lost (Patterson & Grabois, 1986). The reason that there is variation is due to the *extent* of the brain damage in each individual person, because the nerve fibers for all of those things are located close together.

Complete paralysis of the eyes is referred to as *total locked-in syndrome*. This makes communicating the fact that you are actually conscious and not in a coma nearly impossible, and caretakers may not notice that the person is trapped inside, experiencing the world around them but unable to express it. Additionally, there are cases where some movement beyond the eyes is either preserved or recovered over time, which is called *incomplete locked-in syndrome* (Bauer et al., 1979). In an analysis of 139 cases, it was found that 64% were classical locked-in syndrome, 33% were incomplete, and only 2% were total (Patterson & Grabois, 1986). Thus, thankfully, people with this condition are usually left with at least one potential way to communicate.

The Brain Pathology

Locked-in syndrome was named back in the 1960s: "this constellation of alert wakefulness accompanied by mute tetraplegia of brainstem origin we have termed *the locked-in syndrome*" (Plum & Posner, 1966, p. 92). Notice that, even then, it was understood as the result of a damaged brain stem. The most common way to acquire locked-in syndrome is through a stroke called a *pontine infarction*, which is a stroke in a part of the brain stem called the pons (Karatas, 2009). This leads to locked-in syndrome because "traversing the ventral pons are the corticospinal and corticobulbar tracts, hence the voluntary motor supply to the limbs and medullary motor nuclei are disrupted" (Hawkes, 1974, p. 381). In other words, a stroke in that region cuts off the muscle signals that normally pass through, like cutting a power cable, which leads to the symptoms of paralysis.

It's important to note that the brain stem is not responsible for generating the movement signals; the brain stem acts more like a relay station for tracts passing through. Thus, for a person with locked-in syndrome, they may be successfully generating the impulses in the motor cortex of their brain to send to their muscles, but those signals never arrive because they cannot get through to the body. Other damaging events other than a stroke, such as trauma, tumors, and multiple sclerosis can also prevent those signals from getting through, resulting in locked-in syndrome (Halan et al., 2021). As noted above, there are some neural tracts that cross the brain stem in slightly different places, meaning that if the damage is limited in scope, more movements may be possible for that person, such as when the corticofacial tracts are spared, allowing some additional facial movements (Hawkes, 1974).

Because it is possible for some people who seem like they are in comas to actually be experiencing locked-in syndrome, it is essential that caretakers look for signs of *covert cognition*. Covert cognition is a fancy way of saying that the person's brain is experiencing a higher level of consciousness than they are able to express, such as in the case of people with total locked-in syndrome—they are aware of their surroundings but definitely don't appear to be. Identifying covert cognition is difficult: the preserved eye movements are often inconsistent, small, and the person can become easily exhausted from trying to communicate (Laureys et al., 2005). A person may also start out in a coma but then gradually wake up to become locked-in, making covert cognition an evolving and complicated thing to measure. This is why it is recommended that any person that appears to be in a state of disordered consciousness such as a coma should be given multiple opportunities using multiple methods in order to demonstrate covert cognition (González-Lara & Owen, 2018).

It may take multiple months or even years to realize that patients are locked-in rather than in a coma (Laureys et al., 2005). One study found that around one in five people who were thought to be in vegetative states and unaware of the world around them were actually experiencing locked-in awareness, but the medical workers had not looked closely enough—sometimes for total locked-in syndrome you need to look at the brain waves directly to see that the person is able to understand the medical workers (Cruse et al., 2011). As you might expect, it has been reported that such locked-in patients mistaken as being in a coma are "distressed by inappropriate conversation around the bedside" (Hawkes, 1974, p. 379).

Historically, the majority of people with locked-in syndrome passed away within a few months of acquiring the disorder (Patterson & Grabois, 1986). More recently, the majority of people with this condition survive for multiple years (Smith & Delargy, 2005). For those who become stable, it is sometimes possible for them to make slow and partial recoveries—for example, from classic locked-in syndrome to incomplete locked-in syndrome with intense therapy (Pickl, 2002). For those who cannot recover movement, there remains the possibility that they can instead use their brain waves to send messages thanks to brain–machine interfaces that, after surgical implantation, can translate their thoughts into words (Kennedy, 2020).

An interesting question is, do people with locked-in syndrome end up living happy lives? The research in this area is positive. Among those who have the condition for a long time, they generally report being glad to be alive (Laureys et al., 2005). Meaningful life can still be had, and technological advancements are making the prospects for interacting with the world in increasingly complex ways more of a reality every year.

References

Bauby, J. D. (1997). *The diving bell and the butterfly*. Knopf.

Bauer, G., Gerstenbrand, F., & Rumpl, E. (1979). Varieties of the locked-in syndrome. *Journal of Neurology*, *221*(2), 77–91. https://doi.org/dmk9mz

Bleck, T. P. (2003). Levels of consciousness and attention. In C. G. Goetz (Ed.), *Textbook of clinical neurology* (2nd ed., pp. 3–18). Saunders.

Cruse, D., Chennu, S., Chatelle, C., Bekinschtein, T. A., Fernández-Espejo, D., Pickard, J. D., Laureys, S., & Owen, A. M. (2011). Bedside detection of awareness in the vegetative state: A cohort study. *The Lancet*, *378*(9809), 2088–2094. https://doi.org/fq9p94

González-Lara, L. E., & Owen, A. M. (2018). Identifying covert cognition in disorders of consciousness. In C. Schnakers & S. Laureys (Eds.), *Coma and disorders of consciousness* (pp. 77–96). Springer International Publishing. https://doi.org/gttn

Halan, T., Ortiz, J. F., Reddy, D., Altamimi, A., Ajibowo, A. O., & Fabara, S. P. (2021). Locked-in syndrome: A systematic review of long-term management and prognosis. *Cureus*, *13*(7). https://doi.org/hqpk

Hawkes, C. H. (1974). "Locked-in" syndrome: Report of seven cases. *British Medical Journal*, *4*, 379–382. https://doi.org/cpxw8q

Karatas, M. (2009). Internuclear and supranuclear disorders of eye movements: Clinical features and causes. *European Journal of Neurology*, *16*(12), 1265–1277. https://doi.org/dd7dfq

Kennedy, P. R. (2020). *Unlocking Erik: A freedom journey to restore the speech of those with locked-in syndrome*. Nova Science Publishers.

Khanna, K., Verma, A., & Richard, B. (2011). "The locked-in syndrome": Can it be unlocked? *Journal of Clinical Gerontology and Geriatrics*, *2*(4), 96–99. https://doi.org/dtf285

Laureys, S., Pellas, F., Van Eeckhout, P., Ghorbel, S., Schnakers, C., Perrin, F., Berré, J., Faymonville, M.-E., Pantke, K.-H., Damas, F., Lamy, M., Moonen, G., & Goldman, S. (2005). The locked-in syndrome: What is it like to be conscious but paralyzed and voiceless? *Progress in Brain Research*, *150*, 495–611. https://doi.org/ctntgq

Patterson, J. R., & Grabois, M. (1986). Locked-in syndrome: A review of 139 cases. *Stroke*, *17*(4), 758–764. https://doi.org/c2bsww

Pickl, G. B. (2002). Changes during long-term management of locked-in syndrome: A case report. *Folia Phoniatrica et Logopaedica*, *54*(1), 26–43. https://doi.org/bhzw86

Pistorius, M., & Davies, M. L. (2011). *Ghost boy*. Simon and Schuster.

Plum, F., & Posner, J. B. (1966). *The diagnosis of stupor and coma*. FA Davis Co.

Shivji, Z. M., Streletz, L. J., Baeesa, S., & Girvin, J. (2003). Electrophysiological investigations in the locked-in syndrome: A case report. *American Journal of Electroneurodiagnostic Technology*, *43*(2), 60–69. https://doi.org/gttp

Smith, E., & Delargy, M. (2005). Locked-in syndrome. *British Medical Journal*, *330*(7488), 406–409. https://doi.org/cjsr4x

Migraine Headaches

Imagine that you can't tolerate sound or light because your senses have become too sensitive, and you are forced to wait in pain until your brain stops throbbing. The pain comes with nausea, perhaps strong enough that if you are not sitting perfectly still, you will be overcome with the urge to vomit. The pain might be different each time this happens, or you might experience it in a typical way every time—you might even get so good at predicting when the attacks will happen that you can take steps to prevent them from worsening. But truly strange are the other symptoms that plague you: your vision may blur severely, the dizziness may knock you off your feet, and your senses of smell and sound may be exaggerated and become deeply disturbing. What's causing this unpleasant constellation of symptoms?

The Stories

(STORY 1) In the case of a 43-year-old woman who had suffered from two–three painful migraines per month since childhood, her migraines would occasionally break out of that predictable routine during particular events in her life. As the author of this case study wrote, "this is, as it were, a case-history in reverse, showing certain situations in which a patient found herself *free* from life-long migraines" (p. 169). On three occasions of pregnancy, she had no migraines for periods of more than six months. However, on one occasion of pregnancy in which the pregnancy was unwanted and distressing, she continued to experience migraines for the entire nine-month duration and "had more severe attacks than usual for her" (p. 169). On one occasion, she was hospitalized with a severe illness—subacute bacterial endocarditis—for four months and did not experience migraines during that time. Following the death of her father, she had a three-month period of time while in deep mourning during which she did not experience migraines. This case shows the importance of hormonal and psychological factors in the experience of migraines (Sacks, 1992, case 56).

(STORY 2) In a case of migraines inherited genetically through a family bloodline, a grandmother, mother, and son were all seen to have serious cases of "migraine coma syndrome" (p. 59). The son was 6 years old when

DOI: 10.4324/9781003276937-36

hospitalized for the first time with a coma. He recovered after a few days but, after that, he had severe one-sided headaches about twice a week. As he aged, the migraine headaches began to include other severe symptoms, such as the inability to move certain muscles, difficulties in speaking, temporary blindness, temporary hearing loss, and, again, coma. His mother had also shown similar signs, when younger, including temporary muscle paralysis, one-sided headaches, and coma. It was later discovered that the mother of the mother—the son's grandmother—had also shown signs of similar attacks when younger (Münte & Müller-Vahl, 1990, cases 1–3).

(STORY 3) In the case of a 27-year-old woman, *biofeedback* was successfully used in order to help reduce the intensity of her migraines. The patient was a nurse who had a two-year history of migraines that were worsening over time. Because she kept a daily log of how often she had migraines and how long they lasted, she could tell when a treatment was working or not working. One treatment that she tried was temperature biofeedback, where she focused her energy on relaxing and raising the temperature of her fingers as measured by a thermometer on her skin. It is known that some migraines can be made less painful by changing blood flow in and around the brain, and one way to do that is to increase blood flow in other areas of the body. Because increased blood flow in the hands increases their temperature, what this person attempted to do was learn to increase the temperature of her hands to make her migraines more tolerable. She was trained to control the temperature of her hands over the course of several weeks. When the temperature of her hands was hotter, her migraines were less severe (Johnson & Turin, 1975). Biofeedback and similar relaxation techniques have since shown to be effective for at least some other people with recurring migraines (Kropp et al., 2017).

The Features

Migraines are an incredibly important disorder to understand, which is why it's unfortunate that researchers have only recently begun to truly understand them. Migraines are important because they are the most common disabling *headache* disorder (Bahra, 2011), and the sixth most common *overall* disabling disorder (Goadsby et al., 2017). The percentage of people who at least occasionally suffer a migraine is about 14%, which is currently around a billion people (Stovner et al., 2018). So much productivity, and therefore money, is lost every year due to migraines that it's difficult for me to summarize here. If a *cure* for migraines was ever discovered, it would be life-changing for crowds of sufferers. But as of right now, many questions remain.

You might be asking yourself "do migraines belong in a book about brain disorders?" Fortunately for me, the author of this book, the answer is "yes." We'll talk about why migraines count as a brain disorder in just a bit, but first we need to cover what a migraine even is—because it's not just a painful headache like some people believe. Instead, migraines can include a wide variety of symptoms, a fact which has been understood by brain researchers since at least the 19th century: "the headaches known as migraine, may be accompanied by various other symptoms … the functions of the cerebrum are, as you know, vision, sensation, hearing, and motor power … symptoms will ensue whose nature will depend upon the position of the spasm" (Brunton et al., 1899, p. 1242). That is, migraine symptoms depend on location in the brain—let's take a closer look at those symptoms.

A typical migraine attack presents itself in a number of distinct *phases* that a migraine sufferer is all too familiar with, even if they don't know the names for each phase. These phases are the *premonitory* phase, the *aura*, the *headache*, and the *recovery*.

The premonitory phase is the period of time before the actual headache begins, during which other more subtle symptoms may appear. These most commonly include feeling tired, having concentration difficulties, and a feeling like you have a stiff neck (Giffin et al., 2003). The person might also experience mood changes, food cravings, excessive yawning, and sensitivity to light (Dodick, 2018). When asked to track premonitory symptoms, the majority of migraine sufferers report having one or more of these symptoms (Schoonman et al., 2006). Based on brain scans, the premonitory phase lasts around 48 hours, leading up to the aura and headache phases of the migraine (Schulte et al., 2020). Some people can predict that they are going to get a migraine based on their premonitory symptoms (Giffin et al., 2003). That would be a more enviable party trick if it weren't excruciating pain that they were predicting.

The aura is a phase of the migraine that consists of symptoms other than pain that usually show up just before the headache itself (Russell & Olesen, 1996). The three major types of aura symptoms are visual, sensory, and aphasic, and a person can experience more than one type (Eriksen et al., 2004).

Visual aura symptoms are by far the most common. Visual auras may consist of black or white spots, or even linear or zigzag patterns, that a person sees out of one or both eyes (Nye & Thadani, 2015). The spots in the person's vision may resemble a scotoma (see Hemianopsia), and may slowly evolve into different shapes or placement over the course of minutes. Sensory auras are less common. They usually consist of tingling sensations in the hand, arm, face, and possibly other body parts like the tongue, that can spread over time but are generally confined to just one side of the body (Eriksen et al., 2004). Aphasic auras are even less common, and they are when a person temporarily experiences aphasia (see Aphasia) such that they can't understand speech or produce speech.

Beyond those types of auras, a person can also experience motor auras that affect muscle movement, and auras that disrupt senses such as balance (see Vertigo) or hearing. These symptoms are *transient*, which means that they disappear after a while, and they are usually gone in less than an hour (Bahra, 2011).

Not all people with migraines experience auras. In fact, the majority of people with migraines do *not* experience auras (Lipton et al., 2001). For this reason, migraines with auras and migraines without auras are sometimes considered to be separate disorders. The auras that occur with migraines may be similar to auras that occur with seizures (see Seizures), with the difference that migraine auras progress more slowly than seizure auras (Nye & Thadani, 2015).

The headache phase is the part of the migraine that most people are familiar with. This is the painful part. For people who have migraines with auras, the headache most commonly appears during the aura or within 30 minutes of the aura disappearing (Eriksen et al., 2004). The pain of migraine headaches usually lasts between four and 72 hours (Goadsby et al., 2017). Most of the longer attacks belong to women over men, for reasons that we will get into later (Allais et al., 2020).

The pain is "traditionally described as a violent throbbing pain in one temple" (Sacks, 1992). Other symptoms of the headache itself may include light sensitivity, noise sensitivity, movement sensitivity, nausea, and cutaneous allodynia—which is when touches applied to the skin that would generally not be painful are instead painful. Most of these symptoms are, again, more severe in women (Allais et al., 2020).

Finally is the recovery phase—which is also sometimes called the *postdrome*. This phase occurs when the pain finally ends, but don't get too excited, because the brain is still in recovery and therefore still has symptoms. In the postdrome, the person is likely to experience changes in mood, tiredness, difficulties in concentrating, and neck stiffness, similar to the premonitory phase. Think of it like a migraine hangover in which your brain is just trying to pull itself back together. Complete resolution of the postdrome symptoms takes about a day (Bahra, 2011). At least the pain is over.

Rare symptoms of migraines can be quite severe, up to and including severe muscle weakness, temporary blindness, unconsciousness, coma, or, in rare cases, death (Münte & Müller-Vahl, 1990; Russell & Ducros, 2011). Despite the sometimes shockingly severe symptoms of migraine, there is very rarely any noticeable permanent damage, indicating that despite the trouble they cause while they are occurring, migraines seem to generally be benign (Sacks, 1992).

The Brain Pathology

Now let's talk about why migraines count as a neurological disorder of the brain. For a long time, researchers thought that migraines were simply "caused" by blood vessels misbehaving—sometimes called the *vasospastic theory* (Tfelt-Hansen, 2009). The traditional vasospastic view was that the aura is caused by vasoconstriction (blood vessels getting smaller) and the headache by vasodilation (blood vessels getting bigger), but that view has been dismissed as being too simplistic (Ferrari, 1998).

Today's prevailing theories about what causes migraines are much more complex. Researchers have traced the causes to neurological dysfunction in the brain stem and other brain regions, although the precise neuronal mechanisms remain unknown (Goadsby et al., 2017). Importantly, the brain stem dysfunction seems to contribute to *cortical spreading depression*, which is when neurons get excited and then inhibited in a wave pattern, which is what causes the aura symptoms (Tfelt-Hansen, 2009). Depending on where in the brain the cortical spreading depression is happening, the symptoms vary from person to person, leading to those various visual, sensory, and aphasic categories of auras that I elaborated on earlier. It may be a small consolation to those suffering through the pain of a migraine, but it's a cool fact that we can somewhat tell which of your neurons are "doing the wave" based on your aura symptoms.

The headache pain itself is then caused thanks to the trigeminovascular pathway, which includes nerves that sense pain in blood vessels and layers of tissue around the brain (Dodick, 2018). We know that the pain involves these nerves, especially the trigeminal ganglion, because effective treatments of migraine pain target those nerves (Edvinsson et al., 2020).

Women are much more likely to suffer from migraines than are men, with about three times as many women experiencing regular migraines (Lipton et al., 2001). The prevalence in women is at least partially because fluctuating hormone levels during females' monthly cycle—estrogen and progesterone—appear to play a role in migraines (Allais et al., 2020). Sex hormones interact with chemical messengers in the brain such as serotonin, and can affect a person's perception of pain.

The rabbit hole goes much deeper. The mechanisms of migraine also seem to include the blood–brain barrier, the hypothalamus, neuroinflammation, and more (Goadsby et al., 2017). Further work is needed to figure out exactly how these different parts of the migraine puzzle fit together, but one thing is for sure—this is a complicated neurological disorder involving many parts of the brain (Edvinsson et al., 2020). The development of medications and therapies is ongoing, but until we gain a better understanding of migraines, treatment will consist of some trial and error. For far too many people, the symptoms of migraines will continue to visit for the foreseeable future.

References

Allais, G., Chiarle, G., Sinigaglia, S., Airola, G., Schiapparelli, P., & Benedetto, C. (2020). Gender-related differences in migraine. *Neurological Sciences, 41*(s2), s429–s436. https://doi.org/gttq

Bahra, A. (2011). Primary headache disorders: Focus on migraine. *Reviews in Pain, 5*(4), 2–11. https://doi.org/gttr

Brunton, T. L., Grant, D., Allbutt, T. C., Campbell, H., Tyson, J. W., Herschell, G., StClair, T., Pope, F. M., Mullick, S. K., Masters, W. H., & Draffin, D. K. (1899). A discussion on headaches and their treatment. *The British Medical Journal, 2*, 1241–1246.

Dodick, D. W. (2018). A phase-by-phase review of migraine pathophysiology. *Headache: The Journal of Head and Face Pain, 58*(s1) Supplement 1, 4–16. https://doi.org/gdg2zn

Edvinsson, J. C. A., Viganò, A., Alekseeva, A., Alieva, E., Arruda, R., De Luca, C., D'Ettore, N., Frattale, I., Kurnukhina, M., Macerola, N., Malenkova, E., Maiorova, M., Novikova, A., Řehulka, P., Rapaccini, V., Roshchina, O., Vanderschueren, G., Zvaune,

L., Andreou, A. P., & Haanes, K. A. (2020). The fifth cranial nerve in headaches. *Journal of Headache and Pain, 21*(1), 1–17. https://doi.org/gtts

Eriksen, M. K., Thomsen, L. L., Andersen, I., Nazim, F., & Olesen, J. (2004). Clinical characteristics of 362 patients with familial migraine with aura. *Cephalalgia, 24*(7), 564–575. https://doi.org/bm94t2

Ferrari, M. D. (1998). Migraine. *Lancet, 351*(9108), 1043–1051. https://doi.org/b3wgtf

Giffin, N. J., Ruggiero, L., Lipton, R. B., Silberstein, S. D., Tvedskov, J. F., Olesen, J., Altman P. J., Goadsby, A., & Macrae, A. (2003). Premonitory symptoms in migraine: An electronic diary study. *Neurology, 60*(6), 935–940. https://doi.org/gttv

Goadsby, P. J., Holland, P. R., Martins-Oliveira, M., Hoffmann, J., Schankin, C., & Akerman, S. (2017). Pathophysiology of migraine: A disorder of sensory processing. *Physiological Reviews, 97*(2), 553–622. https://doi.org/gh5s8v

Johnson, W. G., & Turin, A. (1975). Biofeedback treatment of migraine headache: A systematic case study. *Behavior Therapy, 6*, 394–397. *https://doi.org/fdb2dc*

Kropp, P., Meyer, B., Meyer, W., & Dresler, T. (2017). An update on behavioral treatments in migraine–Current knowledge and future options. *Expert Review of Neurotherapeutics, 17*(11), 1059–1068. https://doi.org/gmbcsm

Lipton, R. B., Stewart, W. F., Diamond, S., Diamond, M. L., & Reed, M. (2001). Prevalence and burden of migraine in the United States: Data from the American migraine study II. *Headache: The Journal of Head and Face Pain, 41*(7), 646–657. https://doi.org/fgdg57

Münte, T. F., & Müller-Vahl, H. (1990). Familial migraine coma: A case study. *Journal of Neurology, 237*(1), 59–61. https://doi.org/cssfmk

Nye, B. L., & Thadani, V. M. (2015). Migraine and epilepsy: Review of the literature. *Headache: The Journal of Head and Face Pain, 3*(55), 359–380. https://doi.org/f65x2s

Russell, M. B., & Ducros, A. (2011). Sporadic and familial hemiplegic migraine: Pathophysiological mechanisms, clinical characteristics, diagnosis, and management. *The Lancet Neurology, 10*(5), 457–470. https://doi.org/bs987s

Russell, M. B., & Olesen, J. (1996). A nosographic analysis of the migraine aura in a general population. *Brain, 119*(2), 355–361. https://doi.org/cqt6pw

Sacks, O. (1992). *Migraine: Revised and expanded.* Vintage Books.

Schoonman, G. G., Evers, D. J., Terwindt, G. M., Van Dijk, J. G., & Ferrari, M. D. (2006). The prevalence of premonitory symptoms in migraine: A questionnaire study in 461 patients. *Cephalalgia, 26*(10), 1209–1213. https://doi.org/b6gvrw

Schulte, L. H., Mehnert, J., & May, A. (2020). Longitudinal neuroimaging over 30 days: Temporal characteristics of migraine. *Annals of Neurology, 87*(4), 646–651. https://doi.org/gttw

Stovner, L. J., Nichols, E., Steiner, T. J., Abd-Allah, F., Abdelalim, A., Al-Raddadi, R. M., Ansha, M. G., Barac, A., Bensenor, I. M., Doan, L. P., Edessa, D., Endres, M., Foreman, K. J., Gankpe, F. G., Gopalkrishna, G., Goulart, A. C., Gupta, R., Hankey, G. J., Hay, S. I., … & Murray, C. J. L. (2018). Global, regional, and national burden of migraine and tension-type headache, 1990–2016: A systematic analysis for the Global Burden of Disease Study 2016. *The Lancet Neurology, 17*(11), 954–976. https://doi.org/gfjpfq

Tfelt-Hansen, P. C. (2009). History of migraine with aura and cortical spreading depression from 1941 and onwards. *Cephalalgia, 30*(7), 780–792. https://doi.org/d24bwb

Narcolepsy (and Cataplexy)

Imagine that you can't prevent yourself from falling asleep or having your muscles go limp at inconvenient times. When you're eating, you risk snoozing at the table. When you're walking, you risk collapsing on the spot. You can't tell when you're going to be forced to take an inconvenient nap, and you can't seem to fight off the urge when it comes. The attacks of weakness seem tied to your emotional state, such that any strong emotion might be enough to send you tumbling. Perhaps your knees buckle when you laugh, or you drop the things that you are holding when you get excited. Why are your brain and muscles getting so mixed up?

The Stories

(STORY 1) In the case of a 38-year-old who had been hit in the head at least a few times (by a fist, a log, etc.), symptoms of both narcolepsy and cataplexy appeared. During narcoleptic sleep attacks, he would suddenly slump forwards, asleep, but then wake up about a minute later. In addition, he noticed that in situations where he was "laughing out loud or when anticipating a good business deal … he would feel weakness in his legs, which would buckle under him" (p. 308). These cataplexic attacks made actions such as playing a card game difficult, because when he was dealt a good hand of cards he found himself unable to move his arms. Over time the condition seemed to worsen such that even the slightest emotion brought on an attack of sleep, which was quite disruptive to his life. For example, when eating, he would often fall asleep multiple times per meal at the table, causing him to drop his utensils. Sometimes he found himself unable even to finish sentences or answer questions without falling asleep. His doctor wrote about what the attacks felt like: "he merely feels a deep heaviness, an intracranial emptiness, a sort of whirlwind spinning around inside his head" (Gélineau, 1880, case 2, as translated in Schenck et al., 2007).

(STORY 2) In the case of a 21-year-old woman, a doctor made careful notes about her cataplexy and sleep paralysis experiences. Her largest cataplexic attacks seemed to be closely linked to her emotions and would sometimes cause her to fall down. She described this as: "if anything is real funny, I get sort of weak and shaky in the knees—I get all limber and drop everything" (pp. 4–5).

DOI: 10.4324/9781003276937-37

Or, she might have an attack of cataplexy if she became annoyed, such as when her siblings made too much noise while playing. She also had a reaction to fear, during which she would sometimes become unable to move. Occasionally, she had mild attacks where there did not seem to be any particular emotion involved; when reading or writing she would sometimes drop the book or the pen. In the mornings, she would often experience sleep paralysis where, for a few minutes, she was conscious but couldn't move her body. She explained that even though she felt awake, her "body seemed to be dead. Then all of a sudden you limber up, and you're able to move again'" (Levin, 1933, p. 4).

(STORY 3) A 7-year-old boy was having difficulties with schoolwork, sports, and homework, because of excessive sleepiness. While sleeping at night, he experienced scary dreams and hallucinations. He began having episodes of cataplexy as well, causing him to trip while walking or leading to his arms or head suddenly drooping while he was eating. Researchers described him as having "fluctuations of consciousness" as well as "continuous drowsiness" and "sleep attacks" (p. 1577). Several attempted treatments, including for suspected epilepsy, were unsuccessful. Eventually, the parents of the boy saw a television special about narcolepsy, which taught them about the disorder, and were able to get him referred to a specialist. Because his hormone levels were elevated and he seemed to be developing into an adult faster than is typical for a young boy, they diagnosed him with "idiopathic central precocious puberty" (p. 1577). It is a mysterious disorder in which hormones in the pituitary and sex glands are released in unexpected amounts, causing premature puberty, and, in some cases, severe narcolepsy. He began a new course of medication and improvement was reported (Plazzi et al., 2006, case 1).

The Features

Sometimes, the brain shuts parts of itself down, and the body to which it is attached lies more or less still for a period of, ideally, several hours. We all accept this regular behavior as a necessity—everybody sleeps—even though there is a lot left unknown about how it works. According to sleep researchers themselves, we're not even sure *why sleep exists* in the first place. We do have theories, but there doesn't seem to be any particularly clear-cut reason why the human brain *needs* to spend a full third of its time sleeping. Something that we do know is that when sleep goes wrong, it can be extremely disruptive. Sleeping too much (see Sleeping Beauty Syndrome) is bad, and sleeping too little (see Fatal Familial Insomnia) can be deadly. But what about sleeping at times when you don't intend to sleep? When your brain decides to shut down some functions without you intending to do so? That's where narcolepsy comes in.

Chances are that narcolepsy is one of the disorders in this book that you have heard of before now. Unfortunately, popular media often distorts the real symptoms of narcolepsy. To set the record straight, let's go over what a person with narcolepsy might experience. Overall, narcolepsy is a disorder in which the barrier between being awake and being asleep is damaged and thin. Narcolepsy as a disorder includes four major symptoms in its "classic tetrad" of features, even though only around 10% of people with a diagnosis of narcolepsy have all four symptoms at the same time (Akintomide & Rickards, 2011).

The first and most important symptom is *severe sleepiness*, which is sometimes called "somnolence" (Dement, 1993). In order to be diagnosed with narcolepsy, a person must show somnolence during the part of their day when they are trying to be awake and going about their business (Gauci et al., 2017). But it's not just feeling tired—this somnolence involves "irresistible sleep attacks" (Akintomide & Rickards, 2011, p. 507). This means that when they feel sleepy, they are unable to fight off that sleepiness and fall asleep. This is unlike a regular bout of sleepiness in which a person can *resist* the urge to fall asleep. If you've ever driven a car or read a book while extremely tired and forced yourself to stay awake, you have resisted sleepiness, something that a person with narcolepsy cannot do during a sleep attack. That is, narcolepsy is *not* like forgetting a dose of coffee; it's more like forgetting how to be awake for a little while.

But narcolepsy is more than sleepiness, so let's move on. Three other symptoms are not *required* for a person to be diagnosed as narcoleptic, but they are common. The first two optional symptoms are *sleep paralysis* and *hallucinations* at wake-sleep and sleep-wake transitions. They often occur together, so let's discuss them together.

Sleep paralysis occurs when a person can't move or speak at the transition between sleeping and waking up. The person is awake but can't move any voluntary muscles except for the eyes, the diaphragm (to allow breathing), and some small muscles in the ears (Stefani et al., 2019). It may come as a surprise, but this muscle paralysis, scary as it may be, is actually a completely normal thing that your body does when you are sleeping. Seriously, paralysis is normal during a type of sleep called Rapid Eye Movement (REM) sleep. That's typically the part of your sleep cycle where you have dreams. It is believed that your brain paralyzes your muscles in order to prevent you from acting your dreams out in real life and falling out of bed or otherwise injuring yourself. One part of your body that does continue to move during REM sleep is the eyeballs—just like in sleep paralysis. In sleep paralysis, however, this inability to move muscles happens *at the wrong time*, while you are awake instead of during REM sleep.

Sleep paralysis often occurs alongside hallucinations. This makes sense because during REM sleep people often dream, and sleep paralysis is a lot like being awake during REM sleep. Dreams are just hallucinations that we consider to be normal, if you think about it. In other words, a person with narcolepsy sometimes has dreams while they are somewhat awake. There are two major types of hallucinations in narcolepsy: hypnagogic and hypnopompic. The difference is in when they occur. If the hallucination occurs while the person is falling asleep, it is hypnagogic. If it occurs while they are waking up, it is hypnopompic. These hallucinations are more likely to be frightening than regular dreaming, and often seize the person with an extremely unpleasant sensation of fear (Sharpless & Grom, 2016).

It's possible to have sleep paralysis without having narcolepsy. In fact, many people will have at least one attack of sleep paralysis in their lives. One estimate of how many people in the general population will experience at least one attack of sleep paralysis in their life is 7.6% (Sharpless & Barber, 2011). So if you ever wake up, realize that you can't move, and then start hallucinating a scary vision such as something being in the room with you, try to stay calm and focus on slowly moving your fingers or toes. It's just your brain: you'll be able to move in a minute when your brain finishes waking up.

The final major optional symptom of narcolepsy is *cataplexy*, and the majority of people with narcolepsy experience it (Gauci et al., 2017). Cataplexy has been called "the most extraordinary symptom of narcolepsy" (Adamantidis et al., 2020, p. 2). Cataplexy is such a common and dramatic symptom that the name "Type 1 narcolepsy" was given to the form of the condition where a person also has cataplexy, while Type 2 narcolepsy is when a person has somnolence but *doesn't* have cataplexy.

If somnolence is like a switch that turns a person's consciousness off and forces them to sleep, then cataplexy is like a switch for a person's muscles that forces them to relax. During an attack of cataplexy, the person loses the ability to move or *tone* their muscles, resulting in a drooping face, sagging jaw, tongue protrusion, and may cause the person to fall down due to the loss of motor control in the legs (Bassetti et al., 2019). These difficulties in moving muscles are similar to what happens in sleep paralysis, and it has been theorized that cataplexy is similar to REM sleep occurring while you are fully awake (Gauci et al., 2017). Cataplexy doesn't occur during the transition between sleeping and wakefulness like sleep paralysis does—cataplexy happens throughout the course of the person's waking day. Cataplexy attacks can be complete and affect all muscles in the body, or partial, in which they affect only a part of the body such as the face or neck. These attacks usually last for seconds—or a minute or two—and, importantly, the person remains fully awake and conscious the whole time (Adamantidis et al., 2020).

What is truly the standout fact about cataplexy, however, is that the attacks are frequently triggered by strong emotions. More specifically, the emotions that trigger cataplexy tend to be sudden and "triumphant" in nature, such as the feeling of victory when playing sports, feelings of pleasure while having sex, and even laughter due to being tickled (Bassetti et al., 2019). Emotions with a positive valence, like happiness and joy, are more likely to trigger cataplexy attacks than emotions with a negative valence, like anger or sorrow (Sturzenegger & Bassetti, 2004). All kinds of emotions can trigger it. One memorable example was a woman with cataplexy in the 1960s who complained that whenever she tried to discipline her children by spanking them, her muscle tone left her and she could do nothing, leaving her children free to take advantage of the situation and escape from the discipline (Sours, 1963).

Cataplexy remains mysterious as of this writing, and more research is needed to determine exactly how this symptom occurs.

One other important thing to point out about people with narcolepsy is that they don't actually spend more time asleep than people without narcolepsy. This is due to the fact that they often wake up multiple times throughout the night, which counters the extra time they are asleep during the day—this symptom is called *sleep fragmentation* (Bassetti et al., 2019). This means that not only do people with narcolepsy fall asleep in the day when they don't want to, but have trouble *staying* asleep at night when they actually want to be sleeping.

The Brain Pathology

A leading theory about the cause of acquired Type 1 narcolepsy is that the person's immune system attacks and kills cells in the hypothalamus that produce chemicals called hypocretin or orexin (Bassetti et al., 2019). Neurons that produce orexin help to suppress REM sleep (Mahoney et al., 2019). Therefore, the loss of those cells results in the hypothalamus losing the ability to regulate the transitions between being awake and asleep—a rhythm called the sleep-wake cycle. This usually happens in the person's teens or twenties (Dauvilliers et al., 2001).

As for what triggers the immune system to kill off those cells, one theory is that a flu virus sometimes serves as the catalyst. More specifically, a fragment of the flu virus so greatly resembles orexin that, in some people, their immune system goes haywire and destroys not only hypocretin but also the cells that produce it in an attempt to beat the flu virus (Luo et al., 2018). In order to learn more about the interactions between orexin and autoimmune processes, researchers have been studying narcolepsy in dogs and mice, which gives them more control over genetic factors (Mahoney et al., 2019).

As for Type 2 narcolepsy cases without cataplexy—well, that "remains poorly understood" (Bassetti et al., 2019, p. 519). More specifically, researchers have noted that "besides a lack of cataplexy, the symptoms of NT2 are similar to those of NT1, yet almost nothing is known about its neuropathology" because orexin levels in some Type 2 cases appear to be normal (Mahoney et al., 2019, p. 90). In other cases of narcolepsy without cataplexy, there are dips in the person's orexin levels, which can be used to predict the eventual development of cataplexy later on if they get low (Bassetti et al., 2019). Thus, some cases of Type 2 narcolepsy might be due to a milder orexin loss, but it seems to be an oversimplification to say that Type 2 is just less severe than Type 1. As I say: you can have narcolepsy without cataplexy, but you can't have narcolepsy without complexity.

Cases that *might* be linked to the immune system but remain quite mysterious are known as *idiopathic* narcolepsy. Another much more rare type is *familial* narcolepsy, in which the disorder has a clear genetic link to a person's family (Bassetti et al., 2019). There are also reports of narcolepsy following traumatic brain injuries (Lankford et al., 1994). All of those forms of the disorder, and especially the symptom of cataplexy, require more research into exactly how the brain cells are communicating with one another (Adamantidis et al., 2020). Perhaps studying this disorder will finally allow us to unlock the mysteries of sleep. Or, at least, help us learn more about the process of falling asleep and waking up. Imagine a future in which everyone could fall asleep exactly when they intended to.

References

Adamantidis, A. R., Schmidt, M. H., Carter, M. E., Burdakov, D., Peyron, C., & Scammell, T. E. (2020). A circuit perspective on narcolepsy. *Sleep, 43*(5), 1–9. https://doi.org/gttx

Akintomide, G. S., & Rickards, H. (2011). Narcolepsy: A review. *Neuropsychiatric Disease and Treatment, 7*, 507–518. https://doi.org/czdwjj

Bassetti, C. L., Adamantidis, A., Burdakov, D., Han, F., Gay, S., Kallweit, U., Khatami, R., Koning, F., Kornum, B. R., Lammers, G. J., Libra, R. S., Luppi, P. H., Mayer, G., Pollmächer, T., Sakurai, T., Sallusto, F., Scammell, T. E., Tafti, M., & Dauvilliers, Y. (2019). Narcolepsy—Clinical spectrum, aetiopathophysiology, diagnosis and treatment. *Nature Reviews Neurology, 15*(9), 519–539. https://doi.org/ggr86b

Dauvilliers, Y., Montplaisir, J., Molinari, N., Carlander, B., Ondze, B., Besset, A., & Billiard, M. (2001). Age at onset of narcolepsy in two large populations of patients in France and Quebec. *Neurology, 57*(11), 2029–2033. https://doi.org/gkxr73

Dement, W. C. (1993). The history of narcolepsy and other sleep disorders. *Journal of the History of the Neurosciences, 2*(2), 121–134. https://doi.org/bvzhw3

Gauci, S., Hosking, W., & Bruck, D. (2017). Narcolepsy, cataplexy, hypocretin and co-existing other health complaints: A review. *Cogent Medicine, 4*(1), Article 1312791. https://doi.org/gttz

Gélineau, J. B. E. (1880). De la narcolepsie. *Gazette des Hôpitaux, 53*, 626–628.

Lankford, D. A., Wellman, J. J., & O'Hara, C. (1994). Posttraumatic narcolepsy in mild to moderate closed head injury. *Sleep, 17*(s8) Supplement, S25–S28. https://doi.org/gtt2

Levin, M. (1933). The pathogenesis of narcolepsy, with a consideration of sleep-paralysis and localized sleep. *Journal of Neurology and Psychopathology, 14*(53), 1–14. https://doi.org/b293jz

Luo, G., Ambati, A., Lin, L., Bonvalet, M., Partinen, M., Ji, X., Maecker, H. T., & Mignot, E. J.-M. (2018). Autoimmunity to hypocretin and molecular mimicry to flu in type 1 narcolepsy. *Proceedings of the National Academy of Sciences, 115*(52), E12323–E12332. https://doi.org/gjkn3b

Mahoney, C. E., Cogswell, A., Koralnik, I. J., & Scammell, T. E. (2019). The neurobiological basis of narcolepsy. *Nature Reviews Neuroscience, 20*(2), 83–93. https://doi.org/gftxwh

Plazzi, G., Parmeggiani, A., Mignot, E., Lin, L., Scano, M. C., Posar, A., Bernardi, F., Lodi, R., Tonon, C., Barbiroli, B., Montagna, P., & Cicognani, A. (2006). Narcolepsy-cataplexy associated with precocious puberty. *Neurology, 66*(10), 1577–1579. https://doi.org/cx3fv9

Schenck, C. H., Bassetti, C. L., Arnulf, I., & Mignot, E. (2007). English translations of the first clinical reports on narcolepsy and cataplexy by Westphal and Gélineau in the late 19th century, with commentary. *Journal of Clinical Sleep Medicine, 3*(3), 301–311. https://doi.org/gtt3

Sharpless, B. A., & Barber, J. P. (2011). Lifetime prevalence rates of sleep paralysis: A systematic review. *Sleep Medicine Reviews, 15*(5), 311–315. https://doi.org/c4xmnp

Sharpless, B. A., & Grom, J. L. (2016). Isolated sleep paralysis: Fear, prevention, and disruption. *Behavioral Sleep Medicine, 14*(2), 134–139. https://doi.org/3b5

Sours, J. A. (1963). Narcolepsy and other disturbances in the sleep-waking rhythm: A study of 115 cases with review of the literature. *Journal of Nervous and Mental Disease, 137*, 525–542. https://doi.org/b36c5h

Stefani, A., Holzknecht, E., & Högl, B. (2019). Clinical neurophysiology of REM parasomnias. In K. H. Levin & P. Chauvel (Eds.), *Handbook of clinical neurology* (Vol. 161, pp. 381–396). Elsevier. https://doi.org/ghrj77

Sturzenegger, C., & Bassetti, C. L. (2004). The clinical spectrum of narcolepsy with cataplexy: a reappraisal. *Journal of Sleep Research, 13*(4), 395–406. https://doi.org/d5tz2p

Pathological Déjà Vu (and Jamais Vu)

Imagine that you can't shake the feeling that you've experienced something before, even when you clearly haven't. Perhaps you know that feeling as the common form of déjà vu. But pretend that your déjà vu occurred frequently, startlingly, and lasted for long durations. Meeting new people is uncomfortable, because sometimes you feel absolutely certain that you've previously met this total stranger. Visiting new places is unnerving and can make you feel creeped out by combining the definitely new place with the total conviction that the scene is unfolding predictably. You can't shake the feeling that there is something that you can't quite remember about what happens next.

The Stories

(STORY 1) A "highly-educated medical man" wrote a report about his own experiences with "dreamy state" epilepsy back in the late 1800s (p. 200). He wrote that he was waiting around at the bottom of a stairwell for a friend to arrive when suddenly he felt an overwhelming sense of "unexpected 'recollection';—of what, I do not know" (p. 201). That was when his friend showed up and noted that he was pale-looking and leaning up against the wall for support. He reported feeling puzzled and unable to articulate exactly what he had felt he had recollected. This anonymous person went on to describe his own mental condition during these attacks of déjà vu, which recurred at regular intervals over the course of his life along with seizures. He noted that they usually featured that strange feeling of nonspecific recollection, as if his current thought had been thought before "but has been for a time forgotten, and now is recovered" (Hughlings-Jackson 1888, case 5, p. 202).

(STORY 2) A 1994 case series described people who experienced "dreamy states" as part of temporal lobe epilepsy. The researchers recorded some dreamy states using electrodes in and around the patients' brains. This was done as part of epilepsy treatment, as the researchers were determining where the seizures were originating in their brains. These dreamy states included re-experiencing memories as if they were happening again, feelings of fear, feelings of strangeness, and déjà vu. One patient remarked that they experienced the classic *pathological déjà vu* feelings of having previously lived through

DOI: 10.4324/9781003276937-38

a moment in time, with a "feeling of strangeness and often of fear" (p. 78). One patient's seizures always began in the same way: first with a feeling of fear and a constriction around their heart, then with an "indefinable internal feeling of strangeness" that coupled with old or new memories coming back to him, and sometimes with hallucinations of faraway sounds (p. 79). Another patient disclosed "a feeling that what she 'sees, hears and does', she has 'already seen, heard or done exactly the same'" (p. 79). Yet another described "an intensely painful emotional state with a familiar resonance, 'like the memory of an emotion'" during her seizures (p. 80). Feelings of fear and anxiety were frequently reported among other patients, as well (Bancaud et al., 1994, patients 3, 5, 7, and 14).

(STORY 3) An 80-year-old man with memory problems was given the suggestion by his doctor that he should attend a memory clinic to have his memory tested. The man reported that "he had already been" to that memory clinic, which was an impossibility (p. 1364). It turned out that this man had *persistent déjà vu* in which he was almost constantly mistaking new events as repeating events which had already occurred. He would not watch television or read the newspaper because he felt that he'd already seen what they had to offer. When he would go for walks, he would remark that he saw the same bird in the same tree singing the same song or that the people driving by seemed to pass by "at the exact same time every day" (p. 1364). When shopping, he would skip buying certain items on the shopping list because he felt like he had already bought them the day before, even though he had not (Moulin et al., 2005, case 1).

(STORY 4) In a case from France in 1896, a 34-year-old with severe headaches, problems with sleeping, and irritability was admitted to a hospital for the insane. On his first day at the institute, he reacted as if he recognized every object and situation that he encountered. For example, when he met his doctor for the first time, after a few words were exchanged, he suddenly remarked:

> I recognise you now, doctor! It was you who greeted me last year at exactly the same time in the same lounge. You asked me the same questions and I gave the same answers. Everything is very clear to me. You act surprised very well, but you can stop now.
>
> (p. 137)

He also claimed that he recognized the curtains, the sofa, the gardens, and everything else. Of course, he had never actually been there before. Before admission to the institute, he had attended his brother's wedding and made similar outbursts, claiming that he had been to this same event in the previous year and that he didn't understand why they were getting married again at an identical ceremony. When reading newspaper articles, he claimed sometimes that he had read them before, and sometimes they felt so familiar that he claimed that he must have been the one who wrote them. His persistent déjà vu was so severe that he sometimes claimed that he felt his life was repeating over again, as if he were trapped in a cycle of repeating his past events, feelings, and even dreams (Arnaud, 1896; translated by Bertrand et al., 2017).

The Features

Déjà vu is a French term that translates to "already seen." It is a feeling of familiarity for an experience that you are currently having, despite the unfamiliarity of the experience. The experience is new, but it doesn't *feel* new; it feels as though it has already happened. Believe it or not, it's possible to damage your brain such that you *always* feel that uncanny familiarity. Read on to discover how but, first, let's discuss the more common and benign form.

Déjà vu is a global term for "any subjectively inappropriate impression of familiarity of the present experience with an undefined past"—however, there are many different "déjà experiences" with their own names (Neppe, 2010, p. 62). There is *déjà pensé* which is the feeling that you've already thought something that you are currently thinking, even though you haven't. *Déjà lu* is a term used when you believe that you've already read something, but you're actually reading it for the first time. *Déjà raconté* is when you believe that you already told someone something, even though you haven't told them yet. *Déjà lu* is a term used when you believe that you've already read something, but you're actually reading it for the first—wait a minute… Before the French name of "déjà vu" was settled on, the feeling had a bunch of different names, including "sentiment of pre-existence," "promnesia," "illusion of memory," and "Empfindungsspiegelung"—that last one is from 1850s Germany (Sno & Linszen, 1990, p. 1588). I'm not sure why it didn't catch on, but I'm hoping it makes a comeback.

More than half of all people will experience episodes of déjà vu in their lifetime. However, there are two groups of people with especially strong déjà vu: people with seizures (see Seizures), and people with schizophrenia (Brown, 2003). Déjà vu is highly associated with temporal lobe epilepsy—déjà vu in epileptics occurs more frequently, lasts longer, and has more emotional symptoms than in people without epilepsy (Warren-Gash & Zeman, 2014). This *stronger* type of déjà vu that is found in people with disorders of the brain is known as *pathological* déjà vu.

Let's discuss the additional emotional symptoms of pathological déjà vu, because they are quite intense and may differ from what you think of when you imagine déjà vu. Two big emotional symptoms that may occur are intense feelings of *derealization* and *fear*. Derealization is pretty much what it sounds like—you come to feel like your experiences are not real, as if you were dreaming. Feelings of derealization may also happen in non-seizure-related déjà vu.

People with seizure-related pathological déjà vu also frequently report being *frightened* during the episode, something that people experiencing typical non-seizure-related déjà vu do not report feeling. It is sometimes described as a fear in the chest or the throat, as if the fear was giving them breathing difficulties (Bancaud et al., 1994). The feeling of fear is common in epilepsy before the seizure itself happens, so it makes sense for fear to appear along with pathological déjà vu in some people. These emotional differences are big enough that some people with epilepsy claim that they can tell the difference between the kind of pathological déjà vu that accompanies a seizure and the kind of déjà vu that most people experience, because their brains are capable of both kinds (Warren-Gash & Zeman, 2014).

While we are at it, we should also briefly talk about jamais vu. Jamais vu is not only a hit song by the legendary K-pop group BTS; it's also a symptom of a confused brain. Jamais vu is the less commonly discussed sibling of déjà vu and can be thought of as the opposite sensation. Jamais vu is the inappropriate feeling of *unfamiliarity* during a situation that should feel familiar, and it is rarer than déjà vu (Brown, 2003). Imagine walking into your bedroom and feeling like you were seeing it for the first time. More than just not recognizing any of the objects or pieces of furniture, jamais vu is an emotional experience of the unknown at an unexpected time. Jamais vu and déjà vu are both more common in people with temporal lobe epilepsy (Sno et al., 1992).

People with epilepsy can have a variety of *cognitive-dysmnesic phenomena* during seizures, including pathological déjà vu and other ways in which their thinking, memory, and mood is temporarily disrupted (Ardila et al., 1988). Such changes can last anywhere from seconds to hours, depending on the person (Neppe, 2010). They might say, "I feel that I have already dreamed about the things that are happening" or mention a "feeling of repetition of facts, attitudes or words" or even feeling "as if I were in a film" (Ardila et al., 1988, p. 14). What is happening in the brain during these periods when feelings of reality become so strange?

The Brain Pathology

It is widely believed that the parts of the brain involved in pathological déjà vu are in the temporal lobe, including the temporal neocortex, amygdala, and hippocampus (Cleary & Brown, 2021). This makes intuitive sense because the amygdala is involved in generating the feeling of fear, and the hippocampus is involved in processing memories (see Amnesia). Episodes of déjà vu are sometimes triggered by electrically stimulating those parts of the temporal lobe (Bancaud et al., 1994). For example, in a woman with epilepsy, researchers found changes in her hippocampus during electrode-provoked episodes of pathological déjà vu and disturbances to her memory (Kovacs et al., 2009).

There are many dozens of theories about what is happening in the brain during déjà vu, especially because there are multiple types of déjà vu (Neppe, 2010). Many researchers have only recently begun treating déjà vu as a phenomenon worthy of scientific scrutiny, and there are currently no objective criteria for evaluating cases of déjà vu, which makes comparing between cases pretty unscientific at the moment (Cleary & Brown, 2021). And, unfortunately for this particular chapter, the majority of research has focused on examining déjà vu in nonclinical populations—regular old déjà vu. This means that there is much work left before we will understand the pathological form of déjà vu.

In cases of seizure-related pathological déjà vu, the feeling passes with time and the person regains their footing in reality, and probably never fully believed that they truly *were* living through the same moment for a second time. In other words, they were not fooled by their brain into believing that the feeling of déjà vu was correct—they knew that it was just a feeling. In contrast are the rare cases in which the person enters a permanent state of déjà vu—and the intense feelings of familiarity are incorrectly interpreted as genuine memories.

This more or less permanent déjà vu has been called *recollective confabulation* or *persistent déjà vu* (Thompson et al., 2004). This condition can be acquired via brain damage, especially as a consequence of neurodegenerative diseases such as dementia (Moulin, 2013). People with this condition may be bored by the news and television because it feels like they have heard or seen all of it before (Thompson et al., 2004). Indeed, they may find themselves "withdrawing from all novel activities, complaining that they had experienced them before" (Moulin, 2013, p. 1542). This persistent pathological déjà vu is a combination of anosognosia (see Anosognosia) and déjà vu because the person is not aware that their feelings of familiarity are wrong (Thompson et al., 2004).

One theory about what is happening in the brains of people with persistent déjà vu is that, because of brain damage, they are confusing the feeling of encoding a new memory with the feeling of retrieving a memory for that event (O'Connor et al., 2010). In tests where the person is shown pictures, and then later asked to pick out which pictures they have seen before from a group that also includes pictures they have never seen before, people with this disorder show an unusually high false-alarm rate in which they incorrectly identify new pictures as being old pictures (Craik et al., 2014). This shows us that the brain can lose its ability to tell abstract feelings of déjà vu apart from reality. So, the next time that you have a moment when the world doesn't feel real, remember that it's just a trick of your brain and that, most of the time, the feeling will pass.

References

Ardila, A., Botero, M., Gomez, J., & Quijano, C. (1988). Partial cognitive-dysmnesic seizures as a model for studying psychoses. *International Journal of Neuroscience*, *38*, 11–20. https://doi.org/cqfz5p

Arnaud, F. L. (1896). Un cas d'illusion du 'deja vu' ou de 'fausse memoire'. *Annale Medico-Psychologiques*, *3*, 455–471.

Bancaud, J., Brunet-Bourgin, F., Chauvel, P., & Halgren, E. (1994). Anatomical origin of déjà vu and vivid 'memories' in human temporal lobe epilepsy. *Brain*, *117*(1), 71–90. https://doi.org/c8hjs9

Bertrand, J. M., Martinon, L. M., Souchay, C., & Moulin, C. J. (2017). History repeating itself: Arnaud's case of pathological déjà vu. *Cortex*, *87*, 129–141. https://doi.org/f9vm6k

Brown, A. S. (2003). A review of the deja vu experience. *Psychological Bulletin*, *129*(3), 394–413. https://doi.org/bfwb4q

Cleary, A. M., & Brown, A. S. (2021). *The déjà vu experience* (2nd ed.). Routledge. https://doi.org/gtt4

Craik, F. I., Barense, M. D., Rathbone, C. J., Grusec, J. E., Stuss, D. T., Gao, F., Scott, C. J. M., & Black, S. E. (2014). VL: A further case of erroneous recollection. *Neuropsychologia*, *56*, 367–380. https://doi.org/f52r77

Hughlings-Jackson, J. (1888). On a particular variety of epilepsy ("intellectual aura"), one case with symptoms of organic brain disease. *Brain*, *11*(2), 179–207. https://doi.org/dks43x

Kovacs, N., Auer, T., Balas, I., Karadi, K., Zambo, K., Schwarcz, A., Klivenyi, P., Jokeit, H., Horvath, K., Nagy, F., & Janszky, J. (2009). Neuroimaging and cognitive changes during déjà vu. *Epilepsy & Behavior*, *14*(1), 190–196. https://doi.org/c74f2d

Moulin, C. J. A. (2013). Disordered recognition memory: Recollective confabulation. *Cortex*, *49*(6), 1541–1552. https://doi.org/f43xz9

Moulin, C. J. A., Conway, M. A., Thompson, R. G., James, N., & Jones, R. W. (2005). Disordered memory awareness: Recollective confabulation in two cases of persistent déjà vecu. *Neuropsychologia*, *43*(9), 1362–1378. https://doi.org/btscmw

Neppe, V. M. (2010). Déjà vu: Origins and phenomenology: Implications of the four subtypes for future research. *The Journal of Parapsychology*, *74*(1), 61–97.

O'Connor, A. R., Lever, C., & Moulin, C. J. (2010). Novel insights into false recollection: A model of déjà vécu. *Cognitive Neuropsychiatry*, *15*(1–3), 118–144. https://doi.org/c2kp87

Sno, H. N., & Linszen, D. H. (1990). The déjà vu experience: Remembrance of things past? *The American Journal of Psychiatry*, *147*(12), 1587–1595. https://doi.org/gtt5

Sno, H. N., Schalken, H. F. A., & De Jonghe, F. (1992). Empirical research on déjà vu experiences: A review. *Behavioural Neurology*, *5*(3), 155–160. https://doi.org/gcfbrq

Thompson, R. G., Moulin, C. J. A., Conway, M. A., & Jones, R. W. (2004). Persistent déja vu: A disorder of memory. *International Journal of Geriatric Psychiatry*, *19*(9), 906–907. https://doi.org/cg2pp9

Warren-Gash, C., & Zeman, A. (2014). Is there anything distinctive about epileptic déjà vu? *Journal of Neurology Neurosurgery and Psychiatry*, *85*(2), 143–147. https://doi.org/ggwjcg

Phantom Sensations (including Phantom Limb Pain)

Imagine that you can't stop the pain in one of your body parts, despite that body part having been removed. Whether by accident or in an intentional surgery, part of your body is missing, such as an arm, a leg, a breast, or something along those lines. Despite its absence, you still *feel* that it is a part of you. At the worst of times, you feel pain in that missing part. Perhaps you can feel the nails of your missing hand digging into your missing palm. Perhaps there is a constant throbbing in a thigh that you no longer have. Perhaps you can feel shooting pains coming and going in a leg that hasn't been attached to you in years. Is there any way to get these phantoms to leave you alone?

The Stories

(STORY 1) Eight men with phantom pain were interviewed by researchers for a study published in 2014. A man paralyzed from the neck down due to a severed spinal cord reported that "because of the painful itching I know where my legs are" (p. 602). A man with a missing leg due to a motorbike accident shared that he "can feel pain in my 'knee' and down in my 'toes'" (p. 602). One person missing both his right arm and right leg said that sometimes he feels "as if the fingers on my amputated hand are moving uncontrollably, which is both extremely painful and embarrassing" (p. 602). However, despite their pain and mobility setbacks, the men overall found ways to enjoy life and things to look forward to. One of the interviewees who had been injured in a traffic accident was spending time visiting schools to caution children about proper traffic safety. The researchers concluded that "life itself transcends everything, even excruciating and constant pain!" (Nortvedt & Engelsrud, 2014, p. 604).

(STORY 2) A 15-year-old girl had one of her legs amputated above the knee due to cancer. Because she was worried about possible phantom pain before the surgery, she was encouraged to keep a daily log of her pain and sensation experiences in her phantom leg "from her own experience" following the amputation (McGrath & Hillier, 1992, p. 48). On the day following the leg removal, she felt in the phantom limb "itching and tingling sensations … as if her toes were asleep" (McGrath & Hillier, 1992, p. 48). These sensations continued to develop over a period of ten days, eventually covering the

DOI: 10.4324/9781003276937-39

entire phantom limb, such that the whole thing felt itchy and tingly for a few minutes each day. After the 12th day, the phantom episodes began to shorten, until they lasted only a couple of seconds by day 26. The phantom sensations became less frequent, and eventually they disappeared entirely (McGrath & Hillier, 1992). Some researchers believe that the younger a person is when they have a body part removed, the less likely they are to have serious problems with phantoms (Flor et al., 2006).

(STORY 3) A case of supernumerary phantom limb occurred in a 65-year-old man following a severe stroke. He had many symptoms, including somatoparaphrenia (see Somatoparaphrenia), partial vision loss, sensory loss, and limb paralysis. He believed that his left limbs had been amputated—which was not true—and claimed that the arm and leg attached to him were not his limbs. Eventually, the delusions of the non-belongingness of the limbs began to fade, but they were replaced with a belief that he could feel a third arm protruding from his body from the "top left corner of his torso" (p. 160). At one point, he drew its approximate location. When he was asked to elaborate on the appearance of this supernumerary limb, he often requested that the topic of the interview be changed because it disturbed him. However, he did occasionally allow himself to be interviewed about the third arm. He could feel, and reportedly sometimes see, the arm protruding from the middle of his body. It was a left arm, based on the thumb location. He could feel it grow cold, said that it didn't move, and kept "getting in the way" (p. 162). Outside of the third arm, the patient appeared to behave completely rationally. He was even somewhat aware of how irrational believing in a third arm was—when asked what he thought about someone having three hands, he admitted that "it's an odd situation!" (Halligan et al., 1993, p. 162).

(STORY 4) A man who had lost an arm in a motorcycle accident responded to an ad in a newspaper that said "amputees needed" (Doidge, 2007, p. 187). He then found himself, a decade after the accident, in the office of Dr V. S. Ramachandran, participating in a new theoretical therapy for phantom limb pain. After his accident, he lost the ability to move the arm, and it was kept in a sling for about a year until it was amputated. Unfortunately, following the amputation, he developed "a terrible pain in [his] phantom elbow, wrist and fingers" (Ramachandran & Blakeslee, 1998, p. 47). Despite trying to "move" the phantom limb in the hopes of relieving the pain, the patient had never been able to do so. Dr Ramachandran instructed him to use a mirror box to make it *look* like his left arm was still attached to him. By inserting his *right* arm into the mirror box, the reflection made it look like his *left* arm was also in the box, and attached to his body. Amazingly, as he looked at the reflection of his right arm in the mirror, he suddenly felt as if he could move his phantom left arm—but only when his eyes were open and sending visual signals to his brain about how it looked like his left arm was moving. He remarked: "my left arm is plugged in again … I can feel my elbow moving and my wrist moving. It's all moving again" (Ramachandran & Blakeslee, 1998, pp. 47–48). Over time, as he continued using the mirror box, the phantom arm mostly disappeared as his brain restructured itself, although the feeling of the phantom fingers and palm remained. This case was the first known instance of phantom limb amputation (Doidge, 2007).

The Features

Your ability to sense your body parts—where they are currently located, and what they are touching—is possible thanks to nerve cells that run like cables from your body parts all the way up into your brain. The cables then run back down again into each muscle, forming a loop of what is essentially electrical wiring. As examples, you have loops of nerve cell connections that keep track of your leg's placement in space, or whether your hand is bumping up against something dangerous like a hot stovetop. Many of these cells are in your body parts themselves and in your spine, but an important portion of these cells are in a part of your brain located near the very peak of your skull, called the *sensorimotor cortex*. This area is divided between two parts: unsurprisingly, the *sensory* and *motor* parts. The sensory cells are in charge of interpreting incoming sensations from each body part, such as touch. The motor cells are involved in sending out signals that cause each body part to move. It is because of these cells, left behind in the brain when a body part is removed, that phantom sensations are possible.

Each body part has a certain number of sensory cells and a certain number of motor cells that are assigned to it. Body parts that are sensitive to touch—like the lips—take up a relatively large portion of space in the sensory cortex. Body parts that have precise muscular control—like the hands—have many cells representing them in the motor cortex. In contrast, body parts that are relatively insensitive and do not have fine motor control don't have very many cells, such as your trunk. No, I mean the *other* kind of trunk: your chest and abdomen. Unless you're an elephant-person, but in that case, I imagine your trunk would be highly sensitive and have high fine motor skills, so the hypothetical elephant-person's trunk would take up a lot of relative space in the sensorimotor cortex.

When a map of the body parts as they are represented in the brain is drawn out, a creature called a *homunculus* appears. The size of the homunculus' body parts is relative to how many cells our brain has for each body part. This creature has grotesquely exaggerated hands and lips because we have lots of cells dedicated to those parts, and tiny trunks and legs because we have very few cells responsible for those regions. Technically there are two homunculi—one for sensation and one for motor control—and they don't always match. For example, your earlobes are more sensitive than they are movable. The homunculi show us the literal truth of how our body is represented by our brain.

But what happens when a body part goes missing, such as when it is amputated? As it turns out, those brain cells representing that part of the body do not just disappear, nor do they automatically move on to other jobs for other body parts. Because of those sensorimotor cells, a hand that no longer exists at the end of your arm still exists as a *phantom* in your brain. And sometimes, these phantom body parts misbehave.

When a person experiences feelings in a part of their body that no longer exists, they are having *phantom sensations*. Phantom sensations can include feelings of movement, touch, itching, and presence, as if the missing part were occupying physical space. In one study, the most commonly reported phantom sensations were feeling like the phantom was moving, and feelings of cold or electricity moving through the missing part (Kooijman et al., 2000). This may sound unbelievable if you are someone who has never lost a body part, but nearly every amputee reports having some sensations in and/or awareness of their body part that is no longer attached (Sturma et al., 2021). The missing body part can feel so real that surprising mistakes are made, such as a person who tried to use their missing hand to hold onto their horse, while using their one remaining hand to encourage the horse to move, resulting in being thrown to the ground (Mitchell, 1872).

Most commonly, phantom body parts take the form of an arm or a leg, which are referred to as phantom limbs. However, phantoms related to lost body parts are not limited to limbs. A somewhat common phantom body part is the breast following surgical removal, usually as a treatment for breast cancer (Staps et al., 1985). A phantom penis, along with phantom erections, can follow surgeries in which the penis is removed or altered in form (Ramachandran & McGeoch, 2008). Other examples include the phantom uterus, phantom rectum, and phantom bladder—which lead to cases of people having feelings of phantom menstrual cramps, phantom "passing gas," and phantom urinating (Katz & Melzack, 1990, p. 321). The human brain creates all of those perceptions, if you think about it, so it's not as strange as it seems that the brain can create those feelings even in the absence of the respective body part.

Because the feeling of the phantom body part is happening in the brain, sometimes the phantom can be in physically impossible positions (Stankevicius et al., 2021). Perhaps the most extreme example of this is a phenomenon called *telescoping*. Telescoping is a phenomenon in which phantom limbs feel like they have retracted into their stump, like a collapsible telescope. This may result in, for example, a person feeling like they have phantom fingers attached directly to the end of their stump which ends at their elbow (Sturma et al., 2021). Telescoping is rarer than general phantom sensations, with perhaps 15–25% of amputees experiencing it at some point in their life following their amputation (Stankevicius et al., 2021).

Believe it or not, phantom body parts can be mismatched with the reality of the body in other ways, such as in *supernumerary phantom limb*, in which a person's brain represents extra body parts that don't actually exist such as an extra arm or an extra leg. These cases might be similar to phantom limb cases where the person realizes that the limbs are not actually real, or, they may be more serious "delusional" cases (see Anosognosia) where they believe the extra limbs to be real (Halligan et al., 1993). Supernumerary phantom limbs can be combined with the condition of somatoparaphrenia (see Somatoparaphrenia), resulting in people believing that extra limbs are attached to them because they can *feel* them existing, but they believe that the limbs do not actually *belong* to them (e.g., Weinstein et al., 1954, case 1). In contrast, a person who is born without a body part may nonetheless experience a phantom for that absent body part (e.g., Kooijman et al., 2000).

We need to discuss the most troubling phantom symptom, which is that of phantom pain. Phantom pain is feelings of burning, cramping, throbbing, stinging—among other unpleasant sensations—in a body part that is no longer attached to you (Hill, 1999). The pain can come and go in short shocks or be a constant "excruciatingly painful experience"—sometimes the pain begins immediately after the loss of the body part, but it may also appear years later (Flor et al., 2006, p. 873).

Phantom limb pain occurs in 50–80% of limb amputees (Richardson & Kulkarni, 2017). Some amputations occur because of traumatic reasons, such as warfare or car accidents, and some result from nontraumatic disease, like cancer or vascular diseases. Traumatic and nontraumatic amputees are both capable of experiencing phantom pain to a similar degree (Houghton et al., 1994).

The Brain Pathology

Even though phantoms are something that many people experience, researchers still do not have "a widely agreed [upon] and accepted theory" for how phantom pain arises (Sturma et al., 2021, p. 105). There are, however, several avenues of research that have revealed different possible mechanisms of action for phantom pain that, when combined, and with further research, may explain these complex phantom phenomena. The two biggest categories of phantom theories are those of the peripheral nervous system and those of the central nervous system.

Mechanisms of the peripheral nervous system concern themselves with the nerves located near where the body part used to be located, before the electrical messages travel up the spinal cord. Following amputation, the severed nerves toward the end of the stump change shape and size into a sort of bulb called a *neuroma*. Like faulty electrical wiring, neuromas may create unwanted and abnormal electrical activity, possibly due to changes in how sensitive the cells' ion channels are (Flor et al., 2006). These neuromas may then send abnormal electrical messages up through the peripheral nerves and eventually into your brain which interprets those messages as pain (Sturma et al., 2021). However, phantom limb pain often appears even before neuromas have had a chance to form, and the use of anesthesia to numb the peripheral nerves or even the spinal cord itself does not always eliminate the phantom pain (Flor et al., 2006). Which is why we need to look at the brain itself.

As the brain receives fewer sensations from the outside world, it makes changes to the parts of itself that were responsible for processing those sensations in an attempt to adapt to the new situation. This happens in the case of reduced light processed by the eyes (see Charles Bonnet Syndrome), in the case of reduced sound processed by the ears (see Tinnitus), and in the case of phantom sensations, which may be due to reduced sensations of touch. In theory, two important brain phenomena that contribute to phantom pain are *persistent representation* and *cortical reorganization*, both of which seem to occur in the sensorimotor cortex that I mentioned earlier.

Persistent representation is when the cells responsible for representing the missing body part keep doing their old jobs even though the body part is no longer there. Brain scans have revealed phantom fingers still exist in the brain more than three decades following their amputation (Kikkert et al., 2016). As part of persistent representation, phantom pain may result from a change in how many messages the phantom's cells are sending and receiving, called *functional connectivity* (Makin et al., 2013). In other words, in order to understand the pain, it is important to understand when and where the phantom is sending and receiving signals.

Cortical reorganization, on the other hand, is when the cells that were previously used to do jobs for the missing body part are reassigned to do something else. Some research has claimed that more severe phantom pain is associated with more cortical reorganization—as their homunculus increasingly becomes a shape-shifter they increasingly feel pain in their missing parts (Flor et al., 2006). However, more recent research has concluded that "there is no simple relationship between somatosensory map reorganization" and phantom limb pain (Makin & Flor, 2020, p. 7).

It is possible that both persistent representation and cortical reorganization contribute to phantom pain (Sturma et al., 2021). That may sound contradictory, but not if you think of the cells as having part-time jobs. Perhaps some of the brain cells that were representing the amputated arm are now working part-time as cells to represent the person's face, but they are also working part-time to interpret signals as if the arm were still there. As you might imagine, this may result in some confusing sensations such as pain, but more research is needed to fully understand the complexities in the brain during phantom sensations.

When possible, the best approach seems to be preventing the phantom pain from appearing in the first place by ensuring that there is no long-term pain occurring prior to the amputation (Larbig et al., 2019). It has long been shown that sometimes the pain following the loss of the body part is similar to the type of pain that the person felt prior to losing sensation from the body part, such as a person who continued to feel the pain of an ingrown toenail even following a complete break in their spinal cord (Katz & Melzack, 1990). The fact that prior experiences with chronic pain predict a predisposition for phantom limb pain following amputation suggests that proper treatment of chronic pain prior to the removal of the body part can reduce the risk for developing severe phantom pain in the future (Larbig et al., 2019).

But what can be done if the phantom pain already exists? Pharmacological treatments such as painkillers or antidepressants are not very helpful (Flor, 2002). Historically, removing the part of the brain's sensorimotor cortex corresponding to the missing limb was sometimes attempted (e.g., de Gutiérrez-Mahoney, 1944). This psychosurgery is now generally regarded as a bad idea because cutting out parts of the brain has severe side effects. As an interesting sidenote, there are cases of people with phantom pain accidentally becoming cured after acquiring brain damage, allegedly because the part of their brain that was producing the pain was destroyed (e.g., Appenzeller & Bicknell, 1969; Yarnitsky et al., 1988). I absolutely *would not recommend* such a dangerous "treatment."

Fortunately, other treatment options do exist. Mirror box therapy is an interesting alternative in which the visual trickery of mirrors is used to create a reflection as if the person's missing body part was still attached (Ramachandran & Blakeslee, 1998). Apparently, seeing is believing, because some amputees report feeling a reduction in pain and duration of painful episodes after looking at a simulated body part that was not visibly being frozen or electrocuted or telescoping in impossible ways (e.g., Finn et al., 2017). In some cases, if the physician uses a mirror and pretends to touch the phantom limb by stroking the reflection, the amputee may actually feel the touch in the missing limb (Ramachandran & Rogers-Ramachandran, 1996). While mirror therapy doesn't work for all phantom pains, it does seem to help improve quality of life for many people (Campo-Prieto & Rodríguez-Fuentes, 2020). There has also been recent research into neuromodulation techniques, such as electrically stimulating the sensorimotor cortex, and early results have been encouraging (Pacheco-Barrios et al., 2020). Overall, phantoms are a lot less mysterious than they used to be, but even with a scientific explanation, these apparitions may continue to greatly affect the lives of those who experience them.

References

Appenzeller, O., & Bicknell, J. M. (1969). Effects of nervous system lesions on phantom experience in amputees. *Neurology, 19*(2), 141–146. https://doi.org/gtt6

Campo-Prieto, P., & Rodríguez-Fuentes, G. (2020). Effectiveness of mirror therapy in phantom limb pain: A literature review. *Neurología (English Edition)*. https://doi.org/gtt7

de Gutiérrez-Mahoney, C. G. (1944). The treatment of painful phantom limb by removal of post-central cortex. *Journal of Neurosurgery, 1*(2), 156–162. https://doi.org/fh2zx7

Doidge, N. (2007). *The brain that changes itself: Stories of personal triumph from the frontiers of brain science*. Penguin.

Finn, S. B., Perry, B. N., Clasing, J. E., Walters, L. S., Jarzombek, S. L., Curran, S., Rouhanian, M., Keszler, M. S., Hussey-Andersen, L. K., Weeks, S. R., Pasquina, P. F., & Tsao, J. W. (2017). A randomized, controlled trial of mirror therapy for upper extremity phantom limb pain in male amputees. *Frontiers in Neurology, 8*, Article 267. https://doi.org/gbpq4k

Flor, H. (2002). Phantom-limb pain: Characteristics, causes, and treatment. *The Lancet Neurology, 1*(3), 182–189. https://doi.org/bfmqgf

Flor, H., Nikolajsen, L., & Jensen, T. S. (2006). Phantom limb pain: A case of maladaptive CNS plasticity? *Nature Reviews Neuroscience, 7*(11), 873–881. https://doi.org/bf82cx

Halligan, P. W., Marshall, J. C., & Wade, D. T. (1993). Three arms: A case study of supernumerary phantom limb after right hemisphere stroke. *Journal of Neurology, Neurosurgery & Psychiatry, 56*(2), 159–166. https://doi.org/bwp6g4

Hill, A. (1999). Phantom limb pain: A review of the literature on attributes and potential mechanisms. *Journal of Pain and Symptom Management, 17*(2), 125–142. https://doi.org/ct7cp2

Houghton, A. D., Nicholls, G., Houghton, A. L., Saadah, E., & McColl, L. (1994). Phantom pain: Natural history and association with rehabilitation. *Annals of the Royal College of Surgeons of England, 76*(1), 22–25.

Katz, J., & Melzack, R. (1990). Pain "memories" in phantom limbs: Review and clinical observations. *Pain, 43*(3), 319–336. https://doi.org/dm8n5s

Kikkert, S., Kolasinski, J., Jbabdi, S., Tracey, I., Beckmann, C. F., Berg, H. J., & Makin, T. R. (2016). Revealing the neural fingerprints of a missing hand. *eLife, 5*, Article 15292. https://doi.org/f9kt84

Kooijman, C. M., Dijkstra, P. U., Geertzen, J. H., Elzinga, A., & van der Schans, C. P. (2000). Phantom pain and phantom sensations in upper limb amputees: An epidemiological study. *Pain, 87*(1), 33–41. https://doi.org/bxsq27

Larbig, W., Andoh, J., Huse, E., Stahl-Corino, D., Montoya, P., Seltzer, Z. E., & Flor, H. (2019). Pre-and postoperative predictors of phantom limb pain. *Neuroscience Letters, 702*, 44–50. https://doi.org/gjv5jk

Makin, T. R., & Flor, H. (2020). Brain (re)organisation following amputation: Implications for phantom limb pain. *NeuroImage, 218*, Article 116943. https://doi.org/ghmckw

Makin, T. R., Scholz, J., Filippini, N., Henderson Slater, D., Tracey, I., & Johansen-Berg, H. (2013). Phantom pain is associated with preserved structure and function in the former hand area. *Nature Communications, 4*, Article 1570. https://doi.org/f4n5hz

McGrath, P. A., & Hillier, L. M. (1992). Phantom limb sensations in adolescents: A case study to illustrate the utility of sensation and pain logs in pediatric clinical practice. *Journal of Pain and Symptom Management, 7*(1), 46–53. https://doi.org/bskwwv

Mitchell, S. W. (1872). *Injuries of nerves and their consequences.* JB Lippincott.

Nortvedt, F., & Engelsrud, G. (2014). "Imprisoned" in pain: Analyzing personal experiences of phantom pain. *Medicine, Health Care and Philosophy, 17*(4), 599–608. https://doi.org/gtt8

Pacheco-Barrios, K., Meng, X., & Fregni, F. (2020). Neuromodulation techniques in phantom limb pain: A systematic review and meta-analysis. *Pain Medicine, 21*(10), 2310–2322. https://doi.org/gtt9

Ramachandran, V. S., & Blakeslee, S. (1998). *Phantoms in the brain: Probing the mysteries of the human mind.* William Morrow.

Ramachandran, V. S., & McGeoch, P. D. (2008). Phantom penises in transsexuals. *Journal of Consciousness Studies, 15*(1), 5–16.

Ramachandran, V. S., & Rogers-Ramachandran, D. (1996). Synaesthesia in phantom limbs induced with mirrors. *Proceedings of the Royal Society B: Biological Sciences, 263*(1369), 377–386. https://doi.org/fnrnk3

Richardson, C., & Kulkarni, J. (2017). A review of the management of phantom limb pain: Challenges and solutions. *Journal of Pain Research, 10*, 1861–1870. https://doi.org/gbvjbk

Stankevicius, A., Wallwork, S. B., Summers, S. J., Hordacre, B., & Stanton, T. R. (2021). Prevalence and incidence of phantom limb pain, phantom limb sensations and telescoping in amputees: A systematic rapid review. *European Journal of Pain, 25*(1), 23–38. https://doi.org/gtvb

Staps, T., Hoogenhout, J., & Wobbes, T. (1985). Phantom breast sensations following mastectomy. *Cancer, 56*(12), 2898–2901. https://doi.org/cwppjp

Sturma, A., Hruby, L., & Diers, M. (2021). Epidemiology and mechanisms of phantom limb pain. In O. C. Aszmann & D. Farina (Eds.), *Bionic limb reconstruction* (pp. 103–111). Springer, Cham. https://doi.org/gtvc

Weinstein, E. A., Kahn, R. L., Malitz, S., & Rozanski, J. (1954). Delusional reduplication of parts of the body. *Brain, 77,* 45–60. https://doi.org/drf3nv

Yarnitsky, D., Barron, S. A., & Bental, E. (1988). Disappearance of phantom pain after focal brain infarction. *Pain, 32*(3), 285–287. https://doi.org/dp4jb3

Prosopagnosia

Imagine that you can't recognize people that you know when you look at their faces. Pretend that you are approached by someone at a store, and they chat with you for a few minutes about the weather. You politely make small talk, wondering why this person approached you. Then, they specifically ask about a family member of yours. "Oh no," you think in a panic, "do I know this person?" You try looking at their hairstyle and clothing for clues. Finally, they laugh, and you recognize that sound. Relieved, you smile and continue chatting with your old friend that you have just identified, hoping that they didn't notice that you couldn't tell who they were for several minutes.

The Stories

(STORY 1) Dr. Oliver Sacks, a professor of neurology, best-selling author, and a person with prosopagnosia, described an incident of recognition failure when it came to his psychiatrist. Sacks had been seeing this psychiatrist twice a week for several years but had never seen him out of context—that is, outside of a session. A few minutes after leaving a meeting between the two of them, Dr Sacks reported that "a soberly dressed man greeted me in the lobby of the building. I was puzzled as to why this stranger seemed to know me, until the doorman addressed him by name—it was, of course, my own analyst" (p. 84). Sacks noted that the following session with his psychiatrist was awkward. This was not the only instance in his life where he failed to recognize someone right in front of him, including at times his own assistant, and even his own reflection in the mirror (Sacks, 2010).

(STORY 2) A 58-year-old man lost consciousness briefly and, following this, his abilities to identify familiar faces and to identify familiar animals vanished. In the hospital, he failed to recognize his doctor, and then failed to recognize his own wife until she began speaking, at which point he correctly identified her. Each time the hospital staff came in, they seemed completely unfamiliar to him. When he returned to his farm, he found that he could no longer recognize individual cows and calves—something that, before, he had done easily. He had grown up on a farm around animals such as cows and horses, and he continued working on a farm as an adult, so this deficit in animal

DOI: 10.4324/9781003276937-40

recognition worried him. Eighteen months later, he continued to show similar face identification problems, such as being unable to recognize the face of a farmworker who had worked there for over a year (Bornstein et al., 1969).

(STORY 3) In one case, a 38-year-old person with prosopagnosia was shown a picture of himself, and reported that he wasn't sure who the photo featured, although he suspected that it *might* be a picture of himself. Following this, the doctor handed the person with prosopagnosia a picture of the doctor himself. Even though the person with prosopagnosia had met the doctor many times, and was now sitting next to the doctor while looking at the photo, he was unable to identify the person in the picture. In describing this person with prosopagnosia, the authors wrote that when he was approached, he would gaze at the approaching person, and then begin tilting and turning his head in a puzzled way. The patient reported that he would first look at a person's chin and mouth, then the sides of their face, their nose, their eyes, and their forehead—but "according to his own statement, 'could not put it all together'" (p. 238). He would sometimes try using specific features such as clothing, eyeglasses, and body shape in order to identify a person, but even when he was correct, he had no *certainty* of whether he was correct—it felt like guessing. According to the authors of the case study, when he could hear the person's voice or could use some other non-face cue such as clothing, "he was able to identify the person to whom he was speaking, but was unable to do so by simply looking at the face itself" (Cole & Perez-Cruet, 1964, p. 238).

The Features

Being able to recognize people such as friends and family, as well as the ability to realize that you *don't* recognize someone—a potential enemy?—are important survival skills for humans. This is because in our evolutionary history we were social creatures that lived in small groups. If you saw someone from your group, your brain would send a signal of familiarity to let you know that this person was probably safe to hang out with. If you didn't recognize them, your brain would send a signal telling you to be suspicious of the stranger. This won't be a problem for future humans, of course, once we all have facial recognition cameras built into contact lenses. As dystopian as that sounds, it would be very helpful for people with prosopagnosia.

Facial recognition is seemingly automatic in many people, but some struggle to recognize identities from faces. Prosopagnosia was named in 1947, when Joachim Bodamer wrote about some patients that had problems identifying *who* was in a given photograph. For example, one of the patients, when shown a picture of a dog, thought that it was a picture of a person, but with "curious hair" (Bodamer, 1947, as discussed in Bornstein et al., 1969, p. 164). He named this disorder "prosop agnosia" from the Greek words for "face ignorance." In popular culture, prosopagnosia is often called *face blindness*, which is much easier to say. The disorder made some appearances in a few episodes of the television show *Arrested Development* and was depicted more or less accurately, except perhaps for the scene in which Tobias is mistaken as Lindsay (Lorey et al., 2013). People with prosopagnosia often complain about being unable to follow the storyline of television shows and films because they have trouble telling the actors apart, so they would probably find that face-blindness plot from *Arrested Development* to be quite confusing (e.g., Bowles et al., 2009).

In prosopagnosia, the person loses the ability to *recognize* the faces of familiar people. Gazing upon the faces of friends, family, and loved ones doesn't spark that feeling of familiarity that usually lets us know *who* the person is. The person with prosopagnosia can still see every *individual* detail about the person's face: hairstyle, scars, glasses, and so on (Barton, 2011). They might be able to correctly determine a person's age, facial expressions (see Social-Emotional Agnosias), and gender from looking at their face (Tranel et al., 1988). They also can, when looking at a face, correctly say that it is indeed a face—they can *detect* faces (Garrido et al., 2008). But when it comes time to assign an identity to that face, they falter. Why is that? Well, it's complicated, and still a bit of an open question.

There are two main types of prosopagnosia. The first is acquired prosopagnosia, which is when a person originally did possess the ability to recognize people, but then lost it due to a stroke or another type of brain damage. This can cause immediate difficulties when waking up in the hospital because it may require your physicians and nursing staff—as well as any visiting family members—to remind you of their identity every time that you see them. The second type is developmental prosopagnosia, where a person never developed the ability to recognize people in the first place.

Developmental prosopagnosia is more common than was originally thought when the condition was first described. Perhaps around 3% of people qualify as having this condition (Bowles et al., 2009). People with developmental prosopagnosia often adapt to their condition so well that the condition doesn't interfere too much with their day-to-day lives, but you probably know a few people that *really* struggle with identifying people by looking at their faces. Tell them to look into prosopagnosia research, they may find it illuminating.

The acquired type of prosopagnosia is rare and far more severe. Frequently, someone with acquired prosopagnosia also has other deficits in their vision—called "comorbid" symptoms. These frequently include partial colorblindness (see Achromatopsia), difficulties in navigating through space (see Topographical Disorientation), and visual field defects that make them partially blind, usually in the upper part of their vision (Barton, 2011). This is often because people with acquired prosopagnosia develop the disorder during a stroke, and that stroke also damages multiple parts of the brain that are located close together. Speaking of which, let's discuss the brain pathology of prosopagnosia.

The Brain Pathology

The difference between the two types of prosopagnosia that I have mentioned seems to lie in a brain region called the fusiform gyrus, located in the temporal lobe. In people with acquired prosopagnosia, this region is physically and permanently damaged (Barton, 2008). In people with developmental prosopagnosia, research suggests that this brain region has fewer brain cells, leading to a diminished face recognition ability (Garrido et al., 2009). To be a bit more specific, there are at least three different regions of the brain that respond to faces—sometimes called the fusiform face area, the occipital face area, and the face-selective superior temporal sulcus—and when a person looks at faces, those regions respond in somewhat different ways, showing that they have different jobs in the process of face identification (Liu et al., 2010). On average, damage to the right-side fusiform area is more likely to cause prosopagnosia than damage to the left-side fusiform area, and the evidence suggests that there are variants of prosopagnosia depending on the specific location of the damage, such as whether or not it's more of a *vision* or more of a *memory* issue (Albonico & Barton, 2019). That may sound straightforward, but trust me, it is not. While most researchers agree that damage to those brain regions, especially the fusiform gyrus, can lead to prosopagnosia, researchers certainly do *not* agree about the boundaries of the condition. That is: what exactly *is* prosopagnosia?

Prosopagnosia is often defined in encyclopedias as a problem with identifying faces—specifically *human* faces (e.g., Foster & Drago, 2011). However, when you look a bit deeper, there is disagreement over exactly where the boundaries of the recognition problems are. People with acquired prosopagnosia have reported losing their abilities to recognize other categories besides human faces. These reports include a farmer losing the ability to tell apart the cows on their farm, and a bird-watcher losing the ability to differentiate between bird species (Bornstein et al., 1969). Other problematic categories for people with prosopagnosia have included buildings, chairs, fruit and other food, cars, coins, handwriting, clothing, symbols such as ampersands and musical clefs, and other animals (Barton, 2011; Damasio et al., 1982; Meadows, 1974). My own research has found some evidence that a person with prosopagnosia had problems telling apart individual sheep when looking at their extra-fuzzy faces (Toftness, 2019). Overall, many people with prosopagnosia also seem to have some type of more general visual agnosia (see Visual Object Agnosia such that it is not just *human faces* that give them recognition issues.

This raises an important question. Do "pure" cases of prosopagnosia exist—people who *only* have issues recognizing human faces but have no other recognition issues for any other category? Or do all people with prosopagnosia also have some other object recognition problems that are perhaps more subtle than the face blindness part of the disorder? Researchers still disagree about that. One question that may get us closer to answering whether pure prosopagnosia exists is: what is the actual mathematical operation in the brain that is disrupted by prosopagnosia?

Human faces do appear to make use of special processing in the brain. This can be seen in how the brain reacts to looking at upside-down faces (e.g.,

Yin, 1969) or faces that are inverted in color (Galper & Hochberg, 1971). Faces become much more difficult to recognize under those conditions, even more so than objects. Perhaps there is some *extra information* in a face that can be disrupted independently from the rest of your visual abilities. But what is that extra information, exactly? It has been argued that when objects are very similar looking, such as human faces, it is the fine details of the relative position of the parts, like the distance between a person's eyes, that allow identification. Some researchers have referred to this extra information as "coordinate" information (Brooks & Cooper, 2006), while others refer to it as "configural" or "holistic" information (Piepers & Robbins, 2012). Whatever it is, according to such theories, that type of extra information isn't useful for people with prosopagnosia, so instead they just rely on individual features like hair length or facial scars to get hints about identity.

There is some evidence that under certain conditions, such as when a person is an *expert* at identifying a category of objects, that their brain uses this extra "coordinate" information for things other than faces, such as dogs, birds, and cars (Gauthier, 2017). But overall, even if faces are not uniquely special, they are still the *most* special category of object to be disrupted when that extra information is removed. Is that because *everyone* is an expert at recognizing human faces, is it because people are born with a part of the brain dedicated to human faces and only human faces, or is expertise merely one factor in a much more complicated explanation for prosopagnosia? Researchers disagree about that, too.

Because acquired prosopagnosia is so rare, and the brain damage between individuals can vary so much, the question of whether "pure" prosopagnosia exists is incredibly difficult. You can always argue that a person with a case of so-called pure acquired prosopagnosia, and seems to only have issues with recognizing human faces and nothing else, wasn't tested on enough object categories. You could also argue that a person with a so-called case of impure acquired prosopagnosia, and has problems recognizing human faces and other types of objects, actually has brain damage to multiple areas of the brain including brain regions other than the region that specializes in human faces.

So, instead of using people with acquired prosopagnosia, researchers looked at developmental prosopagnosia—are those people also bad at object recognition? When people with developmental prosopagnosia were tested on at least three tests of object recognition, 0% of them performed normally on all three (or more) tests of non-human-face recognition—in other words, no cases of pure prosopagnosia were found in a group of 72 people with prosopagnosia that were tested between the years of 1976 and 2016 by a variety of researchers (Geskin & Behrmann, 2018). Either pure prosopagnosia is exceedingly rare, or it does not exist. That claim is exceedingly contentious, by the way, so I recommend that you drop this book immediately and run away.

Is it possible to help people with prosopagnosia learn how to recognize faces? This probably won't surprise you, but researchers disagree about that too. On the one hand, people with acquired prosopagnosia do sometimes recover, but usually this recovery seems to be spontaneous and not due to effort on the part of the person with prosopagnosia to learn a new way of recognizing faces—historically, when researchers have tried to *help* people with acquired prosopagnosia by teaching them recognition strategies such as which parts of the face to pay attention to, there have been limited successes (DeGutis et al., 2014). On the other hand, a more recent study using people with acquired prosopagnosia found some success in training them to identify faces through an intensive multi-month intervention that made use of highly specific photo manipulations and adaptive training such that the training automatically adjusted to an appropriate level of difficulty as the people with prosopagnosia learned (Davies-Thompson et al., 2017). Taken together, the evidence suggests that recovery from prosopagnosia is at least somewhat possible because face recognition abilities can change over time (Albonico & Barton, 2019).

Living life with prosopagnosia may sound difficult, but people with prosopagnosia are often quite capable of adapting to their face recognition problems by using other characteristics of the people that they need to recognize. For example, their ability to recognize voices remains completely intact, and they are also generally very good at recognizing people simply by the way that they walk and hold themselves, as posture and gait can be very different from person to person (Barton, 2011). If all else fails, they can always ask those most important in their lives to display an unchanging characteristic, such as a unique hat or scarf by which they can be reliably recognized. But even if a person with prosopagnosia told her son to wear a red shirt when he visited, and she saw a man in a red shirt walking toward her, she would still not have the *feeling* of recognition—it would still feel as though she was looking at a stranger because the brain didn't trigger the feeling of familiarity, at least until he spoke or her brain recognized him in some other way. It's that feeling of uncertainty for a person's identity that may especially bother a person with prosopagnosia. However, people tend to find creative ways to face this facial recognition disorder, and may adapt so well that it rarely interferes with their life.

References

Albonico, A., & Barton, J. (2019). Progress in perceptual research: The case of prosopagnosia. *F1000Research*, *8*. https://doi.org/ggfqvv

Barton, J. J. (2008). Structure and function in acquired prosopagnosia: lessons from a series of 10 patients with brain damage. *Journal of Neuropsychology*, *2*(1), 197–225. https://doi.org/bdtzq4

Barton, J. J. (2011). Disorders of higher visual processing. In C. Kennard & R. J. Leigh (Eds.), *Handbook of clinical neurology* (vol. 102, pp. 223–261). https://doi.org/gs46

Bodamer, J. (1947). Die prosop-agnosie. *Archiv für Psychiatrie und Nervenkrankheiten*, *179*(1–2), 6–53. https://doi.org/fq9mdc

Bornstein, B., Sroka, H., & Munitz, H. (1969). Prosopagnosia with animal face agnosia. *Cortex*, *5*(2), 164–169. https://doi.org/gtvd

Bowles, D. C., McKone, E., Dawel, A., Duchaine, B., Palermo, R., Schmalzl, L., Wilson, E., & Yovel, G. (2009). Diagnosing prosopagnosia: Effects of ageing, sex, and participant–stimulus ethnic match on the Cambridge Face Memory Test and Cambridge Face Perception Test. *Cognitive Neuropsychology*, *26*(5), 423–455. https://doi.org/ct4nx4

Brooks, B. E., & Cooper, E. E. (2006). What types of visual recognition tasks are mediated by the neural subsystem that subserves face recognition? *Journal of Experimental Psychology: Learning, Memory, and Cognition*, *32*(4), 684–698. https://doi.org/dfqcvz

Cole, M., & Perez-Cruet, J. (1964). Prosopagnosia. *Neuropsychologia*, *2*(3), 237–246. https://doi.org/c6jdkh

Damasio, A. R., Damasio, H., & Van Hoesen, G. W. (1982). Prosopagnosia: Anatomic basis and behavioral mechanisms. *Neurology*, *32*(4), 331–341. https://doi.org/gtvf

Davies-Thompson, J., Fletcher, K., Hills, C., Pancaroglu, R., Corrow, S. L., & Barton, J. J. S. (2017). Perceptual learning of faces: A rehabilitative study of acquired prosopagnosia. *Journal of Cognitive Neuroscience*, *29*(3), 573–591. https://doi.org/gtvg

DeGutis, J. M., Chiu, C., Grosso, M. E., & Cohan, S. (2014). Face processing improvements in prosopagnosia: Successes and failures over the last 50 years. *Frontiers in Human Neuroscience*, *8*, Article 561. https://doi.org/ghb4jk

Foster, P. S., & Drago, V. (2011). Agnosias. In C. Noggle (Ed.), *The encyclopedia of neuropsychological disorders*. Springer.

Galper, R. E., & Hochberg, J. (1971). Recognition memory for photographs of faces. *The American Journal of Psychology*, *84*(3), 351–354. https://doi.org/dn4k7m

Garrido, L., Duchaine, B., & Nakayama, K. (2008). Face detection in normal and prosopagnosic individuals. *Journal of Neuropsychology*, *2*(1), 119–140. https://doi.org/bqbvng

Garrido, L., Furl, N., Draganski, B., Weiskopf, N., Stevens, J., Tan, G. C. Y., Driver, J., Dolan, R. J., & Duchaine, B. (2009). Voxel-based morphometry reveals reduced grey matter volume in the temporal cortex of developmental prosopagnosics. *Brain*, *132*(12), 3443–3455. https://doi.org/ffhjh2

Gauthier, I. (2017). *The quest for the FFA led to the expertise account of its specialization*. ArXiv. https://arxiv.org/abs/1702.07038

Geskin, J., & Behrmann, M. (2018). Congenital prosopagnosia without object agnosia? A literature review. *Cognitive Neuropsychology*, *35*(1–2), 4–54. https://doi.org/gtvh

Liu, J., Harris, A., & Kanwisher, N. (2010). Perception of face parts and face configurations: An fMRI study. *Journal of Cognitive Neuroscience*, *22*(1), 203–211. https://doi.org/fmd3mz

Lorey, D. (Writer), Rosenstock, R. (Writer), Hurwitz, M. (Director), & Miller, T. (Director). (2013, May 26). Queen B. (Season 4, Episode 10) [TV series episode]. In Hurwitz, M. (Creator), *Arrested Development*. Imagine Entertainment.

Meadows, J. C. (1974). The anatomical basis of prosopagnosia. *Journal of Neurology, Neurosurgery & Psychiatry*, *37*(5), 489–501. https://doi.org/dmnprg

Piepers, D., & Robbins, R. (2012). A review and clarification of the terms "holistic,""configural," and "relational" in the face perception literature. *Frontiers in Psychology*, *3*, Article 559. https://doi.org/gghpp2

Sacks, O. (2010). *The mind's eye*. Knopf.

Toftness, A. R. (2019). *The non-specificity of prosopagnosia: Can prosopagnosics distinguish sheep* (Publication No. 10289373) [Master's thesis, Iowa State University]? Iowa State University Digital Repository.

Tranel, D., Damasio, A. R., & Damasio, H. (1988). Intact recognition of facial expression, gender, and age in patients with impaired recognition of face identity. *Neurology, 38*(5), 690–696. https://doi.org/gk7z9j

Yin, R. K. (1969). Looking at upside-down faces. *Journal of Experimental Psychology, 81*(1), 141–145. https://doi.org/bv77k4

Seizures

Imagine that you occasionally lose control of your body. Every once in a while, you suddenly experience a rush of electrical activity in your brain, resulting in your muscles contracting in wild ways. Or perhaps you experience the exact opposite, a chilling period of absence where your body doesn't move at all until you come out of it. Then, after some time, the aberrant electrical activity vanishes. If it weren't for outside observers that were watching you, you might not even remember that it happened. What is causing you to lose control?

The Stories

(STORY 1) In 1931, a 25-year-old woman described to her physician that since the age of 17 she had experienced fainting attacks upon hearing music. When music was played near her, she would feel weakness, sense that sounds were becoming distant, and then fall to the floor or intentionally lie down to avoid such a fall when fainting. She reported that classical music had the most dramatic effect and that on one occasion she had bitten her tongue and urinated during an attack, both classic signs of seizure. After such attacks she would awaken and feel ill, with a period of lost memory. While in the hospital, the physician tried a few different types of music in order to see what effects they would have. One orchestral record played on a gramophone triggered a seizure, including fainting and convulsions. When she later regained her senses, she described that the music had made her feel a spreading numbness in her body that eventually led to unconsciousness and that she now had a "vile headache" (p. 14). Her musicogenic *epilepsy*, as her physician referred to it, continued despite attempted treatment (Critchley, 1937, case 1).

   (STORY 2) A woman shared her experiences of growing up with *absence seizures*, and those experiences were published in a case study in 1990. She noted that during her childhood she would react erratically to things, either showing great interest or seemingly no interest at all. People around her referred to the differences in the way she acted as "'moods,' 'daydreams' or even 'sulking'" (p. 452). But she wasn't having moods; she was having seizures that caused her to enter "trances" where she was unable to hear the things that were happening around her (p. 452). During the trances, her vision would often make objects

DOI: 10.4324/9781003276937-41

look alien and unfamiliar. Doctors didn't detect an illness, and so she went undiagnosed for a long time. People would accuse her of being rude as a child because she would sometimes not respond to questions. At one point, before her diagnosis, she nearly drowned in a shallow swimming pool during a seizure. She also "many times came close to disaster while crossing roads alone" (p. 455). At the age of 19, when the frequency of her absence seizures was around 50–100 per day, she was diagnosed with a mild form of epilepsy. She went on to try out various ways of controlling the absences, including medication, and found some success in managing them. She went on to become married, and reported that in her adult life "I have felt almost what it must be like to be normal … nonetheless, I have a strong memory of the many times I have found myself suddenly, bewildered and alone, in an alien situation" (Iphofen, 1990, p. 457).

(STORY 3) A man born in 1904 began having seizures at the age of 37. He experienced occasional *tonic-clonic seizures* in which he thrashed his muscles and often bit his tongue, and also frequent absence seizures during which he would stare blankly. He became a bus driver later in life. One day when he was 52 years old, he had a seizure and "drove off the main road and round some back streets" which led to him being demoted to a bus conductor, who was in charge of collecting bus fares (p. 498). In 1955, he had a seizure that led to a religious "conversion experience" while working on the bus: "he was suddenly overcome with a feeling of bliss … he collected the fares correctly, telling his passengers at the same time how pleased he was to be in Heaven" (p. 498). He continued this newfound "exaltation" for two days following the seizure event, claiming that he could hear angelic voices. Years later, in 1958, he again had a major seizure event—this time, "three seizures on three successive days" (p. 498). This led to another religious conversion experience. He stopped being religious altogether, and no longer believed in the afterlife whatsoever. During this second conversion, he showed the same elated mood as he did during the previous conversion, and he claimed that his "mind had 'cleared'" (p. 498). He maintained his newfound agnosticism for religion for at least 18 months following the second set of seizures (Dewhurst & Beard, 1970, case 1).

The Features

Seizures are often depicted in movies and television shows as someone rolling their eyes back into their head, falling to the floor, and violently jerking their muscles. And while some seizures do resemble such scenes, they paint an incomplete picture. In reality, there are many different kinds of seizures, and several different triggers for seizures. Some people have seizures beginning in childhood, while others have their first seizure later in life. Some people have only one seizure in their lifetime while others have multiple seizures every single day. These nuances are difficult to capture completely in a short chapter like this, but hopefully this overview will illuminate the possibilities and intricacies behind the word "seizure."

First, seizures can either be *provoked* or *unprovoked*. Provoked seizures occur because of an injury or change to the brain's chemical composition, including low blood sugar, low sodium, infections, overdosing on drugs, or underdosing on alcohol for someone who is extremely addicted to alcohol—in fact, anyone can have a provoked seizure under certain circumstances (Schoenberg et al., 2011). On the other hand, unprovoked seizures are seizures that take place without being caused by some other brain change. The brain seems to generate the seizure all on its own, hence the name "unprovoked."

It is understandably startling when an unprovoked seizure happens to a person for the first time but, from a neurological perspective, a single unprovoked seizure is not always worrying. However, if a person has two or more unprovoked seizures spread across multiple days, or if they have one seizure and appear to be at great risk for having another one, then they may be diagnosed with *epilepsy*. There are also some types of provoked seizures, such as those caused by flashing lights (i.e., photosensitive seizures) that are considered to be a type of epilepsy called *reflex* epilepsy (Fisher et al., 2014). When diagnosed with epilepsy, it is very important that effort be put into preventing future seizures in order to avoid the side effects discussed below.

Genetics play a role in epilepsy, but it can sometimes be an *acquired* disorder. That is, if the brain changes in particular ways, someone who has never had a seizure before may begin having seizures. This process where the brain becomes capable of generating seizures is called *epileptogenesis* (Thijs et al., 2019). One common event that can lead to epileptogenesis is traumatic brain injury (Ding et al., 2016). This is referred to as post-traumatic epilepsy and, curiously, it often has a "silent period" of months or years between the injury and the onset of the seizures—perhaps up to 20 years in extreme cases (Piccenna et al., 2017, p. 123). More work is needed to understand it, but post-traumatic epilepsy seems to be a relatively common type of epilepsy (Semple et al., 2019). Other types of acquired epilepsy may come from tumors, strokes, parasites, and infections (Thijs et al., 2019). Epilepsy is not just a neurological disorder in which people have seizures however, as it is also affiliated with other less visible changes that may put a person at risk for heart disease, hypertension, migraine, and more (Yuen et al., 2018). But putting those complexities aside, let's focus on the major symptom which is not coincidentally the title of this chapter: seizures.

The number of different types of seizures is staggering. In fact, a seizure can "present clinically as any discrete human experience" (Schoenberg et al., 2011, p. 431). If your brain and body can do it, a seizure can cause it, including laughing without feeling "mirth," smelling burning rubber, uncontrollable swallowing, movements as if pedaling a bicycle, and pelvic thrusting, just to name a few specific examples (Schoenberg et al., 2011, p. 435). Any experience that your brain can have can happen in a seizure. Problematically, some symptoms of seizures overlap with symptoms of migraines (see Migraine Headaches) which may make diagnoses difficult (Mantegazza & Cestèle, 2018; Nye & Thadani, 2015).

The definitions of epilepsy and seizure have changed several times across history, and they will almost certainly change again in the future as our understanding improves (e.g., Falco-Walter et al., 2018; Walker & Kovac, 2015). If you're reading this book in the distant future, it is likely that the definitions below have evolved, and you should take your hoverbike over to the cybrary in order to download the latest classification scheme.

As of this writing, the classification scheme of seizure types was last updated in 2017 (Fisher et al., 2017). Some—but not all—types can be recognized by outward behavioral *signs* in the person, such as when the doctor sees the person's muscles contracting. Other traits are experienced only by the person having the seizure, such as smelling a bad smell—these subjective experiences are called *symptoms*. Together, signs and symptoms help clinicians theorize about where in the brain that person's seizure *focus* might be located—or, to discover that the seizure does not have a focus. The focus is the origin point of the signals from the misbehaving brain cells that lead to the seizure itself and, if it exists, it is located in one place limited to one hemisphere (Fisher et al., 2017). Seizures with a focus are called *focal onset* seizures, and the focus, and therefore brain dysfunction, is often in the cortex or limbic system (Thijs et al., 2019). Seizures without a focus are instead referred to as *generalized onset* seizures, which involve both sides of the brain and especially the thalamic structures (Thijs et al., 2019).

After determining whether the seizure has a focus, the next step in classifying a seizure is to determine whether the person retains awareness during the seizure. When the person remains aware of what is happening to them for the entire duration of the seizure, this is called an *aware* seizure. When awareness is impaired, such as the person falling unconscious, this is called an *impaired awareness* seizure. Focal seizures can be either "aware" or "impaired awareness," but generalized seizures are almost always "impaired awareness."

The next step is all about the signs and symptoms, split into two groups. The *motor* group includes signs of the muscles, while the *non-motor* group involves signs and symptoms having to do with … anything else. Non-motor signs and symptoms can include emotional, sensory, cognitive, and autonomic experiences. The motor group includes tonic, atonic, and clonic characteristics, and other movements that I won't get into.

Let's start with the focal non-motor signs and symptoms. These are incredibly diverse because they can happen in many parts of the brain that are responsible for different functions. Emotional seizures can cause any emotion, including anger, joy, and fear. They may also cause laughing (gelastic seizures) or crying (dacrystic seizures) as part of the sudden emotional change (Fisher et al., 2017). A sensory seizure can include hallucinations such as hearing sounds or seeing colors and shapes that are not there. Focal seizures in the occipital lobe can cause partial blindness (see Hemianopsia). Focal seizures in the posterior parietal lobe may cause illusory perceptions that objects are located further away or located closer than they actually are (see Alice in Wonderland Syndrome). Sensory seizures can also include changes to your smell, taste, balance, and sensations of touch. Cognitive seizures can include changes in language ability or changes in thinking. The person may believe that they have already experienced the moment that is currently happening (see Pathological Déjà Vu), or they may find themselves forced to think about something. Autonomic seizures may include goosebumps, heart palpitations, sexual arousal, changes in breathing, and other reflexive actions of the body's autonomic nervous system. One particularly curious non-motor symptom is that of religious experiences. When the temporal lobe is involved, a person may experience highly emotional religious feelings before, during, or after a seizure (Devinsky & Lai, 2008).

Now let's take a look at the motor signs. Tonic means the stiffening of a muscle, while atonic means the reverse—the loss of stiffness in a muscle. Clonic, on the other hand, refers to rhythmic jerking movements. These movements can occur focally as a single muscle, or generally across many muscles. There are also cases in which clonic movements start with one muscle such as a finger and then move progressively to other muscles such as the entire hand in a sign known as the *Jacksonian March* (Schoenberg et al., 2011). These different movements can also be combined across phases of the same seizure.

A tonic-clonic seizure is probably what you think of when you imagine a seizure. These generalized seizures are often portrayed in movies. The person first experiences the tonic phase where their muscles stiffen, and they fall down. Then, the jerking movements of the clonic phase occur. These seizures usually last less than a few minutes, and the person is typically confused afterwards (Schoenberg et al., 2011). It is possible for a seizure to start out as a non-motor focal seizure with a particular symptom (such as déjà vu) and then evolve into a full-body impaired awareness tonic-clonic seizure. In these cases, called *focal to bilateral tonic-clonic seizures*, the focal symptom may serve as a warning that a motor seizure is coming soon (Fisher et al., 2017).

Another type of seizure is the *absence* seizure, which is considered a generalized non-motor seizure. Absence seizures are seizures in which the person temporarily becomes unresponsive. Typically, an absence seizure doesn't have many obvious signs—it may just seem like the person is daydreaming for a few seconds, or is not paying attention. Absence seizures may occur hundreds of times per day in some people, or perhaps only a few times a day in others, and a typical absence seizure lasts ten seconds or less (Foldvary-Schaefer & Wyllie, 2003).

Another notable phenomenon is called an *epileptic cry* (Schoenberg et al., 2011). This has been described as a "scream of a shrill, unearthly character" (Sieveking, 1861, p. 4). Having worked with epileptics, I can confirm that this sounds a bit like an unearthly moan, but Sieveking may have been embellishing a bit for dramatic effect. It is caused during some seizures when the muscles of the person's core contract, forcing a rush of air against a closed glottis, which is a muscle that is part of your vocal cords. The cry does not indicate pain and is not the same thing as screaming, because the body is mostly producing the sound on its own.

The Brain Pathology

Seizures occur due to *excessive brain activity* or because of *synchronous brain activity* (Fisher et al., 2014). These two components are highly related (Stafstrom, 1998). Excessive brain activity is the easier of the two to understand. To oversimplify a bit, there is too much electricity running through a part of the brain, and so a seizure happens until that electricity can be discharged. More accurately, this excessive brain activity takes the form of *hyperexcitability*, meaning that brain cells are responding to electrical signals with too many of their own electrical signals.

Synchronous brain activity, including the absolutely metal term *hypersynchronous discharge*, occurs when a bunch of neighboring cells recruit each other into firing their electrical impulses in an abnormal pattern. More specifically, synchronous means "at the same time"—the cells are matching each other's firing pattern at the same time, which results in a *spike* of electrical activity in the brain when all of those signals are added together. All brains are capable of having hypersynchronous discharge spikes under provoked circumstances such as low blood sugar, and therefore all people are capable of having seizures (Stafstrom, 1998).

Hyperexcitability and hypersynchonicity are usually the framework through which seizures are understood, although these two ideas alone are not enough to completely explain all seizures (Walker & Kovac, 2015). Researchers still have a lot of work ahead of them.

This probably goes without saying, but seizures are dangerous. Seizures may cause progressive damage to the brain, and even sudden death. This is why it is important to try and prevent seizures. The dangers are most severe for people with prolonged seizures, but milder epilepsies—that some have called benign because there are no obvious signs or symptoms—also show mild negative effects in the brain upon a closer look (Schoenberg et al., 2011). Unfortunately, around 75% of people worldwide with epilepsy are currently untreated (Thijs et al., 2019).

Seizure treatment usually starts with medication. Dozens of medications for seizures exist, and finding one that works can be heavily based on trial and error (Thijs et al., 2019). However, some types of seizures don't seem to respond to medications, especially some focal seizures. After many medication failures, more elaborate treatments may be required (Schoenberg et al., 2011). One option is the implantation of *neuromodulation* devices that can stimulate parts of the brain in order to reduce seizures. Another option is the surgical removal of the seizure focus in the brain. The literal removal of part of the brain may sound extreme, and it does have many risks, but it is often a highly effective treatment. In fact, it has been argued that brain surgery may not be used often enough for people with drug-resistant focal seizures (Thijs et al., 2019). Hopefully, science will advance and eventually prevent the need to resort to partial brain removal. For now, careful observation of signs and symptoms is crucial for discovering how to restore control over a person's seizure-prone brain.

References

Critchley, M. (1937). Musicogenic epilepsy. *Brain*, *60*(1), 13–27. https://doi.org/dn3d6c

Devinsky, O., & Lai, G. (2008). Spirituality and religion in epilepsy. *Epilepsy & Behavior*, *12*(4), 636–643. https://doi.org/c568hj

Dewhurst, K., & Beard, A. W. (1970). Sudden religious conversions in temporal lobe epilepsy. *The British Journal of Psychiatry*, *117*, 497–507. https://doi.org/dwvvz2

Ding, K., Gupta, P. K., & Diaz-Arrastia, R. (2016). Epilepsy after traumatic brain injury. In D. Laskowitz & G. Grant (Eds.), *Translational research in traumatic brain injury* (pp. 299–313). https://doi.org/gtvj

Falco-Walter, J. J., Scheffer, I. E., & Fisher, R. S. (2018). The new definition and classification of seizures and epilepsy. *Epilepsy Research*, *139*, 73–79.

Fisher, R. S., Acevedo, C., Arzimanoglou, A., Bogacz, A., Cross, J. H., Elger, C. E., Engel, J., Forsgren, L., French, J. A., Glynn, M., Hesdorffer, D. C., Lee, B. I., Mathern, G. W., Moshé, S. L., Perucca, E., Scheffer, I. E., Tomson, T., Watanabe, M., & Wiebe, S. (2014). ILAE Official Report: A practical clinical definition of epilepsy. *Epilepsia*, *55*(4), 475–482. https://doi.org/f24dp7

Fisher, R. S., Cross, J. H., D'Souza, C., French, J. A., Haut, S. R., Higurashi, N., Hirsch, E., Jansen, F. E., Lagae, L., Moshé, S. L., Peltola, J., Roulet Perez, E., Scheffer, I. E., Schulze-Bonhage, A., Somerville, E., Sperling, M., Yacubian, E. M., & Zuberi, S. M. (2017). Instruction manual for the ILAE 2017 operational classification of seizure types. *Epilepsia*, *58*(4), 531–542. https://doi.org/f9s9vj

Foldvary-Schaefer, N., & Wyllie, E. (2003). Epilepsy. In C. G. Goetz (Ed.), *Textbook of clinical neurology* (2nd ed., pp. 1155–1185). Saunders.

Iphofen, R. (1990). Coping with a 'perforated life': A case study in managing the stigma of petit mal epilepsy. *Sociology*, *24*(3), 447–463. https://doi.org/cc5nkd

Mantegazza, M., & Cestèle, S. (2018). Pathophysiological mechanisms of migraine and epilepsy: Similarities and differences. *Neuroscience Letters*, *667*, 92–102. https://doi.org/gc736q

Nye, B. L., & Thadani, V. M. (2015). Migraine and epilepsy: Review of the literature. *Headache: The Journal of Head and Face Pain*, *3*(55), 359–380. https://doi.org/f65x2s

Piccenna, L., Shears, G., & O'Brien, T. J. (2017). Management of post-traumatic epilepsy: An evidence review over the last 5 years and future directions. *Epilepsia Open*, *2*(2), 123–144. https://doi.org/gtvk

Schoenberg, M. R., Werz, M. A., & Drane, D. L. (2011). Epilepsy and Seizures. In M. R. Schoenberg & J. G. Scott (Eds.), *The little black book of neuropsychology: A syndrome-based approach*. https://doi.org/dv3n2j

Semple, B. D., Zamani, A., Rayner, G., Shultz, S. R., & Jones, N. C. (2019). Affective, neurocognitive and psychosocial disorders associated with traumatic brain injury and post-traumatic epilepsy. *Neurobiology of Disease*, *123*, 27–41. https://doi.org/gtvm

Sieveking, E. H. (1861). *On epilepsy and epileptiform seizures, their causes, pathology, and treatment*. Savill and Edwards.

Stafstrom, C. E. (1998). The pathophysiology of epileptic seizures: A primer for pediatricians. *Pediatrics in Review*, *19*(10), 342–351. https://doi.org/dz5h9f

Thijs, R. D., Surges, R., O'Brien, T. J., & Sander, J. W. (2019). Epilepsy in adults. *The Lancet*, *393*(10172), 689–701. https://doi.org/gft4r7

Walker, M. C., & Kovac, S. (2015). Seize the moment that is thine: How should we define seizures? *Brain*, *138*(5), 1127–1128. https://doi.org/gf28h6

Yuen, A. W. C., Keezer, M. R., & Sander, J. W. (2018). Epilepsy is a neurological and a systemic disorder. *Epilepsy and Behavior*, *78*, 57–61. https://doi.org/gh7hrf

Sleeping Beauty Syndrome (Kleine-Levin Syndrome)

Imagine that you begin sleeping much more than usual, perhaps over 18 hours per day. Your life is completely disrupted and, try as you might, you can't seem to overpower the extreme tiredness that has come over you. You can be woken up if someone is determined to do so, but it isn't long before you fall back to sleep. You may get up occasionally to eat a meal, and perhaps you feel very hungry at those times but other than that you are mostly confined to your bed for days or weeks at a time. Then, one day, you wake up and feel relatively back to normal—at least, that is, until the *next* time you find yourself getting drowsier than you can stand.

The Stories

(STORY 1) A series of Kleine-Levin syndrome attacks were described in a teenage boy, beginning with his first attack in 1948. It lasted three days, during which he was extremely drowsy, irritable, and seemed confused and unable to understand what was said to him. He showed excessive eating, and even sold his bicycle and then spent all of the money on "preserved fruits" which he ate in a single sitting (p. 379). He was found to have urinated in a pair of boots for two nights in a row, "and was quite unashamed and apathetic when his family commented thereon" (p. 379). In 1949, he had a second attack which lasted four days. He was again drowsy and irritable with an unending appetite and even resorted to stealing the food rations of another boy at his boarding school. In 1950, he was admitted to a hospital for an attack that lasted for about four days, during which he slept for most of each day. He complained that he felt "'out of touch' with his surroundings" and of apathy and extreme drowsiness (p. 378). During the attack, he was described as confused, irritable, and hostile, with an excessive appetite. He made lewd remarks to the nuns working at the hospital and urinated in front of one of them in the garden. When he recovered from the Kleine-Levin attack, he had amnesia for the events of the previous few days and was embarrassed to learn the details of his actions. His personality seemed entirely different after recovery, and he was described as respectful and well mannered (Robinson & McQuillan, 1951).

DOI: 10.4324/9781003276937-42

(STORY 2) A man was admitted to a hospital in 1941 after several years where he experienced strange bouts of sleepiness. Every six months to a year, he would suddenly have a period of a few days where he would experience excessive sleepiness and hunger. During these sleepy periods, he would be easy to wake up, but would fall back to sleep quickly. He would spend most of the day sleeping, although he sometimes tried to keep himself awake through physical activity. He reported that during his sleepiness attacks that his thoughts felt unconnected, as if thinking was more difficult. It seemed as if he had difficulties translating thoughts into speech. But when he was in his periods between attacks of sleepiness, he showed none of these symptoms for months at a time. While he was under observation at the hospital, it was noted that he slept "almost the whole of the time" except when he woke up to have meals, during which he displayed an excessive appetite (Critchley & Hoffman, 1942, case 1, p. 137).

(STORY 3) An atypical case of Kleine-Levin syndrome occurred in a 40-year-old man around 1972. The case was unusual because the man was much older than the average Kleine-Levin patient. When admitted to the hospital, he was found to sleep all day if not woken up. When woken up, he would become very angry. He also exhibited two other classic signs of Kleine-Levin syndrome: hypersexuality and hyperphagia. The hypersexuality was especially problematic for the female nurses attending him and for nearby female patients, because he threatened them with sexual attacks and would run naked through the ward of the hospital. His hyperphagia was problematic for him, because he would eat excessively and gained a large amount of weight. In between attacks of Kleine-Levin syndrome, he was described as cooperative and polite. At one point he had a serious choking fit while eating and needed rescuing. Eventually, he died of aspiration pneumonia, probably because of his hyperphagia habits, most likely due to food or liquid entering his lungs (Carpenter et al., 1982).

The Features

The tale of *Sleeping Beauty* is a story that dates back to at least the 1300s and features a princess who is cursed to fall into a deep sleep lasting for an unnaturally long time. It may be just a story, but it's easy to see why this tale lends its name to a rare disorder of excessive sleeping.

Sleeping beauty syndrome, which is called Kleine-Levin syndrome (KLS) in the medical literature, is a rare neurological condition. KLS is a disease that mostly affects teenagers, and more boys are affected than girls (Miglis & Guilleminault, 2014). The major clinical symptom of KLS is *hypersomnia*, wherein the person sleeps for an abnormally long amount of time. If that wasn't enough, there are often additional life-disrupting symptoms. KLS may involve *cognitive disorders*, including feelings that the world isn't real or of being trapped in dreams (see Pathological Déjà Vu), feelings of confusion, memory loss (see Amnesia), and apathy, which is a general lack of interest in everything

(Arnulf et al., 2018). A symptom of extreme hunger, sometimes called "morbid hunger," *hyperphagia*, or *megaphagia*, is also commonly associated with KLS (Arnulf et al., 2005). Another possible symptom is *hypersexuality* in which the person's sexual drive increases (Lavault et al., 2015).

The main symptom of hypersomnia is where the less formal name "sleeping beauty syndrome" comes from. Hypersomnia means that the affected person sleeps an increased amount, making it the opposite of insomnia (see Fatal Familial Insomnia). The amount of time that a person with KLS spends asleep per day varies, but it is typically around 16–18 hours per day (Lavault et al., 2015). As such, the disorder generally upends the person's plans, as most of their time is spent unconscious instead of living their lives. According to Levin, a person with this disorder "can always be roused," meaning that they can always be woken up if needed, but "when roused he usually is irritable and wants to be let alone so that he can go back to sleep" (Levin, 1936, p. 494).

Even when a person with KLS is conscious, their experiences of life may be diminished due to their other symptoms. The extreme apathy and mental confusion may cause them to lose interest in all activities including speaking to others and maintaining hygiene, and instead they may simply lie in bed even when awake (Arnulf et al., 2018).

Along with hypersomnia, hyperphagia and hypersexuality are sometimes considered to be main symptoms of KLS, but fewer than half of people with KLS appear to have all three of these symptoms (Arnulf et al., 2018). When hyperphagia occurs, people with KLS tend to compulsively eat large amounts of food, especially sweet food (Miglis & Guilleminault, 2014). Hypersexuality may take the form of inappropriate sexual advances, frequent masturbation, and exposing themselves (Arnulf et al., 2018). However, some people end up doing the opposite behaviors—eating less and showing less interest in sex—possibly as a result of the emotional apathy associated with this disorder (Lavault et al., 2015). Instead, it is generally agreed that hypersomnia and cognitive symptoms make up the major expected symptoms of this disorder, and that hyperphagia and hypersexuality are less likely and harder to predict.

KLS symptoms appear periodically in episodes before disappearing and then reappearing, in a cycle of relapse and remittance (Arnulf et al., 2018). In between the KLS episodes, the person sleeps and behaves in more or less expected patterns for a healthy person. During these periods without symptoms, people with KLS are often embarrassed about their behavior during their episodes, especially if hypersexuality was one of their symptoms. These periods without symptoms are just one of the factors that make KLS very different from narcolepsy (see Narcolepsy), even though both are associated with excessive sleepiness.

An episode of KLS can last a variable amount of time depending on the person and on the specific episode itself, but typically it lasts one or more weeks. The median number of days that an episode lasts was found to be ten days in one study, although episodes lasting much longer are possible (Arnulf et al., 2005). It has been found that around 28% of people diagnosed with KLS experience episodes lasting longer than 30 days at a time (Arnulf et al., 2018). In between episodes of KLS, the interval of health before the next attack has a median interval of about three months, although much longer durations are possible (Arnulf et al., 2005).

The Brain Pathology

KLS is not understood to the point that it may be one of the least understood disorders in this entire book. In most KLS cases, scanning the brain to look for *structural* abnormalities turns up nothing unusual (Engström et al., 2018). However, there are many studies that have claimed to find *functional* differences in the brains of people with this disorder—that is, their brains are more or less active in specific brain regions. For example, there seems to be less blood flow in certain parts of the brain in a person with KLS, including the hypothalamus, thalamus, and regions of the cortex (Kas et al., 2014). However, depending on how you take measurements of brain activity, there is evidence for many different brain regions and brain networks involved in this disorder, including frontotemporal regions, thalamocortical networks, the temporoparietal junction, and sleep-wake networks in the deeper parts of the brain (Engström et al., 2018). That is to say, either huge portions of the brain are involved in generating this disorder, or researchers have some serious narrowing down to do.

There may be factors that trigger KLS symptoms, such as head trauma, viral infections, menstruation, and alcohol use, but some people with this disorder have not identified a particular triggering factor (Afolabi-Brown & Mason II, 2018). Of these triggering factors, perhaps the most commonly blamed is viral infection (Arnulf et al., 2018). KLS is also believed to have a genetic component in at least some cases, with recent research finding genetic variants that will be studied further (Ambati et al., 2021). So, not only is the pathology of this disorder unclear, but so is the origin of that pathology. Still, what we do know so far is better than simply filling up this section of the book with a long series of question marks.

Several different classes of drugs have been used to treat KLS, including lithium, but no drug has yet shown to be effective across many patients in a properly designed medical study (Afolabi-Brown & Mason II, 2018). The American Academy of Sleep Medicine has a "conditional" recommendation for lithium to be used to treat KLS because it *sometimes* seems to reduce disease severity, but much more research is needed (Maski et al., 2021). Fortunately, most people with KLS eventually recover from the disorder after a median of 15 years, and begin having fewer or no attacks of hypersomnia, although a minority continue to show symptoms even after multiple decades (Arnulf et al., 2018). Just like sleeping beauty, most people with KLS do eventually wake up.

References

Afolabi-Brown, O., & Mason II T. B. A. (2018). Kleine-Levin syndrome. *Paediatric Respiratory Reviews, 25,* 85–87. https://doi.org/gc32d4

Ambati, A., Hillary, R., Leu-Semenescu, S., Ollila, H. M., Lin, L., During, E. H., Farber, N., Rico, T. J., Faraco, J., Leary, E., Goldstein-Piekarski, A. N., Huang, Y. S., Han, F., Sivan, Y., Lecendreux, M., Dodet, P., Honda, M., Gadoth, N., Nevsimalova, S., … Mignot, E. J. M. (2021). Kleine-Levin syndrome is associated with birth difficulties and genetic variants in the TRANK1 gene loci. *Proceedings of the National Academy of Sciences of the United States of America, 118*(12), 1–11. https://doi.org/gjrpb6

Arnulf, I., Zeitzer, J. M., File, J., Farber, N., & Mignot, E. (2005). Kleine–Levin syndrome: A systematic review of 186 cases in the literature. *Brain, 128*(12), 2763–2776. *https:// doi.org/frch93*

Arnulf, I., Groos, E., & Dodet, P. (2018). Kleine–Levin syndrome: A neuropsychiatric disorder. *Revue Neurologique, 174*(4), 216–227. https://doi.org/gddt5c

Carpenter, S., Yassa, R., & Ochs, R. (1982). A pathologic basis for Kleine-Levin syndrome. *Archives of Neurology, 39*(1), 25–28. https://doi.org/dhscpv

Critchley, M., & Hoffman, H. L. (1942). The syndrome of periodic somnolence and morbid hunger (Kleine-Levin syndrome). *British Medical Journal, 1*(4230), 137–139. https://doi .org/dgp2b3

Engström, M., Latini, F., & Landtblom, A. M. (2018). Neuroimaging in the Kleine-Levin syndrome. *Current Neurology and Neuroscience Reports, 18*(9). https://doi.org/gd8hv7

Kas, A., Lavault, S., Habert, M. O., & Arnulf, I. (2014). Feeling unreal: A functional imaging study in patients with Kleine-Levin syndrome. *Brain, 137*(7), 2077–2087. https://doi .org/ggwhmz

Lavault, S., Golmard, J. L., Groos, E., Brion, A., Dauvilliers, Y., Lecendreux, M., Franco, P., & Arnulf, I. (2015). Kleine–Levin syndrome in 120 patients: Differential diagnosis and long episodes. *Annals of Neurology, 77*(3), 529–540. https://doi.org/gtvp

Levin, M. (1936). Periodic somnolence and morbid hunger: A new syndrome. *Brain, 59*(4), 494–504. https://doi.org/bnccpm

Maski, K., Trotti, L. M., Kotagal, S., Auger, R. R., Rowley, J. A., Hashmi, S. D., & Watson, N. F. (2021). Treatment of central disorders of hypersomnolence: An American academy of sleep medicine clinical practice guideline. *Journal of Clinical Sleep Medicine.* https://doi.org/gtvq

Miglis, M. G., & Guilleminault, C. (2014). Kleine-Levin syndrome: A review. *Nature and Science of Sleep, 6*, 19–26. https://doi.org/gfsz5g

Robinson, J. T., & McQuillan, J. (1951). Schizophrenic reaction associated with the Kleine-Levin syndrome. *Journal of the Royal Army Medical Corps, 96*(6), 377–381.

Social-Emotional Agnosias

Imagine that you can't recognize emotions. Looking at a person's face as they react to the words that you are saying doesn't reveal their inner emotional state—are they happy, sad, or angry? You can see the wrinkles in their face flexing, the corners of their mouth moving, and their eyebrows dancing, but assigning meaning to any of that is no longer automatic and easy. Why can you no longer read how people are feeling?

The Stories

(STORY 1) In the case of a 21-year-old man who had suffered a motorcycle accident with a head injury, anger-related issues developed. He reported that he had problems identifying "the feelings he was experiencing"—which in turn led him to experience depression as well as frustration (p. 637). His "emotional blindness," or *alexithymia*, seemed to have been acquired from the accident due to damage to the frontal and parietal lobes of his brain (p. 633). He experienced increased social isolation as a result of his anger management and emotional confusion issues. His "inability to identify and describe his feelings" led him to seek therapy as well as education about anger (p. 642). For example, he was instructed how to identify the changes that happened to him when he was angry, both psychologically and physiologically, such that he could better identify the emotion. Following therapy, he showed progress in controlling angry outbursts (Becerra et al., 2002).

(STORY 2) A 68-year-old woman developed problems with recognizing emotions on other people's faces due to extensive damage to her brain, including to the amygdala. When she was shown pictures of faces as a test, she had the most trouble with recognizing anger and fear but also showed signs of trouble with identifying the emotions of sadness and happiness when compared to other people. Her perception of eye-gaze direction was also impaired, meaning that she had trouble telling when the eyes of a person were looking directly at her versus when they were looking off to the right or left. In contrast, she had an above-average performance on intelligence tests and as-expected performance on some memory tests for words and the recognition of names. When her results were considered alongside the results of other people with amygdala

DOI: 10.4324/9781003276937-43

damage, researchers found clear evidence that amygdala damage changes the ability of a person to read the emotion of fear on another person's face (Broks et al., 1998, patient JC).

(STORY 3) An 83-year-old man who had previously suffered a stroke in his seventies was given neurological exams at a rehabilitation center for victims of stroke. His wife pointed out that since his stroke his voice had changed such that it was "quieter, and 'that everything sounded the same no matter how he was feeling'" (p. 412). He was given a series of tests to demonstrate his *prosody* abilities, such as injecting the emotions of sadness, happiness, fear, and anger into his spoken sentences. He had the most difficulty when the emotion he was supposed to convey with his words did not match the emotional context of the words that he was asked to say—a common example of this task is saying "all the puppies are dead" in a cheerful voice (p. 413). Similarly, he also showed difficulty in identifying the emotions that were being conveyed by someone speaking to him. He could, however, accurately determine which emotions were being displayed on pictures of faces, showing that he could interpret emotion under some circumstances (Heilman et al., 2004).

(STORY 4) A woman had parts of both of her amygdalae intentionally damaged in an attempt to treat epilepsy that wasn't responding to medication. Years later, at 51 years old, she still had "six or seven [seizures] per day" which was less frequent than before her brain damage, but at the apparent cost of some of her ability to read facial expressions (Young et al., 1995, p. 16). Her ability to determine which direction a person was looking (gaze direction) and her abilities to match or recognize facial expressions were both impaired. When she watched video clips of people making various facial expressions, she had a hard time figuring out which emotions those people were experiencing. Interestingly, she behaved in a way that was usually upbeat and cheerful, and it was reported that "she does not easily get upset or complain of pain, even when she falls and injures herself" (Young et al., 1995, p. 17). This suggests that the amygdala damage may have changed her ability to process her own emotions as well (Young et al., 1995; Young et al., 1996).

The Features

The ability to quickly read a person's emotions by looking at their face for a fraction of a second is a superpower that most people have—but a superpower that you probably haven't really thought about before. Think about it: facial expressions are really just tiny muscle movements on a person's face. Then, in order to correctly interpret the facial expression, you need to combine your reading of those tiny muscle movements with your prior knowledge of the situation and of that specific person's historical moods. Despite this complexity, the average person is pretty good at interpreting human emotions, probably because it was evolutionarily helpful to be able to quickly figure out whether a person you saw was in a friendly mood or in a murderous mood. Presumably, if aliens were asked to read the emotions from a human's face, they'd have a pretty difficult time. For people with various forms of social-emotional agnosias, emotions have become a bit alien to them as well.

Social-emotional agnosias come in several different forms, and the underlying brain differences and recommended treatments vary as a result (Lane et al., 2020). All of the forms are disruptive to the brain processes used to decode and encode the social world known as *social cognition* (Beer & Ochsner, 2006). Essentially, social cognition requires abilities of *other-perception*, abilities of *self-perception*, and a collection of brain-dwelling facts such as *scripts*, which are expectations for what is likely to happen next in a given situation.

Other-perception is a term that refers to using your senses like your vision and hearing to extract cues such as facial expressions and vocal tone from a social situation and then using your brain to process those cues into meaningful categories like happy, sad, or angry. Sometimes this is straightforward, such as when a person frowns, furrows their brow, and says that they are mad. That person is probably mad. Other situations are more complex, such as a person smiling with only their mouth but not their eyes, and saying "I'm fine." That person may not be fine. In order to better find out, we can use the other two pieces of social cognition.

Self-perception refers to knowledge about yourself, including recognizing that the emotions that you are feeling may be different from what others are feeling. You might realize that sometimes you say that you are fine when you are not fine, and that may give you a clue about how the other person is truly feeling. The final piece is the script and the other facts of the situation—if this person has a history of saying that they are fine when they really aren't, then that prior knowledge can help you suss out the truth. Or, if you know that it's relatively common in the English language to say "I'm fine" when you're actually doing poorly, then that is also a clue. Putting these pieces of social cognition together happens automatically in the brains of many, but not all, people. Difficulties with putting together the pieces of social cognition are sometimes associated with autism spectrum disorder, but such difficulties can also be acquired through brain damage.

Difficulty in other-perception, specifically in recognizing the emotions of other people, is sometimes called *expressive agnosia*, or emotional agnosia (Broicher & Jokeit, 2011). It isn't the most frequently reported symptom, but many people with traumatic brain injuries struggle with recognizing emotions from facial expressions and tone of voice (McDonald & Flanagan, 2004). When a person specifically loses the ability to read emotions from facial expressions it is sometimes called *prosopo-affective agnosia* (Kurucz & Feldmar, 1979). People who lose the ability to read facial expressions do not necessarily lose the ability to perceive faces (see Prosopagnosia). For example, they may be able to recognize people's faces, or tell people's ages and genders from their faces—the problem can be specific to gleaning emotions from facial expressions (Adolphs, 2002). The problems with recognizing emotions after brain injury seem to be especially apparent for negative emotions and for complex emotions, such as guilt or admiration (McDonald & Flanagan, 2004).

One interesting way that researchers have been able to measure expressive agnosia is through the use of electrodermal activity. Electrodermal activity refers to measuring the electrical conductivity of the skin as it changes over time, usually due to the production of small amounts of sweat. Essentially, when the average person views an image of a person making a negative facial expression such as fear, their skin sweats a little bit, causing electrodermal activity to increase slightly. However, in some people with brain injuries their skin does not react in this way to negative facial expressions, indicating that perhaps they are not fully understanding the fear on the fearful person's face (Hopkins et al., 2002).

A person may also lose the ability to inject emotion into their own speech (Ross & Mesulam, 1979) or lose the ability to understand emotion in others' speech patterns such as tone of voice (Dimoska et al., 2010). These speech patterns are sometimes called *prosody*. They are a collection of changes to "pitch, amplitude, tempo, and rhythm" (Heilman et al., 2004, p. 411). Using prosody can mean the difference between making a statement or asking a question—or between an angry accusation and a calm clarification. Losing the ability to put emotion into speech due to the loss of prosody may be called *affective aprosodia* (Heilman et al., 2004) and losing the ability to understand emotion in others' voices may be called *auditory affective disorder* (Heilman et al., 1975). One possible difficulty with vocal tones takes the form of losing the ability to understand sarcasm in speech (McDonald & Pearce, 1996), which is a super awesome problem to have.

Besides facial expressions and tone of voice, it's also possible to lose the ability to *interpret* the emotions of oneself. In other words, to lose self-perception of your own emotions. When a person loses the ability to recognize emotions in themselves, it is called *alexithymia*, or sometimes affective agnosia (Lane et al., 2015). These people cannot, for example, easily tell the difference between when they are feeling a positive emotion like happiness or a negative emotion like sadness. This disorder can be caused by traumatic brain injury (Becerra et al., 2002; Henry et al., 2006), or it can exist without brain injury, such as in psychiatric patients (Lane et al., 2015). Being unable to effectively interpret one's own emotions seems to be related to the inability to recognize emotions from other people's facial expressions and tone of voice—in other words, alexithymia and trouble with interpreting the emotions of others seem to be tied together in the same brain injuries for some people (Henry et al., 2006).

The Brain Pathology

As you would probably guess, the different symptoms associated with social-emotional agnosias, such as an inability to recognize the emotions of other people in expressive agnosia or a lack of prosody in affective aprosodia, seem to have different origins in the brain. That is, there are at least a few different places in the brain that can be damaged in order to produce social-emotional agnosias, including damage to the frontal parts of the brain or to the amygdala

(McDonald & Flanagan, 2004). More broadly speaking, social cognition as an ability involves "a large number of different brain areas and their connectivity" which spans pretty much all across the brain (Adams et al., 2019, p. 401). This diverse brain involvement is pretty good evidence that social interactions have been very important for the survival of our species across evolutionary history. Keep that in mind the next time someone engages you in seemingly pointless small talk—friendly interactions are something that the brain is built to do.

Much like damage to the left hemisphere seems most important for disorders of aphasia (see Aphasia), it instead appears to be damage to the *right* hemisphere that is most likely to produce some of the social-emotional agnosias (Joseph, 1988). As examples, it is believed that damage to the right-sided insula, anterior supramarginal gyrus, and somatosensory cortices can lead to impaired recognition of emotions from facial expressions, while damage to the right-sided posterior-superior temporal region can lead to difficulties in recognizing emotion from prosody (Adams et al., 2019). However, the ability to *produce* prosody using your own tone of voice seems to involve both hemispheres of the brain, and damage to just one side of the brain often isn't enough to cause affective aprosodia (Ross et al., 2013).

Many interventions and treatments have been proposed for social emotional agnosias, especially alexithymia, but because there are so many individual differences in where the brain is tripping up in its interpretation of social cognition, there is no one perfect treatment for all of these forms of emotional difficulties (Lane, 2020). Therefore, the approach for each person needs to be personalized in order for emotions to begin making sense again.

References

Adams, A. G., Schweitzer, D., Molenberghs, P., & Henry, J. D. (2019). A meta-analytic review of social cognitive function following stroke. *Neuroscience and Biobehavioral Reviews, 102*, 400–416. https://doi.org/gkvs8s

Adolphs, R. (2002). Recognizing emotion from facial expressions: Psychological and neurological mechanisms. *Behavioral and Cognitive Neuroscience Reviews, 1*(1), 21–62. https://doi.org/brpxcf

Becerra, R., Amos, A., & Jongenelis, S. (2002). Organic alexithymia: A study of acquired emotional blindness. *Brain Injury, 16*(7), 633–645. https://doi.org/bj6w88

Beer, J. S., & Ochsner, K. N. (2006). Social cognition: A multi level analysis. *Brain Research, 1079*(1), 98–105. https://doi.org/b8b4sv

Broicher, S., & Jokeit, H. (2011). Emotional agnosis and theory of mind. In M. R. Trimble & B. Schmitz (Eds.), *The neuropsychiatry of epilepsy* (2nd ed., pp. 109–123). Cambridge University Press.

Broks, P., Young, A. W., Maratos, E. J., Coffey, P. J., Calder, A. J., Isaac, C. L., Mayes, A. R., Hodges, J. R., Montaldi, D., Cezayirli, E., Roberts, N., & Hadley, D. (1998). Face processing impairments after encephalitis: Amygdala damage and recognition of fear. *Neuropsychologia, 36*(1), 59–70. https://doi.org/dvmwtq

Dimoska, A., McDonald, S., Pell, M. C., Tate, R. L., & James, C. M. (2010). Recognizing vocal expressions of emotion in patients with social skills deficits following traumatic brain injury. *Journal of the International Neuropsychological Society*, *16*(2), 369–382. https://doi.org/dxf6hx

Heilman, K. M., Leon, S. A., & Rosenbek, J. C. (2004). Affective aprosodia from a medial frontal stroke. *Brain and Language*, *89*(3), 411–416. https://doi.org/fdkzf3

Heilman, K. M., Scholes, R., & Watson, R. T. (1975). Auditory affective agnosia. Disturbed comprehension of affective speech. *Journal of Neurology Neurosurgery and Psychiatry*, *38*(1), 69–72. https://doi.org/bqmxdd

Henry, J. D., Phillips, L. H., Crawford, J. R., Theodorou, G., & Summers, F. (2006). Cognitive and psychosocial correlates of alexithymia following traumatic brain injury. *Neuropsychologia*, *44*(1), 62–72. https://doi.org/d9c4w7

Hopkins, M. J., Dywan, J., & Segalowitz, S. J. (2002). Altered electrodermal response to facial expression after closed head injury. *Brain Injury*, *16*(3), 245–257. https://doi.org/cmjj6d

Joseph, R. (1988). The right cerebral hemisphere: Emotion, music, visual–spatial skills, body-image, dreams, and awareness. *Journal of Clinical Psychology*, *44*(5), 630–673. https://doi.org/fpv8bp

Kurucz, J., & Feldmar, G. (1979). Prosopo-affective agnosia as a symptom of cerebral organic disease. *Journal of the American Geriatrics Society*, *27*(5), 225–230. https://doi.org/gtvs

Lane, R. D., Weihs, K. L., Herring, A., Hishaw, A., & Smith, R. (2015). Affective agnosia: Expansion of the alexithymia construct and a new opportunity to integrate and extend Freud's legacy. *Neuroscience & Biobehavioral Reviews*, *55*, 594–611.

Lane, R. D., Solms, M., Weihs, K. L., Hishaw, A., & Smith, R. (2020). Affective agnosia: A core affective processing deficit in the alexithymia spectrum. *BioPsychoSocial Medicine*, *14*(1), 1–14. https://doi.org/gtvt

McDonald, S., & Flanagan, S. (2004). Social perception deficits after traumatic brain injury: Interaction between emotion recognition, mentalizing ability, and social communication. *Neuropsychology*, *18*(3), 572–579. https://doi.org/dktbdq

McDonald, S., & Pearce, S. (1996). Clinical insights into pragmatic theory: Frontal lobe deficits and sarcasm. *Brain and Language*, *53*(1), 81–104. https://doi.org/cwfkqb

Ross, E. D., & Mesulam, M. M. (1979). Dominant language functions of the right hemisphere?: Prosody and emotional gesturing. *Archives of Neurology*, *36*(3), 144–148. https://doi.org/cx37vh

Ross, E. D., Shayya, L., & Rousseau, J. F. (2013). Prosodic stress: Acoustic, aphasic, aprosodic and neuroanatomic interactions. *Journal of Neurolinguistics*, *26*(5), 526–551. https://doi.org/hrbg

Young, A. W., Aggleton, J. P., Hellawell, D. J., Johnson, M., Broks, P., & Hanley, J. R. (1995). Face processing impairments after amygdalotomy. *Brain*, *118*(1), 15–24. https://doi.org/ffdmr5

Young, A. W., Hellawell, D. J., Van de Wal, C., & Johnson, M. (1996). Facial expression processing after amygdalotomy. *Neuropsychologia*, *34*(1), 31–39. https://doi.org/dgmrcr

Somatoparaphrenia

Imagine that you can't figure out to whom the arm attached to you belongs. Maybe it belongs to your brother, or a neighbor? But why is it in your hospital bed with you? Perhaps looking at it makes you feel sick, or you feel like you hate the arm. Doctors seem to keep asking you the same questions about it, insisting that you're wrong about who it belongs to. But you know that the arm can't be yours, because it doesn't *feel* like your arm.

The Stories

(STORY 1) A 79-year-old woman developed a severe case of *misoplegia* around the time that she was diagnosed with a brain tumor. She called her left leg names and would occasionally beat it with her hands. She referred to her left leg as a "bugger" and as her enemy that she wished to be rid of (p. 1099). She told people that if her left leg "were just dead" that it would make her happier (p. 1099). Reportedly, she was found crying on occasion with presumably self-inflicted bruises on her leg after having fights with it. After her tumor was surgically operated on, she began to alternate between showing affection for her left leg and cursing at it. She ultimately died around six weeks following her brain surgery due to worsening brain cancer (Loetscher et al., 2006).

(STORY 2) In 1980, a 65-year-old woman was admitted to a hospital's emergency room after developing weakness in the limbs on the left side of her body. She was cooperative and spoke to the medical workers, but she claimed that she was feeling weakness on the right side of her body, not the left. In fact, she insisted that the arm on her left did not belong to her at all, but had been left in the ambulance by another patient. When she was asked if her left shoulder was a part of her body, "she admitted without hesitation" that it was (p. 32). She was then led down the logical path that because her upper arm and elbow were attached to her shoulder, they probably belonged to her. She accepted this, given the "evident continuity of those members" (p. 32). However, she was elusive about the forearm and insisted on denying ownership of the left hand. When asked, she was unable to explain why rings belonging to her were being worn by the hand that she claimed did not belong to her (Bisiach & Geminiani, 1991, case L.A.-O.).

DOI: 10.4324/9781003276937-44

(STORY 3) A 61-year-old woman began to develop a number of symptoms including weakness and clumsiness in her left-sided limbs, throbbing headaches, a propensity for losing her way even in familiar places, and impairment of vision. Additionally, sometimes she felt like her left hand did not belong to her. While in the hospital, she was constantly getting lost and walking into the wrong rooms and even climbing into the wrong hospital beds—the doctor hypothesized that this was due to her failure to turn left at particular junctures. She also "tended to ignore events occurring to the left of her" in a classic sign of neglect (p. 91). She frequently complained that she could not find her left hand when she was looking for it, and was, on several occasions, observed while she was trying to find it. She remarked that "it feels as if someone had stolen it" (p. 91). The delusions about her arm continued to grow more severe. At later dates, she had extreme weakness in her left arm and left leg, but rather than admitting that anything was wrong with her limbs, she began insisting that she couldn't move her arm properly for a variety of false reasons, including that she had been sleeping on it or that it was too cold to move. At one point she said "a few days ago that arm was broken, but it is quite all right again, thank you" (p. 92). These confabulations were classic signs of anosognosia (see Anosognosia). Eventually, she was diagnosed with an inoperable brain tumor, and her symptoms continued up until the day that she died (Roth, 1949, case 1).

The Features

Have you ever fallen asleep on top of your arm for so long that when you woke up it seemed more like an object than a part of your body? Perhaps you've sat in an awkward position for so many minutes that you lost literally all feeling in the tips of your toes and could poke them and play with them as if they belonged to someone else. Usually, we're pretty good at feeling like we have ownership over our bodies—in these scenarios your limb will wake back up with restored sensitivity in a matter of minutes and you'll feel whole again. But imagine if that feeling of the limb not belonging to you was permanent, and whenever you looked at that body part it felt like it belonged to … someone else. Welcome to the world of somatoparaphrenia.

Somatoparaphrenia is closely related to neglect (see Hemispatial Neglect) and is considered a subtype of asomatognosia, which is the feeling of disownership of a limb such that it feels like it doesn't belong to you (Feinberg et al., 2010; Romano & Maravita, 2019). What makes somatoparaphrenia different, however, is the addition of a *delusional* component. According to Gerstmann, somatoparaphrenia cases are "cases in which with the experience of absence of the affected limbs or side of the body are associated illusional, confabulatory or delusional ideas of a peculiar nature" (Gerstmann, 1942, p. 909). Many times, people with somatoparaphrenia not only lose track of where their limb is located in space, but they also lose track of *who* the limb belongs to.

The typical person with somatoparaphrenia has at least one paralyzed limb, although in rare cases the limb is not paralyzed (Romano & Maravita, 2019). It usually overlaps with anosognosia (see Anosognosia) for paralysis in that limb such that the person does not believe that their own limb is paralyzed (Ardila, 2016). In other words, they frequently believe that their own limb can move, but the paralyzed limb that is in bed with them *is not their limb*.

They often mistake their limb as belonging to somebody else, oftentimes a family member, such as their mother, husband, brother, or niece (Feinberg & Venneri, 2014). For example, one patient insisted that the arm that was attached to his left side was not his arm, and that the doctors had mistakenly "given him the arm of another patient who was admitted to the hospital on the same day" (Moro et al., 2004, p. 439). They may otherwise claim that the paralyzed limb is a different object such as a piece of wood, a baby, or a fake limb (Vallar & Ronchi, 2009).

The person may also mistake *other people's* limbs as *belonging to themselves* (e.g., Jenkinson et al., 2018; Vallar & Ronchi, 2009). For example, this may happen when a physician asks the patient to close their eyes, the physician holds his hand in front of the patient's face, and when the patient opens their eyes the patient misidentifies the physician's hand as the patient's hand (Romano & Maravita, 2019).

There is also a name given to the specific situation in which a person displays hatred of their own limb: *misoplegia* (Loetscher et al., 2006). This sometimes occurs along with somatoparaphrenia, but they can be separate as well. In people with misoplegia, the person often treats their limb as a separate object from themselves, and they may even give it a made-up identity and/or name, which is called *personification* of the limb (Baier & Karnath, 2008). The person with misoplegia may verbally abuse the limb and even physically attack it, such as by violently striking it (Loetscher et al., 2006). At the least severe end, a person may merely express negative feelings about the limb, such as: "I was troubled the day this hand appeared" (Moro et al., 2004, p. 439). In severe cases, the person may abuse the limb, and talk about it as if it were a creature. One person called theirs Zodoquio, hit it several times, and said "it does not obey me" while claiming that it belonged to a nearby person (Starkstein et al., 1990, p. 1381).

In extreme cases of somatoparaphrenia, misoplegia, and similar disorders like alien hand syndrome (see Alien Hand Syndrome), there is sometimes a wish to remove the limb. This desire to amputate a limb is called *xenomelia* in the medical literature (Hilti et al., 2013). While this symptom is not yet fully explained by science, there is evidence that the person has reduced feelings of touch in the limb that they desire to be amputated, suggesting that their brain's understanding of their body does not include that particular limb (McGeoch et al., 2011). In other words, people with xenomelia may feel "overcomplete" such that a piece of flesh is attached to them that doesn't feel like it should be attached (Fornaro et al., 2020).

The Brain Pathology

Somatoparaphrenia may sound like a psychiatric disorder in which the person is altogether delirious, but that is often not the case—rather, this disorder seems to be partly due to a disruption to a person's conscious awareness of part of their body (Romano & Maravita, 2019). For whatever reason, the person's brain has lost the ability to put together a coherent body representation—merging the position of the limb in space with the person's recognition and feeling of ownership for that limb. Somatoparaphrenia seems to be related to delusional misidentification syndromes (see Capgras Syndrome), and may even be considered to be a delusional misidentification syndrome itself in which the person's brain has lost the ability to assign the appropriate identity to the limb (Kakegawa et al., 2020).

This disorder occurs from time to time in people who acquire brain damage due to strokes, tumors, or other damaging events, and while it usually goes away on its own relatively quickly, there have been reports of somatoparaphrenia lasting for years (Vallar & Ronchi, 2009). Somatoparaphrenia is most strongly associated with damage to the right hemisphere of the brain, leading to feelings of disownership of limbs on the left side of the person's body (Vallar & Ronchi, 2009). Damage or dysfunction in some specific areas such as the orbitofrontal region are associated with this disorder, but damage to other areas is usually also present (Feinberg & Venneri, 2014).

Overall, people with somatoparaphrenia tend to have more extensive brain damage than comparable people with neglect, which makes sense, because somatoparaphrenia is sort of like advanced neglect to the point of delusion. Recent work suggests that there isn't just one damage point in the brain that produces this disorder but, rather, there is an entire network of regions in your brain that help you to determine ownership of your own limbs—it is the disruption to the transfer of information between these networked brain regions that produces somatoparaphrenia (Moro et al., 2021). One way to think of this is that the person's mental representation of where their limb is supposed to be doesn't match the actual location of the limb in real physical space—this results in the delusion that the limb that they can see does not belong to them because it is in an unexpected location (Romano & Maravita, 2019). Count yourself lucky every time that you wake up in bed with an assortment of limbs and correctly identify that they are, in fact, yours.

References

Ardila, A. (2016). Some unusual neuropsychological syndromes: Somatoparaphrenia, akinetopsia, reduplicative paramnesia, autotopagnosia. *Archives of Clinical Neuropsychology*, *31*(5), 456–464. https://doi.org/gkx9s3

Baier, B., & Karnath, H. O. (2008). Tight link between our sense of limb ownership and self-awareness of actions. *Stroke*, *39*(2), 486–488. https://doi.org/cgfgzj

Bisiach, E., & Geminiani, G. (1991). Anosognosia related to hemiplegia and hemianopia. In G. P. Prigatano & D. L. Schacter (Eds.), *Awareness of deficit after brain injury: Clinical and theoretical issues* (pp. 17–39). Oxford University Press.

Feinberg, T. E., & Venneri, A. (2014). Somatoparaphrenia: Evolving theories and concepts. *Cortex*, *61*, 74–80. https://doi.org/f6wrcp

Feinberg, T. E., Venneri, A., Simone, A. M., Fan, Y., & Northoff, G. (2010). The neuroanatomy of asomatognosia and somatoparaphrenia. *Journal of Neurology, Neurosurgery & Psychiatry*, *81*(3), 276–281. https://doi.org/cq235q

Fornaro, S., Patrikelis, P., & Lucci, G. (2020). When having a limb means feeling overcomplete. Xenomelia, the chronic sense of disownership and the right parietal lobe hypothesis. *Laterality*, *0*(0), 1–20. https://doi.org/gtvv

Gerstmann, J. (1942). Problem of imperception of disease and of impaired body territories with organic lesions. *Archives of Neurology and Psychiatry* *48*(6), 890–913. https://doi.org/gts2

Hilti, L. M., Hänggi, J., Vitacco, D. A., Kraemer, B., Palla, A., Luechinger, R., Jäncke, L., & Brugger, P. (2013). The desire for healthy limb amputation: Structural brain correlates and clinical features of xenomelia. *Brain*, *136*(1), 318–329. https://doi.org/kb6

Jenkinson, P. M., Moro, V., & Fotopoulou, A. (2018). Definition: Asomatognosia. *Cortex*, *101*, 300–301. https://doi.org/gc8zbv

Kakegawa, Y., Isono, O., Hanada, K., & Nishikawa, T. (2020). Incidence and lesions causative of delusional misidentification syndrome after stroke. *Brain and Behavior*, *10*(11), 1–10. https://doi.org/gtvw

Loetscher, T., Regard, M., & Brugger, P. (2006). Misoplegia: A review of the literature and a case without hemiplegia. *Journal of Neurology, Neurosurgery & Psychiatry*, *77*(9), 1099–1100. https://doi.org/fr29nq

McGeoch, P. D., Brang, D., Song, T., Lee, R. R., Huang, M., & Ramachandran, V. S. (2011). Xenomelia: A new right parietal lobe syndrome. *Journal of Neurology, Neurosurgery and Psychiatry*, *82*(12), 1314–1319. https://doi.org/dz57tn

Moro, V., Zampini, M., & Aglioti, S. M. (2004). Changes in spatial position of hands modify tactile extinction but not disownership of contralesional hand in two right brain-damaged patients. *Neurocase*, *10*(6), 437–443. https://doi.org/bfbhvx

Moro, V., Pacella, V., Scandola, M., Rossato, E., & Jenkinson, P. (2021). *A fronto-insular-parietal network for the sense of body ownership*. Research Square. https://doi.org/gtvx

Romano, D., & Maravita, A. (2019). The dynamic nature of the sense of ownership after brain injury. Clues from asomatognosia and somatoparaphrenia. *Neuropsychologia*, *132*, Article 107119. https://doi.org/ghmtkv

Roth, M. (1949). Disorders of the body image caused by lesions of the right parietal lobe. *Brain*, *72*(1), 89–111. https://doi.org/cr6gpx

Starkstein, S. E., Berthier, M. L., Fedoroff, P., Price, T. R., & Robinson, R. G. (1990). Anosognosia and major depression in 2 patients with cerebrovascular lesions. *Neurology*, *40*(9), 1380–1382. https://doi.org/gtvz

Vallar, G., & Ronchi, R. (2009). Somatoparaphrenia: A body delusion. A review of the neuropsychological literature. *Experimental Brain Research*, *192*(3), 533–551. https://doi.org/cw8spn

Synesthesia

Imagine that your senses are intertwined. Sensations that for the average person would evoke only a single sound, color, or taste, instead produce a multimedia experience for you. Whenever you hear a certain noise, you see a certain burst of light. Or perhaps whenever you think about numbers, you can physically experience them in the space in front of you, greatly assisting in your calculations. Whatever your ability, you feel pieces of your experience connected in ways that others can only imagine.

The Stories

(STORY 1) A man went blind at the age of 40 after progressive loss of his vision from retinitis pigmentosa. He acquired touch-to-vision synesthesia a couple of years later around the age of 42. For example, when he would attempt to read Braille using his fingertips, he would also experience visual perceptions at the same time, even though he couldn't see. These visual perceptions included "vividly colored dots" and visual perceptions of movement such as "swirling" or "jumping" of the whole visual field (p. 294). He also experienced flashes of images in his head whenever he touched the edges of objects such as chairs or walls. He would sometimes feel like he was seeing the wall as he was touching it, but the wall that he imagined wouldn't look like it actually looked in reality and would instead be exaggerated or at a strange angle. By tapping on this person's fingers, the researchers were able to evoke sensations of flashing and jiggling in the patient's visual field (Armel & Ramachandran, 1999).

(STORY 2) A man was hit in the back of the head during an assault, and afterwards he developed a number of symptoms including the fact that he would see "complex geometrical figures and figures with fragmented boundaries" (p. 2). Visions of these figures could be induced by witnessing motion, such as watching a moving object. Following the development of seeing these shapes, he took a math class that taught him the ability to read mathematical formulas—after which, he began to see complex figures while viewing mathematical equations as well. These figures are automatic responses of his brain to the moving objects or mathematical equations, and when retested using the same equation or object, he reported seeing (and can draw) the same complex

DOI: 10.4324/9781003276937-45

figure. When he drew the figures that he saw, he did so "with great precision," demonstrating the intensity of the synesthesia that he was experiencing (Brogaard et al., 2013, p. 567).

(STORY 3) A man began regularly experiencing seizures following an infection that caused a long fever. His seizures were frequently accompanied by an unusual synesthetic experience. The experience came in three parts. He would feel "intense shooting facial pain" while at the same time both hearing and seeing a word (p. 1050). He reported, for example, hearing words such as "five" or "fist" and at the same time he saw that number or word appear as mental imagery (p. 1050). The attacks were very predictable to him, and before beginning treatment he experienced them around ten times each month. He developed a habit of grabbing his right wrist with his left hand and holding it during his seizures, believing that it would help to end them. What makes these experiences unusual when compared to the typical hallucinations that may occur with a seizure is that the senses of vision, hearing, and pain were all involved at the same time, and in a predictably linked way (Jacome & Gumnit, 1979).

(STORY 4) A man who went blind late in his life at the age of 52 due to damage to his optical nerves behind his eyes went on to develop a curious sort of mixed-sensory experience involving seeing flashes of light whenever he heard certain noises. These imaginary lights were especially common when the noise that he heard was loud and unexpected. It was shown in a laboratory setting that his brain was indeed responding to things that he heard by producing flashes of light that he could see. Sounds such as "jangling keys, banging on a metal bin, hand-clap, whistle, shout, or coughing" as well as noises that reminded him of car crashes or war, would produce bursts of light (p. 295). He would always see the light appear directly in front of him, even if the sound came from a different direction (Rao et al., 2007).

The Features

Before we can talk about synesthesia, we need to discuss *qualia*. Qualia are conscious experiences that a person has, such as seeing the color red, or feeling the rough texture of sandpaper on their fingertips. To someone who experiences them, they are familiar and obvious, but they are utterly impossible to describe to someone who cannot experience them. For example, imagine trying to describe the qualia of seeing the colors red and blue to someone who has never been able to see. You literally cannot do it because colors are concepts in your brain that you generate as part of your conscious experience of the world— nobody has access to your specific experience of colors except for you (see Achromatopsia). In people with synesthesia, the qualia that their brains create are *even more unique* because they contain *extra* information.

Synesthesia takes many different forms—in fact, new forms are still being described—so let's start with a general definition. Synesthesia is when one attribute of a stimulus (the *inducer*) leads to the conscious experience of an additional attribute (the *concurrent*), and this relationship is generally *automatic* (Ward, 2013). The attributes that make up the inducer and the concurrent can be any sort of conscious experience, such as hearing a sound or tasting a taste. Most typically, however, inducers are linguistic in nature such as letters and digits, while concurrents are visual in nature such as experiencing a color (Ward, 2013). A typical synesthesia pairing is that whenever a person sees a letter or number, their brain also generates a color, and therefore reading the letter or number and seeing the color are experienced *together* as linked qualia.

By that second part of the definition, automatic, I mean that the person cannot prevent the second attribute from being provoked even if they try. They have no control over what the concurrent is, or when it is triggered in the brain (Ward, 2013). The inducer–concurrent pairing is relatively stable across time such that if hearing jazz music makes you see the color orange, those two things will likely continue to be paired in your brain for years to come. Notably, a group of researchers gave nine synesthetes a list of 130 words, phrases, and letters, and asked them which color sensations were provoked (Baron-Cohen et al., 1993). Then, they retested them a year later. On the second test, 92.3% of their responses matched the responses from the year before. In comparison, the researchers also tested nine people without synesthesia, but instead of waiting a year, they only waited one week. For these people without synesthesia, only 37.6% of their responses matched their responses from the original test from the prior week. This is evidence for automatic and relatively stable inducer–concurrent pairings.

The most common type of synesthesia is developmental, which is synesthesia that exists from childhood onward. Many people with developmental synesthesia don't find out that they are experiencing the world differently from others until later in life and are reportedly often shocked to find out that other people do not perceive things the way that they do (Hubbard, 2007). Synesthesia changes across a person's life span, with children typically experiencing the most vivid qualia such as bright colors compared to drabber colors in adults, and with inducer–concurrent pairings declining in consistency over time as the person ages (Meier et al., 2014).

Developmental synesthesia can take a staggering number of different forms, but let's focus on some well-established varieties (Ward, 2013). Some common types are *spatial forms*, such as calendar→space, which is seeing the days of a calendar physically represented in space whenever you think about them. Another is vision→touch, which is also called *mirror touch* because when you see someone get touched, you may also feel the touch. One that is often discussed is grapheme→color, which is experiencing colors whenever you encounter letters and numbers. Other somewhat common forms include music→color, and taste→shape.

However, because this book is about changes that can happen to people's brains, we are mostly interested in the other major type of synesthesia, which is the acquired kind. Acquired synesthesia sometimes develops after an event that damages sensory organs or nerves. This most commonly takes the form of damage to the visual pathways leading from the eyes to the brain, such as the retina and optic nerve (Ward, 2007). Other known but less common causes of acquired synesthesia include stroke (Ro et al., 2007), brain tumor (Vike et al., 1984), and epilepsy (Jacome & Gumnit, 1979). Certain drugs can also cause you to temporarily experience synesthesia, but this tends to be tightly coupled with illusions and pseudohallucinations, and the associations can be highly variable rather than automatic (Sinke et al., 2012). So, even if the sound of your own voice tasted like citrus the first time that you took a drug trip, it is unlikely to taste that way on your second trip.

Importantly, acquired synesthesia seems to be different from developmental synesthesia at the level of the brain. While developmental synesthesia may include complicated connections between complex stimuli, acquired synesthesia seems to involve more basic sensory information (Ward, 2013). By basic sensory information, I mean things like brief flashes of light that are caused by something other than light entering the eye. Those flashes are called *phosphenes*, and they show up in acquired synesthesia quite frequently (e.g., Page et al., 1982).

The most common form of acquired synesthesia is probably audio→visual synesthesia following vision loss, in which partially blind or blind people experience phosphenes when they hear noises (Afra et al., 2009). Experiencing touch in response to sounds has also been reported (Ro et al., 2007). There has also been an account of acquired touch→vision synesthesia, where a blind person saw things when their skin was touched (Armel & Ramachandran, 1999). People who are deaf from a very young age who receive cochlear implants later in life sometimes experience sensations of touch on their bodies when they hear sounds using their new implant (McFeely Jr et al., 1998). Phantom sensations of pain and touch in amputated body parts when someone touches near the previous location of that body part (see Phantom Sensations) and ringing in the ears triggered by various other sources following inner ear damage (see Tinnitus) also sometimes fit the definition of synesthesia, because they can include automatic pairings of sensory experiences (Ward, 2013).

The Brain Pathology

One theory about developmental synesthesia is that it may be a relatively normal part of brain development but, as the person grows older, the brain connections that cause the synesthesia are "pruned" away (e.g., Hubbard, 2007). In people with synesthesia, then, perhaps this *pruning* process is simply reduced, leaving behind some neural paths that most people do not keep, allowing those complicated qualia to occur (Ramachandran & Hubbard, 2001).

Acquired synesthesia is trickier to explain at the level of the brain, and it is still quite mysterious. We do have some clues about how it works, though. Notably, after the damage happens, the impaired sense such as vision or hearing typically acts as the concurrent—the triggered qualia—in the resulting synesthesia (Ward, 2013). In theory, this is because the previous inducer of that qualia has gone missing and the brain is compensating by looking for other inputs to trigger that qualia.

For example, let's say that a person has new damage to their optic nerve. Now, their eyes are sending less information to their brain for processing. But the part of their brain that processes vision is still *there*, it is just hungry for input signals so that it can do its job and produce some vision (see Charles Bonnet Syndrome). So, that part of your brain starts looking for signals to interpret from elsewhere in your brain. In people who develop acquired synesthesia, their brains find some new information to interpret as vision, such as sound. How does the visual part of the brain find the sound to interpret it as vision? Researchers don't really know yet. Two possibilities stand out, however. These possibilities depend upon the concept of brain *reorganization* thanks to *neuroplasticity*, which is the ability of the brain to *change old connections* or *form new connections* between areas of the brain (Pascual-Leone et al., 2005).

First, maybe the synesthesia is due to changing old connections. Maybe the synesthesia was always there—perhaps their brains already had existing underlying structural connections that were not pruned away as a child, and when their brain got quieter because of the damage, those preexisting connections between sound and vision that they hadn't noticed before got a chance to "unmask" themselves because they were no longer being inhibited (Yong et al., 2017).

Alternatively, perhaps the brain created new connections. This is a slow process, but the brain can reorganize itself over time such that underutilized parts of the brain begin to be used in a different way, such as how the brains of people who acquire blindness or deafness begin to use those less active areas of the brain to process other sensory information instead, such as touch (Merabet & Pascual-Leone, 2010).

Because acquired synesthesia can happen just days after brain damage, or it can happen years later, both of these ideas may be supported—with the first explanation explaining the quick synesthesia while the second explanation explains the slow synesthesia (Afra et al., 2009; Ward, 2013). Regardless, people with synesthesia often have difficulty fully describing their experiences, and may even find it difficult to convince people that the experiences are really happening. But the evidence shows us that synesthesia is real, and it may be hidden in more brains than we realize, only to be occasionally revealed by unlucky instances of brain damage.

References

Afra, P., Funke, M., & Matsuo, F. (2009). Acquired auditory-visual synesthesia: A window to early cross-modal sensory interactions. *Psychology Research and Behavior Management, 2*, 31–37. https://doi.org/fsr8x8

Armel, K. C., & Ramachandran, V. S. (1999). Acquired synesthesia in retinitis pigmentosa. *Neurocase, 5*(4), 293–296. https://doi.org/dq32jp

Baron-Cohen, S., Harrison, J., Goldstein, L. H., & Wyke, M. (1993). Coloured speech perception: Is synaesthesia what happens when modularity breaks down? *Perception*, *22*(4), 419–426. https://doi.org/brz4kn

Brogaard, B., Vanni, S., & Silvanto, J. (2013). Seeing mathematics: Perceptual experience and brain activity in acquired synesthesia. *Neurocase*, *19*(6), 566–575. https://doi.org/gs5f

Hubbard, E. M. (2007). Neurophysiology of synesthesia. *Current Psychiatry Reports*, *9*(3), 193–199. https://doi.org/fcx9mn

Jacome, D. E., & Gumnit, R. J. (1979). Audioalgesic and audiovisuoaglesic synesthesias: Epileptic manifestation. *Neurology*, *29*(7), 1050–1053. https://doi.org/gs5g

McFeely Jr., W. J., Antonelli, P. J., Rodriguez, F. J., & Holmes, A. E. (1998). Somatosensory phenomena after multichannel cochlear implantation in prelingually deaf adults. *The American Journal of Otology*, *19*(4), 467–471.

Meier, B., Rothen, N., & Walter, S. (2014). Developmental aspects of synaesthesia across the adult lifespan. *Frontiers in Human Neuroscience*, *8*, Article 129. https://doi.org/drvv

Merabet, L. B., & Pascual-Leone, A. (2010). Neural reorganization following sensory loss: The opportunity of change. *Nature Reviews Neuroscience*, *11*(1), 44–52. https://doi.org/cshg3c

Page, N. G. R., Bolger, J. P., & Sanders, M. D. (1982). Auditory evoked phosphenes in optic nerve disease. *Journal of Neurology, Neurosurgery, and Psychiatry*, *45*(1), 7–12. https://doi.org/dhjrjc

Pascual-Leone, A., Amedi, A., Fregni, F., & Merabet, L. B. (2005). The plastic human brain cortex. *Annual Review of Neuroscience*, *28*, 377–401. https://doi.org/bqdq3h

Ramachandran, S., & Hubbard, E. M. (2001). Synaesthesia—A window into perception, thought and language. *Journal of Consciousness Studies*, *8*(12), 3–34.

Rao, A., Nobre, A. C., Alexander, I., & Cowey, A. (2007). Auditory evoked visual awareness following sudden ocular blindness: An EEG and TMS investigation. *Experimental Brain Research*, *176*(2), 288–298. https://doi.org/bdhpgt

Ro, T., Farnè, A., Johnson, R. M., Wedeen, V., Chu, Z., Wang, Z. J., Hunter, J. V., & Beauchamp, M. S. (2007). Feeling sounds after a thalamic lesion. *Annals of Neurology*, *62*(5), 433–441. https://doi.org/dr6m27

Sinke, C., Halpern, J. H., Zedler, M., Neufeld, J., Emrich, H. M., & Passie, T. (2012). Genuine and drug-induced synesthesia: A comparison. *Consciousness and Cognition*, *21*(3), 1419–1434. https://doi.org/f39fg8

Vike, J., Jabbari, B., & Maitland, C. G. (1984). Auditory-visual synesthesia: Report of a case with intact visual pathways. *Archives of Neurology*, *41*(6), 680–681. https://doi.org/d7dmm9

Ward, J. (2007). Acquired auditory-tactile synesthesia. *Annals of Neurology*, *62*(5), 429–430. https://doi.org/c7btvm

Ward, J. (2013). Synesthesia. *Annual Review of Psychology*, *64*, 49–75. https://doi.org/gf5286

Yong, Z., Hsieh, P. J., & Milea, D. (2017). Seeing the sound after visual loss: Functional MRI in acquired auditory-visual synesthesia. *Experimental Brain Research*, *235*(2), 415–420. https://doi.org/f9q54c

Tinnitus

Imagine that you cannot stop a noise from playing over and over inside of your brain. It makes sleeping difficult; it makes concentrating a chore, and, overall, you find it to be excruciatingly annoying. Perhaps you can only experience silence while you are unconscious, and the first thing you hear every time you wake up is the noises whining in your own head. Or perhaps you are luckier and the noises come and go throughout the day, but whenever they come back your stomach drops in dread. Where are these noises coming from?

The Stories

(STORY 1) A reduction of stress may help in some cases of tinnitus. As Dr. MacNaughton Jones wrote back in 1890, working long nights and "excessively hard work" made his tinnitus worse (p. 667). He wrote that the tinnitus often prevented him from sleeping and was worse when his head was pressing on the pillow. He wrote that the noises sounded exactly like a heartbeat in his left ear, and in a later bout of tinnitus, like the "rustling sound of waving trees" (p. 667). Pressure on a particular part of his upper jaw partially relieved the problem, but tinnitus continued to prove annoying. Fortunately, he found that the relaxing atmosphere of country air eased it. "Switzerland, I think, cured me," he noted in his lecture on the topic, where he sought to further the quest for understanding and a cure for tinnitus for himself and his patients (Jones et al., 1890, p. 667).

(STORY 2) A celebrity who has been vocal about tinnitus is William Shatner, who has spoken about how on the set of *Star Trek* he acquired tinnitus after finding himself too close to a special effects explosion (Shatner, 2012). He described the condition as being "tormented" by "screeching" inside of his own head. He coped by using a white noise machine to mask the noise, and has since found his condition much improved. In one informal interview in 2013, an internet commenter wrote to Shatner that "sleeping with a fan helps," suggesting a common coping mechanism—a rotating fan that blows air and generates white noise to mask the tinnitus—but Shatner either mistakenly or intentionally took the comment as a flirty double entendre (Burlingame,

DOI: 10.4324/9781003276937-46

2017). Shatner is a supporter of the American Tinnitus Association, which raises money and awareness for tinnitus.

(STORY 3) People with tinnitus often tell their doctors that the annoyance is worse in the mornings, when the tinnitus takes the form of a "morning roar" (Probst et al., 2017, p. 6). A group of researchers set out to determine whether the time of day had an effect on the severity of tinnitus. They developed an app called Track Your Tinnitus that asked people throughout the day, at random times, to report how loud the tinnitus was at that moment, how much the tinnitus was distressing them, and their current overall stress level. In this way, they were able to look into the lives of 350 people as they went about their regular days, interrupted occasionally by their phone asking them about the current state of their tinnitus. Powered by such technology, this method proved useful in finding conclusive evidence that tinnitus is rated as louder and more disturbing during the night and early morning when compared to the daytime. More specifically, the period from 12 AM to 8 AM was rated as more unbearable for the tinnitus sufferers than any other time of day (Probst et al., 2017). Additionally, a study that asked people with tinnitus to write about their experiences also found that the early morning hours were the worst in terms of tinnitus severity (Flor et al., 2004). There is still much to learn about why tinnitus is sometimes worse at certain times of day, but this discovery may help sufferers target their various tinnitus coping mechanisms by using them at specific times.

The Features

Tinnitus is often thought of as ringing in the ears that occurs after hearing loud noises. However, tinnitus can be caused by a variety of things (e.g., loud noise, infections, brain tumors, a misaligned jaw, etc.) and may take a variety of phantom noise-forms. In an old but fascinating collection of tinnitus noise descriptions, one doctor wrote that the noise may resemble a "bee humming; noise of shell; horse out of breath, puffing; thumping noise; continual beating; crackling sounds in the head … furnace blowing; constant hammering; rushing water … railway whistling; distant thunder; chirping of birds; kettle boiling; waterfall; mill wheel; music; bells" (Jones et al., 1890, p. 668). Thus, pitch, volume, and annoyingness can all vary, with rare forms of tinnitus even resembling low voices or music. You know how annoying it is to be able to hear someone speaking, but to not be able to hear exactly what they are saying? Now imagine that happening all of the time, inside of your brain. There are milder forms of tinnitus from which you generally recover in short order and, as we will see, those cases are the lucky ones. Here, in this particular book, we will be discussing the more severe sort of tinnitus—that is, haunting noise that repeats over and over and over.

Interestingly, tinnitus can occur subjectively or objectively. In *subjective* tinnitus, only the sufferer can hear the noise. In *objective* tinnitus, using the right instruments, an outside observer such as a doctor can hear the noise too.

Objective tinnitus is much rarer than subjective tinnitus, and often is caused by mechanics in vascular, skeletal, respiratory, or muscular systems (Henry et al., 2014). For example, a malformation of an artery in the head can lead to a pulsating objective tinnitus as the person's heartbeat forces blood through in an absolutely metal-sounding event called "blood turbulence" (Sismanis, 1998, p. 474). However, because this book focuses on the brain, I will focus on the kind of tinnitus found in the brain itself: subjective tinnitus.

Tinnitus most often results from damage to the *hair cells* located in a structure of your inner ear called the *cochlea* that are together responsible for the sensation of sound. A common way that this hair cell damage happens is that a person has too much exposure to loud noise, such as explosions or heavy machinery. Tinnitus can also be associated with head injuries, neck injuries, certain medications, and oftentimes tinnitus just kind of shows up and the person doesn't know why—this last mysterious category is known as *idiopathic tinnitus* (Henry et al., 2005). Tinnitus may also occur when a person hasn't experienced hearing loss, but that is significantly more rare and may even involve different problematic areas in the brain when compared to the more common type associated with hearing loss (Vanneste & De Ridder, 2016).

It is difficult to know exactly how many people experience tinnitus across their lives. Part of the problem is that there is currently no established standard diagnostic criterion, which means that different doctors may diagnose tinnitus differently. This is why estimates of the prevalence of tinnitus range from 5–43% of the adult population, with 3–31% of those affected reporting that it negatively impacts their quality of life (McCormack et al., 2016).

Severe tinnitus may have an enormous emotional impact, but physicians have a history of not taking the problem seriously. This ranges from distant history, where in 1880 a lecturer on the topic remarked that "of the various forms and kinds of noises, the descriptions given by patients are often perplexing, and not seldom ludicrous" (Hemming, 1880, p. 505)—and continues into the present day, where some doctors continue to tell patients to simply ignore the noises. But for many sufferers, ignoring simply isn't an option. People with tinnitus may be kept awake by the noise, causing severe insomnia (Asnis et al., 2018). And first thing in the morning, many of them are greeted by a severe *morning roar*, which is a time period during which the sound is particularly loud and disruptive (Probst et al., 2017). The sounds of tinnitus may be intermittent with periods of respite, or may be persistent with no silence to be found. There is no shortage of emotional tinnitus stories, with descriptions of years of maddening noises and the desperate quest for peace and quiet. In a survey of 150 people with especially severe tinnitus, some of them were so desperate that they reported that if it would stop the noise, they would have accepted not only surgical treatment, but the permanent loss of their hearing in exchange for silence (House, 1981).

When measured clinically, people with tinnitus are more likely to suffer from anxiety and depression (Trevis et al., 2018). Stress, depression, and insomnia often result from tinnitus and also seem to *contribute* to tinnitus, in a vicious cycle (Henry et al., 2005). But there is also a cognitive toll as well, meaning that general thinking, reaction time, and accuracy of short-term memory may be disrupted by tinnitus (Clarke et al., 2020). My point is that tinnitus can be a severe problem that should be taken seriously, and not dismissed as merely "ringing in the ears."

The Brain Pathology

The phantom noise, even though it is often experienced as if it were happening in the ears, is actually happening in the brain itself (Eggermont & Roberts, 2004). Thanks to neuroimaging studies such as those using fMRI machines, we know that tinnitus is "not just a problem of the ear," it is a problem of the brain: evidence for brain differences in people with tinnitus have been found in the temporal lobes, the prefrontal cortex, and in the limbic system (Melcher, 2012, p. 180). There are several competing theories as to how tinnitus actually arises in the brain at the neural level (Henry et al., 2014). The following is a leading theory of how tinnitus comes to be.

Following inner ear damage, the amount of neural signals being sent from a person's snail-shaped inner ear structure—called the *cochlea*—to the person's brain becomes lower (Henry et al., 2014). Therefore, the brain cells that used to interpret the incoming signals from the cochlea suddenly start having less work to do. When the brain cells in these areas aren't doing much of anything, a few changes occur.

First, the brain reorganizes its *tonotopic map*. The tonotopic map is a way of dividing the parts of your brain that process sound into regions that respond to different sound waves, such as 20 Hz (a very low-pitched noise) versus 20,000 Hz (a very high-pitched noise). Typically, the neurons in this part of your brain, the primary auditory cortex, are tuned to specific levels and frequencies of sounds, but in tinnitus the tuning of the brain changes as it reorganizes which sounds it responds to in the regions of the tonotopic map (Eggermont, 2012).

Next, the brain cells become hyperexcitable—meaning that cells that connect to one another have an easier time spreading brain activation to each other. They do this because they are trying to make up for the damage that is making it harder for hearing sensations such as signals from the cochlea to reach them, so the cells begin to react as a group to weaker signals (Schaette & McAlpine, 2011). Firing together like this is called *neural synchrony*.

Thirdly, the brain cells begin firing somewhat randomly, even in the absence of noise, and maintain a baseline level of activity because they are told to fire a certain amount by the brain stem (Schaette & McAlpine, 2011). These random firings, when counted, are called *spontaneous firing rates*. Because the brain cells are already hyperexcitable and synchronized, the random firings are amplified and can potentially be perceived as the noise of tinnitus.

Overall, the thalamus and the cortex especially seem to play an important role in generating tinnitus thanks to reorganization of the tonotopic map, increased neural synchrony, and increased spontaneous firing rates (Eggermont, 2012). Then, the prefrontal cortex and the limbic system decide which noises picked up by the auditory system should be attended to consciously by the person. In a person experiencing tinnitus, the phantom noise is let through a sort of noise filter instead of being tuned out—a decision assisted by the limbic system's thalamic reticular system (Leaver et al., 2011). In theory, this whole process is similar to that for phantom vision (see Charles Bonnet Syndrome) and phantom pain (see Phantom Sensations).

There are dozens of different possible treatment recommendations for tinnitus. These include active music therapy, cognitive behavioral therapy, and several experimental electromagnetic procedures (Zenner et al., 2017). For example, using repetitive transcranial magnetic stimulation—which is repeatedly turning an electromagnet on and off near the brain—can sometimes lead to a temporary reduction in the tinnitus symptoms (Lefaucheur et al., 2020). Unfortunately, no treatment is a guaranteed cure for this excruciating disorder.

References

Asnis, G. M., Majeed, K., Henderson, M. A., Sylvester, C., Thomas, M., & La Garza, R. De. (2018). An examination of the relationship between insomnia and tinnitus: A review and recommendations. *Clinical Medicine Insights: Psychiatry*, 9, 1–8. https://doi.org/gs5c

Burlingame, R. (2017, September 6). *William Shatner joins Reddit, answers fan questions.* Comicbook. https://bit.ly/3zEXtAM

Clarke, N. A., Henshaw, H., Akeroyd, M. A., Adams, B., & Hoare, D. J. (2020). Associations between subjective tinnitus and cognitive performance: Systematic review and meta-analyses. *Trends in Hearing*, 24, 1–23. https://doi.org/gtv2

Eggermont, J. J. (2012). Cortex: Way station or locus of the tinnitus percept? In J. J. Eggermont, F.-G. Zeng, A. N. Popper, & R. R. Fay (Eds.), *Springer handbook of auditory research* (pp. 137–162). Springer. https://doi.org/gtv3

Eggermont, J. J., & Roberts, L. E. (2004). The neuroscience of tinnitus. *Trends in Neurosciences*, 27(11), 676–682. https://doi.org/bdc5rp

Flor, H., Hoffmann, D., Struve, M., & Diesch, E. (2004). Auditory discrimination training for the treatment of tinnitus. *Applied Psychophysiology and Biofeedback*, 29(2), 113–120. https://doi.org/c8j9jz

Hemming, W. D. (1880). The forms, causes, and treatment of tinnitus aurium. *British Medical Journal*, 2(1030), 505–507. https://doi.org/cpq9k3

Henry, J. A., Dennis, K. C., & Schechter, M. A. (2005). General review of tinnitus: Prevalence, mechanisms, effects, and management. *Journal of Speech, Language, and Hearing Research*, 48(5), 1204–1235. https://doi.org/d6nhvd

Henry, J. A., Roberts, L. E., Caspary, D. M., Theodoroff, S. M., & Salvi, R. J. (2014). Underlying Mechanisms of Tinnitus: Review and Clinical Implications. *Journal of the American Academy of Audiology*, 25(1), 5–22. https://doi.org/f5vtm3

House, P. R. (1981). Personality of the tinnitus patient. In D. Evered & G. Lawrenson (Eds.), *Tinnitus* (pp. 193–203). Pitman.

Jones, H. M., Turnbull, L., Cousins, J. W., & Grant, J. D. (1890). A discussion on the etiology of tinnitus aurium. *The British Medical Journal*, 667–672.

Leaver, A. M., Renier, L., Chevillet, M. A., Morgan, S., Kim, H. J., & Rauschecker, J. P. (2011). Dysregulation of limbic and auditory networks in tinnitus. *Neuron, 69*(1), 33–43. https://doi.org/fwkc26

Lefaucheur, J. P., Aleman, A., Baeken, C., Benninger, D. H., Brunelin, J., Di Lazzaro, V., Filipović, S. R., Grefkes, C., Hasan, A., Hummel, F. C., Jääskeläinen, S. K., Langguth, B., Leocani, L., Londero, A., Nardone, R., Nguyen, J. P., Nyffeler, T., Oliveira-Maia, A. J., Oliviero, A., … Ziemann, U. (2020). Evidence-based guidelines on the therapeutic use of repetitive transcranial magnetic stimulation (rTMS): An update (2014–2018). *Clinical Neurophysiology, 131*(2), 474–528. https://doi.org/ggvmz3

McCormack, A., Edmondson-Jones, M., Somerset, S., & Hall, D. (2016). A systematic review of the reporting of tinnitus prevalence and severity. *Hearing Research, 337*, 70–79. https://doi.org/f8td66

Melcher, J. R. (2012). Human brain imaging of tinnitus. In J. J. Eggermont, F.-G. Zeng, A. N. Popper, & R. R. Fay (Eds.), *Springer handbook of auditory research* (pp. 163–185). Springer. https://doi.org/gtv4

Probst, T., Pryss, R. C., Langguth, B., Rauschecker, J. P., Schobel, J., Reichert, M., Spiliopoulou, M., Schlee, W., & Zimmermann, J. (2017). Does tinnitus depend on time-of-day? An ecological momentary assessment study with the "TrackYourTinnitus" application. *Frontiers in Aging Neuroscience, 9*, Article 253. https://doi.org/gs5d

Schaette, R., & McAlpine, D. (2011). Tinnitus with a normal audiogram: physiological evidence for hidden hearing loss and computational model. *Journal of Neuroscience, 31*(38), 13452–13457. https://doi.org/d39z9b

Shatner, W. (2012). *Message from William Shatner to you*. American Tinnitus Association. https://bit.ly/3zKEy7K

Sismanis, A. (1998). Pulsatile tinnitus. A 15-year experience. *The American Journal of Otology, 19*(4), 472–477.

Trevis, K. J., McLachlan, N. M., & Wilson, S. J. (2018). A systematic review and meta-analysis of psychological functioning in chronic tinnitus. *Clinical Psychology Review, 60*, 62–86. https://doi.org/gdff3h

Vanneste, S., & De Ridder, D. (2016). Deafferentation-based pathophysiological differences in phantom sound: tinnitus with and without hearing loss. *Neuroimage, 129*, 80–94. https://doi.org/gktk8r

Zenner, H. P., Delb, W., Kröner-Herwig, B., Jäger, B., Peroz, I., Hesse, G., Mazurek, B., Goebel, G., Gerloff, C., Trollmann, R., Biesinger, E., Seidler, H., & Langguth, B. (2017). A multidisciplinary systematic review of the treatment for chronic idiopathic tinnitus. *European Archives of Oto-Rhino-Laryngology, 274*(5), 2079–2091. https://doi.org/f95b5g

Topographical Disorientation

Imagine one day that you are walking to the store to buy some goods or services. But on your way there, something strange happens. You suddenly feel … lost. Despite having walked this path numerous times, and despite the fact that you can clearly see all of the landmarks around you—the building with the red roof, the park bench on the corner—the place has lost all meaning to you. Defeated, you turn around to walk back home. Unfortunately, you're not sure where exactly that is either …

The Stories

(STORY 1) A 49-year-old cyclist was pedaling around a city in 1898 when he suddenly had a minor vascular event in his brain that caused him to go partially blind. He got off of his bike and called for help, but none came. He tried to find his way around and wandered for about six hours, all while carrying his bicycle. By following the sound of the wind and brightly burning street lamps, he made his way back into a somewhat familiar area, but not before falling into several ditches. Eventually, a police officer helped him return home. When he was checked out by physicians later, he found that his ability to navigate was gone. He could answer questions about which street a particular building was located on, but when he was actually walking around, he was helplessly lost. While he was in the hospital for 14 days, he was consistently getting lost. He had a room that he shared with another patient on the first floor of the hospital. Each day, he was taken to the ground floor for tests and questions and then was asked to try and find his way back to his room. He was so unable to navigate correctly that sometimes he ended up in the basement. When he did make it back to his floor, he used a strategy of entering each and every room and looking for something that he recognized. His roommate had a big black beard, and whenever he saw a black beard he would report that he had found his room—but he was often wrong. He would also try to use his personal possessions that he kept on his bedside table to judge whether he had found his room. But when the table was moved, he no longer knew that it was his room. When the physician took him on a walk, the patient was extremely disoriented, and when the physician asked him where he thought he was, he would desperately look

DOI: 10.4324/9781003276937-47

for a street sign to help him. Over the course of many months, with the help of his wife on long walks, he became better able to orient himself, but never felt completely sure of his location, even years later (Meyer, 1900, case 1).

(STORY 2) A 58-year-old woman suddenly developed *landmark agnosia* while on her way to work. She was on public transportation when she felt that she no longer knew where she was, even though the driver announced a stop at a street that was well known to her. She found it necessary to ask for directions to a store that she had visited many times before. When she made it home, her apartment that she had lived in for 20 years seemed completely unknown to her—eerily unfamiliar. When she went to the doctor, she had some issues with her vision as well as the gait of her walk. In the hospital, she navigated by memorizing and paying careful attention to turns and which doors to go into, but she never felt that the hospital ward had grown familiar to her. That is, as she navigated around, it did not feel like she had been there before, even though she definitely had been there many times. Years later, she continued to rely on memorization tricks such as mnemonics for street names because she still felt that her surroundings were unfamiliar (Landis et al., 1986, case 2).

(STORY 3) A 60-year-old man developed *anterograde disorientation* following a pair of strokes. His overall memory was decent, but it was almost impossible for him to learn and remember new topographical information. While being tested by researchers, he never learned the layout of the laboratory's rooms even though he was there across several days. When he moved to a neighborhood that had many similar-looking homes, he had to rely on street signs and then examine each house in detail in order to find his own home. Later on, he and his wife moved to a different home that was also in a different country. He described the new home as a "haunted house" because he was never able to learn the layout (p. 485). As one example, his bedroom had a balcony attached to it, but he always forgot that fact, so he would constantly surprise himself when he discovered the existence of the balcony. Despite this, he could navigate through environments that he knew from before the stroke, he could recognize famous landmarks that he knew from before the stroke, and he could follow directions marked on a map. He could even draw a map of the house that he had lived in before the stroke. Eventually, after several months, he did learn the layout of the so-called haunted house enough to navigate through it—let's hope he never had to move again (Epstein et al., 2001, case 1).

The Features

Navigation is a skill that many people struggle with at least a little bit. Overall, it's pretty common to get turned around and lost in your environment every now and again. But some people with brain damage find themselves afflicted with much more severe navigation problems, getting lost on familiar streets and while walking through familiar rooms.

Like many of the conditions in this book, there is a *developmental* form of topographical disorientation in which a person grows up with extremely poor navigational abilities (Iaria & Barton, 2010). However, I will be focusing on the *acquired* kind, which is when some type of brain-damaging event causes a person to lose their navigational abilities.

As you may expect, navigating through disorders of navigation can be tricky. This is because topographical disorientation is actually a collection of different disorders. One prominent classification scheme for types of topographical disorientation sorts them into four types (Aguirre & D'Esposito, 1999). In order to successfully navigate, you need to either be very good at keeping track of your own *position*, your own *orientation*, or at least be very good at using *landmarks* to find your way to your destination. It's also helpful to be able to form *memories* about the navigational paths that you are following, so that you can follow them again later on. Those four key things represent four different ways that your brain can lose the ability to navigate, because different parts and pathways in the brain contribute to processing those different types of information (Aguirre, 2003).

When the brain damage is in the posterior parietal lobe, it can cause a form of topographical disorientation called *egocentric disorientation* (Aquirre & D'Esposito, 1999). These people cannot represent their own body's relative position to the locations of objects around them. In other words, their brain can't seem to calculate where they themselves are located in space. When their eyes are open, they can often correctly point in the direction of objects. But when their eyes are closed, they struggle to point in the direction of the objects now that they cannot be seen (Aguirre, 2003). For example, if asked to touch something while their eyes are closed, they may "grope aimlessly" and be unable to find where the object is positioned, even though they were just looking at it a moment ago (Stark et al., 1996, p. 485). These people may not be able to describe a route from one location to another, even if it is a route that they follow regularly, because they struggle with concepts like left or right, near or far, and above or below (Levine et al., 1985). People with egocentric disorientation are therefore lost in space.

Somewhat similarly, if an area of the brain called the posterior cingulate is damaged, it may produce *heading disorientation* (Aquirre & D'Esposito, 1999). These people are not lost in space themselves, but they cannot use positional relationships. This means that the person becomes unable to derive directional information from their environment such that they no longer know, for example, which way is north or which way is the way towards home. When shown photographs of buildings, these people may be unable to decipher *where* the photograph was taken, and they may also be completely unable to determine in which compass direction they are facing when looking at a map (Suzuki et al., 1998). They may also struggle to explain how two locations are located relative to one another, such as describing that a restaurant is located north of the shopping mall (Takahashi et al., 1997). Overall, their sense of heading is disrupted when it comes to the world around them.

Those first two types were problems with spatial processing: where am I? This next one is a recognition problem: what am I looking at? Damage to the lingual gyrus can lead to *landmark agnosia*, which is the inability to recognize places. It is also sometimes called topographagnosia or topographic agnosia, and it is similar to other agnosias (see Visual Object Agnosia). Of the four, this is the type of topographical disorientation that appears to be most common and has been studied the most (Aguirre, 2003).

People with landmark agnosia can use spatial abilities and can still follow directions such as "turn right" or "go east" when following a map or GPS instructions (Farah, 2004). Where they struggle is with identifying which building they are looking at, and whether it is their house or their neighbor's house. If the person perfectly memorized their route such as where and how many times to turn left or right, they may be able to follow that route—but when they arrive, they still don't *feel* like they are in the correct place because it is unrecognizable to them and feels unfamiliar (Pallis, 1955).

Sometimes the problems are mostly with new buildings they have not seen before, but sometimes the problems extend also to buildings that they have seen many times before (van der Ham et al., 2017). In some cases, they have difficulties recognizing familiar landmarks from photos (della Rocchetta et al., 1996). They may even be unable to identify a photograph of their own house even if they have lived there for many years (McCarthy et al., 1996).

However, people with landmark agnosia often retain the ability to recognize small features such as mailboxes and doorways—at least when they are examined closely (Landis et al., 1986). Small environmental signs and symbols are commonly reported as the biggest thing that these people look for as a strategy to find their way around (Aguirre, 2003). One person with this condition noted that he could see and describe buildings, but, "if he looks away and then looks back again, it looks different as though someone had put another unfamiliar building in its place" (Whiteley & Warrington, 1978, p. 575).

Now, the question becomes: why can't these people recognize large environmental landmarks like buildings, but they can identify small things like individual objects? One possibility is that they have lost the ability to represent *multiple* visual objects in different points in space at the *same time* in their brain, leading to difficulties with large scenes with many features such as buildings (Mendez & Cherrier, 2003). The distribution of windows, the pattern of bricks, the slope of the roof: all of those things *together* can tell a person which building they are looking at, but not for people with landmark agnosia. The region of the brain that is damaged in landmark agnosia might represent certain *groups of features* that the person *learns* to use as landmarks, and once that part of the brain is gone they have to rely on a new strategy of examining just one object at a time (Aguirre, 2003).

Finally, damage to the parahippocampus can cause *anterograde disorientation*. If that word anterograde looks familiar, you probably remember it from the amnesia chapter (see Amnesia). Anterograde disorientation is a sort of amnesia, but it is specific to a certain kind of information—specifically, people with this disorder struggle to form new memories about environments. Areas that were familiar to them before the brain damage are not a problem—they can even sketch maps of previously known places (Epstein et al., 2001). They can orient themselves and navigate through *familiar* places, but have extreme difficulties in learning to navigate through *unfamiliar* places like hospital corridors or newly visited streets (Habib & Sirigu, 1987). By using specific information like room numbers and street names, these people may navigate new places somewhat successfully, but they understandably prefer to travel within well-known places.

The Brain Pathology

Generally speaking, topographical disorientation seems most likely to arise following damage to the "posterior parietal region," and this is generally true in people with brain lesions and in studies where the brains of monkeys were intentionally damaged, wherein the monkeys ended up with problems such as difficulty finding their way back to their cages or trouble solving a "stylus maze" that they had previously learned (De Renzi, 1982, pp. 231–232). However, as noted in the previous section, because there are a variety of different types of disorientation, there are also a variety of underlying damage types.

I don't want to make it sound like there are exactly four types of topographical disorientation and that all researchers agree about that. There are other proposed ways to classify topographical disorientation disorders, such as with a recent "navigation impairment" taxonomy (Claessen & van der Ham, 2017). Using a group of 77 stroke patients with navigation problems, researchers showed that their problems could be sorted into three categories of things that they struggled with: landmarks, locations, and paths—and they found subcategories of people who struggled with both old locations and new locations versus people who struggled only with new locations (Claessen et al., 2017). However, that classification scheme didn't work as well in a science communication book like this one, and so I stuck with the classic four-part classification above and a basic explanation of a place in the brain that can be damaged in order to cause each one. It's also worth pointing out that there is not a clean line of division between "agnosia" and "amnesia" in these cases—there is usually some impairment to both recognition ability and memory (Barrash, 1998). The overall lesson remains the same: your brain can lose the ability to navigate in many different ways.

Topographical disorientation often occurs with other types of difficulties such as trouble with face recognition (see Prosopagnosia) or acquired color-blindness (see Achromatopsia), probably because the parts of the brain that process those types of information are located close to one another (Aguirre, 2003). It's also notable that topographical disorientation seems to be more common in right hemisphere brain damage (Claessen & van der Ham, 2017). Most people with these types of disorders make some improvements in their abilities to navigate over time, but mostly this seems to be due to coming up with new strategies for navigation rather than recovering their lost abilities (Barrash, 1998). However, many people with this disorder continue to receive messages from their brain that they've gone astray, even when they are right where they belong.

References

Aguirre, G. K. (2003). Topographical disorientation: A disorder of way-finding ability. In M. D'Esposito (Ed.), *Neurological foundations of cognitive neuroscience* (pp. 89–108). MIT Press.

Aguirre, G. K., & D'Esposito, M. (1999). Topographical disorientation: A synthesis and taxonomy. *Brain, 122*(9), 1613–1628. https://doi.org/bxrd75

Barrash, J. (1998). A historical review of topographical disorientation and its neuroanatomical correlates. *Journal of Clinical and Experimental Neuropsychology, 20*(6), 807–827. https://doi.org/bxnch6

Claessen, M. H. G., & van der Ham, I. J. M. (2017). Classification of navigation impairment: A systematic review of neuropsychological case studies. *Neuroscience and Biobehavioral Reviews, 73*, 81–97. https://doi.org/f9p7vj

Claessen, M. H. G., Visser-Meily, J. M. A., Meilinger, T., Postma, A., de Rooij, N. K., & van der Ham, I. J. M. (2017). A systematic investigation of navigation impairment in chronic stroke patients: Evidence for three distinct types. *Neuropsychologia, 103*, 154–161. https://doi.org/gbwn9x

De Renzi, E. (1982). *Disorders of space exploration and cognition*. John Wiley & Sons.

della Rocchetta, A. I., Cipolotti, L., & Warrington, E. K. (1996). Topographical disorientation: Selective impairment of locomotor space? *Cortex, 32*(4), 727–735. https://doi.org/gs5b

Epstein, R., DeYoe, E. A., Press, D. Z., Rosen, A. C., & Kanwisher, N. (2001). Neuropsychological evidence for a topographical learning mechanism in parahippocampal cortex. *Cognitive Neuropsychology, 18*(6), 481–508. https://doi.org/c4rprb

Farah, M. J. (2004). *Visual agnosia* (2nd ed.). MIT Press.

Habib, M., & Sirigu, A. (1987). Pure topographical disorientation: A definition and anatomical basis. *Cortex, 23*(1), 73–85. https://doi.org/gtv5

Iaria, G., & Barton, J. J. S. (2010). Developmental topographical disorientation: A newly discovered cognitive disorder. *Experimental Brain Research, 206*(2), 189–196. https://doi.org/b5tg2j

Landis, T., Cummings, J. L., Benson, D. F., & Palmer, E. P. (1986). Loss of topographic familiarity: An environmental agnosia. *Archives of Neurology, 43*(2), 132–136. https://doi.org/dqpvjc

Levine, D. N., Warach, J., & Farah, M. (1985). Two visual systems in mental imagery: Dissociation of "what" and "where" in imagery disorders due to bilateral posterior cerebral lesions. *Neurology, 35*(7), 1010–1018. https://doi.org/gtv6

McCarthy, R. A., Evans, J. J., & Hodges, J. R. (1996). Topographic amnesia: Spatial memory disorder, perceptual dysfunction, or category specific semantic memory impairment? *Journal of Neurology Neurosurgery and Psychiatry, 60*(3), 318–325. https://doi.org/bt5fbn

Mendez, M. F., & Cherrier, M. M. (2003). Agnosia for scenes in topographagnosia. *Neuropsychologia, 41*(10), 1387–1395. https://doi.org/c4vbr9

Meyer, O. (1900). Ein- und doppelseitige homonyme Hemianopsie mit Orientierungsstörungen. *European Neurology, 8*(6), 440–456.

Pallis, C. A. (1955). Impaired identification of faces and places with agnosia for colours: Report of a case due to cerebral embolism. *Journal of Neurology, Neurosurgery, and Psychiatry, 18*(3), 218–224. https://doi.org/c4v5mb

Stark, M., Coslett, H. B., & Saffran, E. M. (1996). Impairment of an egocentric map of locations: Implications for perception and action. *Cognitive Neuropsychology, 13*(4), 481–524. https://doi.org/dmq78v

Suzuki, K., Yamadori, A., Hayakawa, Y., & Fujii, T. (1998). Pure topographical disorientation related to dysfunction of the viewpoint dependent visual system. *Cortex, 34*(4), 589–599. https://doi.org/c86djc

Takahashi, N., Kawamura, M., Shiota, J., Kasahata, N., & Hirayama, K. (1997). Pure topographic disorientation due to right retrosplenial lesion. *Neurology, 49*(2), 464–469. https://doi.org/gtv7

van der Ham, I. J. M., Martens, M. A. G., Claessen, M. H. G., & van den Berg, E. (2017). Landmark agnosia: Evaluating the definition of landmark-based navigation impairment. *Archives of Clinical Neuropsychology, 32*(4), 472–482. https://doi.org/f964w8

Whiteley, A. M., & Warrington, E. K. (1978). Selective impairment of topographical memory: A single case study. *Journal of Neurology, Neurosurgery & Psychiatry, 41*(6), 575–578. https://doi.org/ccg9hd

Vertigo

Imagine that you can't balance. Your sense of balance is probably something that you take for granted, except on those rare occasions when you get dizzy or disoriented. But what if you were always dizzy and disoriented? Your brain can't seem to compute all of the necessary information to find out where "up" is and, as a consequence, you spend a lot of time lying down or falling down. Where has up gone, and why can't you seem to find it?

The Stories

(STORY 1) In his classic book about migraines, Edward Liveing described a patient who sometimes experienced severe vertigo when he quickly turned his head to look at something. Liveing wrote:

> one day, when speaking to a friend who was standing behind him, and turning his head to look towards him, he was seized with such an instantaneous and violent giddiness as almost to deprive him of consciousness, yet not to such a degree as to prevent his thinking at the time that it was a cerebral hæmorrhage, and feeling thankful that his will was made and other matters arranged. Since then … he has had two similar attacks of sudden vertigo of the same severe character, and brought on in each case by circumstances singularly alike—namely, suddenly changing the direction in which he was looking … these attacks of vertigo lasted some time, and the whirl of objects, even when lying down, he describes as most extraordinary.
>
> (Liveing, 1873, p. 126)

(STORY 2) A 32-year-old woman experienced occasional periods of vertigo that were strongly associated with feelings that things weren't real and that she wasn't herself. She also had a history of migraines, which may help explain both vertigo and depersonalization. Her vertigo was described as dizzy spells, including light-headedness. She would sometimes feel as if she were bouncing up and down while standing still. Other times, she would feel as if she were bouncing all the way to the ceiling and then back down to the floor.

DOI: 10.4324/9781003276937-48

She also described a feeling of being trapped in a twirl, with the world spinning around her. These vertigo symptoms would occur a few times monthly, but she was free of them for most of the time (Grigsby & Johnston, 1989, case 1).

(STORY 3) In a case that he called *The Disembodied Lady*, Oliver Sacks reported on a 27-year-old woman who almost entirely lost her sense of proprioception due to neural inflammation. Her muscle, tendon, and joint senses, which were supposed to report the position of her body parts to her brain, were unable to correctly do their jobs. She reported that "I may 'lose' my arms. I think they're one place, and I find they're another. This 'proprioception' is like the eyes of the body ... *it's like the body's blind*" (p. 47). When her eyes were open, she could use them to help her guide her muscle movements, but as soon as her eyes were closed, she tended to collapse into a heap. Following the catastrophic inflammation event, Sacks reported that "for about a month afterwards, [she] remained as floppy as a ragdoll, unable to even sit up" (p. 49). But over the ensuing months and years, she retrained her brain to adopt certain movements and postures that looked a bit more natural—including walking—although she did not recover her proprioceptive sense and had to carefully pay attention to her positioning (Sacks, 1998, pp. 43–54).

The Features

If you've ever felt dizzy after spinning around, or when looking down from a large height, or if you've ever become motion sick from riding on something that was moving a bit too wildly, then you already have some idea of what vertigo is like. In fact, dizziness and vertigo are often used as synonyms because medical patients usually describe their vertigo in terms of dizziness (Gurr & Moffat, 2001). Vertigo is more strictly defined as the illusion or hallucination of movement—most commonly, rotation—of either the environment around you or of your own body (Hanley et al., 2001). Reynolds wrote all the way back in 1854 that it's "the sensation of motion independent of its real existence ... the apparent motion is by some referred to external objects, and by others to their own person" (Reynolds, 1854, p. 545). That is, you literally feel like the room is spinning, or that you yourself are spinning. Usually this is temporary and the feeling goes away on its own. However, the types of vertigo that are considered disorders are more severe; they may feel like sudden violent tilts of the ground beneath you, or a long-lasting spinning.

There are at least three brain systems that contribute to your balancing abilities (see also Environmental Tilt). They include your vision, your proprioception systems, and your vestibular systems, and when two or more of them disagree—when they are mismatched—vertigo can be the result (Brandt, 2003). For example, vertigo in the form of motion sickness may happen to you in a vehicle when your eyes report that you are not moving very much, but your other balance systems report that you are moving quickly. Similarly, you can get motion sickness when using a virtual reality headset because the opposite is true: your eyes tell your brain that you are moving quickly, but your other balance systems report that you are not moving.

Your vision is useful for balancing because it allows you to see the position of your own body. Some people with vertigo only notice a balance problem when their eyes are closed, and physicians can use this as a test—comparing your balance with your eyes open to your balance when your eyes are closed—to narrow down the possible types of brain dysfunction (Killeen et al., 2019). Proprioception is a person's ability to use feedback from the nerves in their body parts to determine what position those body parts are currently occupying—such as being able to tell whether your arm is currently by your side or above your head. Proprioception can be involved in other disorders, as well (see Somatoparaphrenia).

The vision and proprioception systems are important for balance, but the focus will be on the vestibular systems, because they are usually the most directly related to vertigo (Brandt, 2003). The vestibular systems create your sense of balance through the clever use of some mechanisms in your inner ear. One of the mechanisms is a series of three looped tubes called the *semicircular canals* that contain liquid that sloshes around as you move. The three canals measure three dimensions of rotation in space: pitch (bending forwards or backwards), yaw (spinning around), and roll (tilting to the side). The sensors inside of your semicircular canals can sense the liquid sloshing in these three dimensions, and then send that information to your brain to help you balance. Another mechanism uses gravity—essentially, your brain figures out where "up" is located based on the position and pull of calcium crystals called *otoconia* that are deep inside of your ears. Perhaps when you were a kid, you were taught that the body has five senses: seeing, hearing, tasting, smelling, and touching. Well, you also have others, including liquid slosh and crystal maneuvers.

There are two main categories of vertigo: peripheral and central. Peripheral vertigo is a collection of vertigo types that are caused by problems in the inner ear, such as problems with the vestibular mechanisms that were mentioned above. The nerve that sends signals from your inner ear into your brain is called the vestibular nerve, and all kinds of peripheral vertigo warp the signals being sent through that nerve such that the signals end up being incorrect. Once the signals make it into your brain they don't make sense when compared to what your visual and proprioceptive systems are reporting, and this causes the sensation of spinning. Peripheral vertigo is usually temporary and may depend on the position that your body is in such as whether you are standing, lying down, or if your head is moving—if you have ever experienced temporary vertigo, it was probably caused by a peripheral change (Brandt et al., 2013). One potential cause of peripheral vertigo is that the otoconia crystals become misaligned in your semicircular canals and disrupt the movement of fluid. This results in a condition called *benign paroxysmal positional vertigo*, which usually shows up mysteriously but can sometimes be linked to anything from head trauma to viral infections, to the position that you sleep in at night, and many other factors (Yetiser, 2019). So yes, crystal misalignment can make you dizzy. That's just science.

Central vertigo, on the other hand, can be a much more constant sensation wherein you can't find a way to stop the spinning. Central vertigo occurs due to damage to the brain itself, usually the cerebellum, the brain stem, or the eighth cranial nerve (Lawal & Navaratnam, 2019). Strokes and tumors commonly result in central vertigo (Brandt, 2003). Let's get deep into the brain pathology below.

The Brain Pathology

Because the brain stem, cerebellum, and the inner ear are all supplied by closely connected arteries, and because interruption of blood supply to any one of those areas is enough to cause vertigo, it can be difficult to figure out the specific mechanism for a specific person's long-term vertigo (Lawal & Navaratnam, 2019). Thus, it takes some work to figure out *why* you are feeling dizzy all of the time, because of the many possible ways to cause vertigo. To an expert, the variety of vertigo syndromes may be "surprisingly easy to diagnose" due to key differences between the syndromes (Brandt, 2003, p. vii). Unfortunately for the dizzy people themselves, everything from a cerebellar infarct to a glioma on the brain stem, to the Miller Fisher variant of Guillain-Barré acute demyelinating polyneuropathy leads to feeling dizzy—so it is up to a skilled physician to evaluate the evidence to determine where the problem lies (Lawal & Navaratnam, 2019).

Another common cause of vertigo is traumatic brain injury, including vehicle accidents, falls, and sports injuries (Lan & Hoffer, 2019). Traumatic brain injuries may cause peripheral vertigo such as benign paroxysmal positioning vertigo, or they may cause more direct brain damage (Maskell et al., 2006). In some cases, people feel continuously unsteady after a traumatic brain injury and discover that the sensation of unsteadiness is worse whenever they are not moving at all or when they are moving quickly, leading to the adoption of a strategy of moving slowly at a constant rate in order to alleviate the off-balance feeling (Lan & Hoffer, 2019). In one study, five years after the traumatic brain injury, the majority of patients were still experiencing vertigo (Berman & Fredrickson, 1978).

Migraines can also be associated with vertigo in a condition called vestibular migraine (see Migraine Headaches). People with this condition lose their sense of balance while they are experiencing migraine attacks, finding themselves off-balance before, during, or even after the headache (Schettino & Navaratnam, 2019). These attacks can vary in length from minutes to days (Neuhauser et al., 2001). Vertigo is also affiliated with seizures, which is sometimes called epileptic vertigo (see Seizures). In fact, vertigo or dizziness is a frequently reported symptom of epilepsy in general (Lawal & Navaratnam, 2019).

Rehabilitation for vertigo is often a lengthy process, but many people with this condition do improve over time. One frequently used treatment is called *vestibular rehabilitation therapy* which is a series of exercises that helps people experiencing vertigo to partially recover—although it is possible that the treatment will be less effective for someone with central vertigo compared to someone with peripheral vertigo (Han et al., 2011). Depending on where the damage is that caused the central vertigo, there can still be a benefit to physical therapy to retrain balance, such that the person feels more able to balance after the therapy (Brown et al., 2006).

More experimental treatments also exist, such as sensory augmentation. Sensory augmentation is when more sensory information is given to a person about some specific sense, in this case balance, but in a way that avoids that damaged sense. This is accomplished by converting that sensory information into information that can be interpreted by a different sense. For example, a device can translate information about the position of a person's head into electrical signals that are zapped into a person's tongue (Danilov et al., 2015). Or, a belt containing vibrating motors wrapped around a person's waist can buzz as the person's balance shifts, giving them physical signals about their position that their brain wouldn't otherwise receive (Bao et al., 2018). More work is needed to understand when and how such devices are useful for vertigo, but some preliminary work shows that, at least for some people, balance is restored.

References

Bao, T., Carender, W. J., Kinnaird, C., Barone, V. J., Peethambaran, G., Whitney, S. L., Kabeto, M., Seidler, R. D., & Sienko, K. H. (2018). Effects of long-term balance training with vibrotactile sensory augmentation among community-dwelling healthy older adults: A randomized preliminary study. *Journal of NeuroEngineering and Rehabilitation, 15*(1), 1–13. https://doi.org/gdwstf

Berman, J. M., & Fredrickson, J. M. (1978). Vertigo after head injury—a five year follow-up. *The Journal of Otolaryngology, 7*(3), 237–245.

Brandt, T. (2003). *Vertigo: Its multisensory syndromes* (2nd ed.). Springer-Verlag London.

Brandt, T., Dieterich, M., & Strupp, M. (2013) *Vertigo and dizziness: Common complaints* (2nd ed.). Springer London. https://doi.org/gtv8

Brown, K. E., Whitney, S. L., Marchetti, G. F., Wrisley, D. M., & Furman, J. M. (2006). Physical therapy for central vestibular dysfunction. *Archives of Physical Medicine and Rehabilitation, 87*(1), 76–81. https://doi.org/b6zk5n

Danilov, Y., Kaczmarek, K., Skinner, K., & Tyler, M. (2015). Cranial nerve noninvasive neuromodulation: New approach to neurorehabilitation. In F. H. Kobeissy (Ed.), *Brain neurotrauma: Molecular, neuropsychological, and rehabilitation aspects*, (pp. 605–628). Taylor & Francis. https://doi.org/gtv9

Grigsby, J. P., & Johnston, C. L. (1989). Depersonalization, vertigo and Meniere's disease. *Psychological Reports, 64*(2), 527–534. https://doi.org/d9nq79

Gurr, B., & Moffat, N. (2001). Psychological consequences of vertigo and the effectiveness of vestibular rehabilitation for brain injury patients. *Brain Injury, 15*(5), 387–400. https://doi.org/d3fvsz

Han, B. I., Song, H. S., & Kim, J. S. (2011). Vestibular rehabilitation therapy: Review of indications, mechanisms, and key exercises. *Journal of Clinical Neurology (Korea), 7*(4), 184–196. https://doi.org/fx77wg

Hanley, K., O'Dowd, T., & Considine, N. (2001). A systematic review of vertigo in primary care. *British Journal of General Practice, 51*(469), 666–671.

Killeen, D. E., Isaacson, B., & Walter Kutz, J. (2019). History and physical examination of the dizzy patient. In S. Babu, C. A. Schutt, & D. I. Bojrab (Eds.), *Diagnosis and treatment of vestibular disorders* (pp. 27–44). Springer. https://doi.org/gtwb

Lan, D. & Hoffer, M. E. (2019). Post-traumatic dizziness. In S. Babu, C. A. Schutt, & D. I. Bojrab (Eds.), *Diagnosis and treatment of vestibular disorders* (pp. 301–309). Springer. https://doi.org/gtwc

Lawal, O., & Navaratnam, D. (2019). Causes of central vertigo. In S. Babu, C. A. Schutt, & D. I. Bojrab (Eds.), *Diagnosis and treatment of vestibular disorders* (pp. 363–375). Springer. https://doi.org/gtwd

Liveing, E. (1873). *On megrim, sick-headache, and some allied disorders: A contribution to the pathology of nerve-storms.* Churchill.

Maskell, F., Chiarelli, P., & Isles, R. (2006). Dizziness after traumatic brain injury: Overview and measurement in the clinical setting. *Brain Injury, 20*(3), 293–305. https://doi.org/cf23vm

Neuhauser, H., Leopold, M., Von Brevern, M., Arnold, G., & Lempert, T. (2001). The interrelations of migraine, vertigo, and migrainous vertigo. *Neurology, 56*(4), 436–441. https://doi.org/gtwf

Reynolds, R. (1854). On the pathology of vertigo. *Lancet, 63*(1603), 545–546. https://doi.org/ff4bnx

Sacks, O. (1998). *The man who mistook his wife for a hat and other clinical tales.* Touchstone.

Schettino, A., & Navaratnam, D. (2019). Vestibular migraine. In S. Babu, C. A. Schutt, & D. I. Bojrab (Eds.), Diagnosis and treatment of vestibular disorders (pp. 255–276). Springer. https://doi.org/gtwg

Yetiser, S. (2019). Review of the pathology underlying benign paroxysmal positional vertigo. *Journal of International Medical Research, 48*(4), 1–12. https://doi.org/gtwh

Visual Object Agnosia

Imagine that you can't understand shapes. Pretend that you are grocery shopping, and you need to buy some onions for a stew. But as you walk along the various displays at the market, you encounter a problem. You cannot tell any of the fruits and vegetables apart from one another in the usual way by simply looking at the item's form. In fact, you really can't tell what shape the items are at all. The edges and lines of the objects look bizarre or are missing. Instead, you are forced to find the onions with your other senses, such as by picking up the various produce items and feeling them. But even when you think you've found what you want to buy, you just aren't entirely sure that what you're holding is correct. After all, it doesn't *look* like an onion to you. You bring the onion up to your nose and sniff—yes, that's an onion, all right!

The Stories

(STORY 1) A 25-year-old soldier was admitted to the hospital many months after suffering carbon monoxide poisoning, where at the time he had been "found stuporous on the bathroom floor after having been exposed to leaking gas fumes while showering" (pp. 82–83). It was discovered that he could no longer recognize physical objects, images of objects, letters, numbers, geometrical figures, or body parts while he was looking at them. However, he was able to recognize objects when he was allowed to use his other senses such as touch, hearing, or smell. As part of his assessment by the physician, the patient was given a picture of a scantily clad cover girl from a magazine in order to see if he could recognize what he was looking at. After studying the image carefully, this person with visual object agnosia was able to guess that the picture was of a woman based on the presence of a large amount of her skin color and the lack of hair on her arms. But when he was asked to point to her eyes, he pointed to her breasts instead. Had she not been a photograph, there would never have been a more appropriate moment to respond with "my eyes are up here" (Benson & Greenberg, 1969).

(STORY 2) A curious case of visual object agnosia inspired the title of the book *The Man Who Mistook His Wife for a Hat and Other Clinical Tales*, by Oliver Sacks. In this book, Dr Sacks described an individual who confused

DOI: 10.4324/9781003276937-49

his foot for his shoe and his shoe for his foot. Dr Sacks wrote that "it was the strangest mistake I had ever come across," before helping the man to put on his shoe (p. 10). Even though the man had decent vision and was able to see a pin when it was placed on the floor, he made mistakes in identifying the things at which he was looking. He could not immediately identify a glove or a rose, for example. At one point, when he was looking around for his hat, he "took hold of his wife's head, tried to lift it off, to put it on" (Sacks, 1998, p. 11).

(STORY 3) In a classic case of *apperceptive visual agnosia*, an 80-year-old man was unable to tell the difference between objects by looking at them. His guesses about the object he was looking at were often wildly incorrect: "for example, an umbrella would be seen as a plant with leaves … a coloured apple was taken for the portrait of a lady" (p. 173). He often confused different articles of clothing, such as by mixing up his pants and his jacket. When eating, he would sometimes mix up the utensils or use the wrong end of the spoon. As noted by the author of the case study, the reactions of the patient, when confused, seemed unjustifiably confident. For instance, "rarely did he say outright that he did not know what it was" and would often "give a definite but wrong response" (Lissauer, 1890, translated in Lissauer & Jackson, 1988, pp. 172–173).

(STORY 4) In a classic case study of *associative visual agnosia*, a 47-year-old man was shown to be unable to identify objects. For example, when shown a piece of soap, he identified it as something to eat. He was able to draw the outlines of objects, which showed that the problem was not with perception but with identification. When the experimenter showed him an object and said the name of the object, the patient would nod and agree, saying, "yes, I see it now" (p. 309). However, when the experimenter brought the identity of the object into question by saying, "suppose I told you that the last object was not really a pipe, what would you say?"—the man admitted that "I would take your word for it," indicating that he remained unsure of object names even after claiming to have recognized them (p. 309). This person frequently complained that something was wrong with his eyes and frequently chose to keep his eyes closed or sleep to avoid the problem (Rubens & Benson, 1971).

The Features

Agnosia is a term that you have seen many times throughout this book, assuming that you read the chapters in order. In general, that term means an inability to recognize, such as an inability to recognize faces (see Prosopagnosia), an inability to recognize locations (see Topographical Disorientation), or an inability to recognize emotions (see Social-Emotional Agnosias). But there is a type of agnosia that is even more "quintessential" than those specific types: agnosia for *objects* themselves (Kirshner, 2021, p. 128).

Humans are excellent at object recognition. We can recognize an endless number of pieces of furniture even though they are mostly just variations of rectangle combinations. We can identify black and white line drawings of objects even though, if you think about it, a drawing of a bucket looks very little like an actual bucket. Shapes give way to meaning in our brains almost automatically, letting us organize the endless squares, triangles, and ellipses of various sizes and orientations into a coherent universe of objects. This is a skill at which computers are noticeably inferior, being unable to reliably tell the difference between a pig, dog, or loaf of bread. So, how is it that our brains can accomplish this feat in a split second while advanced mechanical minds repeatedly fail? Not to disappoint, but researchers still do not completely agree on exactly *how* the human brain accomplishes this marvelous feat. What we *do* know is that there are a lot of ways that this process can break down.

Object agnosia is usually referred to as *visual* object agnosia, because people with such disorders often retain the ability to recognize objects through other senses such as touch or hearing (Barton, 2014). The term visual object agnosia is an umbrella term that refers to a wide variety of disorders that all have something to do with problems recognizing objects using vision. Many attempts have been made to classify these similar-but-different visual form-processing problems into neat groups (Unzueta-Arce et al., 2014). However, there always seems to be some overlap or edge cases or additional degree of specificity to a person's individual recognition problems that make these categories muddy. Let's discuss them anyway, because that's what we're here to do.

The most notable clinical difference in object agnosia cases is between people who lose the ability to recognize *form* and the people who lose the ability to *associate* object names with their forms. Respectively, these are the *apperceptive* and *associative* versions of visual object agnosia, and they help to describe the phase of the object recognition process that the person is struggling with. Please keep in mind, as Barton notes, "it is probable that this apperceptive/associative distinction is rarely encountered in a pure form" (Barton, 2011, p. 226).

A person with apperceptive object agnosia cannot perceive objects in a way that leads them to correctly recognize those objects—they do not *look* like familiar objects. There are three major subtypes of apperceptive object agnosia, the most prominent of which is *shape agnosia* (Barton, 2011).

In shape agnosia, the person cannot perceive the form of an object, such as how rounded the edges of a shape are, but they can still see its color, size, and other non-form characteristics (Marotta & Behrmann, 2002). Thus, they would not be able to tell apart a square from a hexagon, for example, because they simply could not *see* the difference in shape. One way to diagnose shape agnosia is by having the person try to draw a copy of an object. People with shape agnosia cannot draw copies of objects because they cannot see the form of the object or detect the similarities and differences between the forms of multiple objects (Tikhomirov et al., 2019).

Another subtype of apperceptive object agnosia is *integrative agnosia*, which includes people who struggle to perceive objects that are made up of multiple parts even though they can perceive each individual part (Haque et al., 2018). These people have great difficulties with understanding overlapping figures such as one shape on top of another shape and telling drawings of real objects apart from drawings of fake objects that are made up of jumbled parts (Barton, 2011). For example, if you showed them a drawing of a kangaroo but with its tail replaced with a human foot, someone with integrative agnosia would have trouble deciding whether that was a realistic whole object or not (Riddoch & Humphreys, 1987). That may sound like a wild example, but that's a real drawing that was shown to a person with this condition.

Finally, there is *transformational agnosia*, which is a subtype of apperceptive object agnosia in which a person struggles to recognize common objects when seen from unusual viewpoints (Haque et al., 2018). For example, people with this condition may struggle to identify a fire hydrant when seen from above, a car when seen from below, or any other unusual visual angle. People with this condition may find it less disruptive to their lives than the other kinds of apperceptive object agnosia (Barton, 2011). This is because most of the time that you encounter a given object, it is in a particular orientation, such as a coffee cup having an opening at the top or a tree having its roots pointing down. And because these people can recognize those objects from their common viewpoints, most of the time their recognition abilities can function quite well.

In contrast, a person with associative object agnosia can perceive the form of the object that they are looking at, but they simply cannot identify what the object is or what it is used for. If you ask one of these people to draw an object or to copy a drawing of an object, they can generally do so almost perfectly (Farah, 2004). Therefore, they are not having trouble *perceiving* the object, unlike a person with apperceptive agnosia. However, these people cannot make *meaning* out of what they are perceiving and therefore do not recognize the object. It's important to also ask the person to try to name the objects as well as describe their functions, because sometimes the person can do the latter but not the former, which is a condition called object *anomia* (Tikhomirov et al., 2019).

Even more specific deficits are possible to define as well. For example, there are differences between people who lose the ability to recognize shapes and people who fail to recognize *textures* (Cavina-Pratesi et al., 2010). It also seems possible to lose the ability to recognize one *category* of objects, such as living creatures, while retaining the ability to recognize nonliving creatures (Barton, 2011). It also appears to be possible to have problems recognizing line drawings of objects but not with recognizing real objects (Hiraoka et al., 2009). In other words, because your brain does a lot of different work while attempting to recognize objects, there are a lot of brain areas involved in object recognition and, therefore, there are a bunch of different, often subtle, differences between each individual person when it comes to their visual object agnosia symptoms. Let's take a closer look at the brain's role in these symptoms.

The Brain Pathology

Much of the visual information processing that happens in your brain occurs in the back of your cortex, called the occipital lobe. Overall, visual object agnosias can result from a variety of different types of brain damage to the occipital lobe, including strokes, tumors, Creutzfeldt-Jakob disease (see Creutzfeldt-Jakob Disease), and carbon monoxide poisoning (Tikhomirov et al., 2019). Areas outside of the occipital lobe can also be involved. The more specific symptoms depend on which regions are damaged or disrupted.

For example, in various cases of apperceptive visual agnosia, the medial occipital cortex contributes especially to perceiving texture, while the lateral occipital cortex contributes especially to perceiving shapes (Kirshner, 2021). In contrast, a person with the typical case of associative object agnosia may have their symptoms because the visual area of their brain has been disconnected from the verbal area of their brain due to damage to the brain's white matter, which is sort of like the wires that connect one area of the brain to another area (Pelak, 2019). This disconnection means that the visual and verbal areas can no longer effectively share information, and so even though the person can both see and speak, they have trouble speaking about what they are seeing. Because so many visual information processing systems are located close together in the brain, visual object agnosia frequently seems to occur in conjunction with other disorders, especially other agnosias such as face blindness (Haque et al., 2018).

Automatic recovery from visual object agnosia is very rare, so some people try special training sessions to relearn how to recognize objects—although the focus is usually on using compensatory techniques to make up for the lost ability, such as using touch and sound, rather than recovering the visual ability of object recognition (Tikhomirov et al., 2019). These compensatory strategies seem to be helpful for many people, although more work is needed in order to better understand the extent to which such rehabilitation is helpful for different types of visual object agnosia (Heutink et al., 2019). I hope that learning about agnosia has made you appreciate your brain for all of the unrecognized recognition labor that it does throughout the background of your life.

References

Barton, J. J. S. (2011). Disorders of higher visual processing. In C. Kennard & R. J. Leigh (Eds.), *Handbook of clinical neurology* (Vol. 102, pp. 223–261). Elsevier. https://doi.org/gs46

Barton, J. J. S. (2014). Higher cortical visual deficits. *Continuum, 20*(4), 922–941. https://doi.org/gs47

Benson, D. F., & Greenberg, J. P. (1969). Visual form agnosia: A specific defect in visual discrimination. *Archives of Neurology, 20*(1), 82–89. https://doi.org/dktdrc

Cavina-Pratesi, C., Kentridge, R. W., Heywood, C. A., & Milner, A. D. (2010). Separate channels for processing form, texture, and color: Evidence from fMRI adaptation and visual object agnosia. *Cerebral Cortex, 20*(10), 2319–2332. https://doi.org/bqc3mf

Farah, M. J. (2004). *Visual agnosia* (2nd ed.). MIT Press.

Haque, S., Vaphiades, M. S., & Lueck, C. J. (2018). The visual agnosias and related disorders. *Journal of Neuro-Ophthalmology, 38*(3), 379–392. https://doi.org/gfq3xf

Heutink, J., Indorf, D. L., & Cordes, C. (2019). The neuropsychological rehabilitation of visual agnosia and Balint's syndrome. *Neuropsychological Rehabilitation*, *29*(10), 1489–1508. https://doi.org/gjs4wj

Hiraoka, K., Suzuki, K., Hirayama, K., & Mori, E. (2009). Visual agnosia for line drawings and silhouettes without apparent impairment of real-object recognition: A case report. *Behavioural Neurology*, *21*(3–4), 187–192. https://doi.org/gcd8wn

Kirshner, H. S. (2021) Agnosias. In J. Jankovic, J. C. Mazziotta, S. L. Pomeroy, & N. J. Newman (Eds.), *Bradley and Daroff's neurology in clinical practice* (8th edition, pp. 127–133). Elsevier.

Lissauer, H. (1890). Ein Fall von Seelenblindheit nebst einem Beitrage zur Theorie derselben. *Archiv für Psychiatrie und Nervenkrankheiten*, *21*(2), 222–270. https://doi.org/cpp2s3

Lissauer, H., & Jackson, M. (1988). A case of visual agnosia with a contribution to theory. *Cognitive Neuropsychology 5*(2), 157–192. https://doi.org/fxcd5p

Marotta, J. J., & Behrmann, M. (2002). Agnosia. In V. S. Ramachandran (Ed.), *Encyclopedia of the human brain* (pp. 59–70). Elsevier Science & Technology.

Pelak, V. S. (2019). Disorders of higher cortical visual function. In G. T. Liu, N. J. Volpe, & S. L. Galetta (Eds.), *Liu, Volpe, and Galetta's Neuro-Ophthalmology* (3rd ed., pp. 341–364). Elsevier. https://doi.org/gs49

Riddoch, M. J., & Humphreys, G. W. (1987). A case of integrative visual agnosia. *Brain*, *110*(6), 1431–1462. https://doi.org/c578x9

Rubens, A. B., & Benson, D. F. (1971). Associative visual agnosia. *Archives of Neurology*, *24*(4), 305–316. https://doi.org/ctsmrq

Sacks, O. (1998). *The man who mistook his wife for a hat and other clinical tales*. Touchstone.

Tikhomirov, G. V., Konstantinova, I. O., Cirkova, M. M., Bulanov, N. A., & Grigoryeva, V. N. (2019). Visual object agnosia in brain lesions. *Medical Technologies in Medicine/Sovremennye Tehnologii v Medicine*, *11*(1), 46–52. https://doi.org/gs48

Unzueta-Arce, J., García-García, R., Ladera-Fernández, V., Perea-Bartolomé, M. V., Mora-Simón, S., & Cacho-Gutiérrez, J. (2014). Visual form-processing deficits: A global clinical classification. *Neurología*, *29*(8), 482–489. https://doi.org/f2vfdt

Index

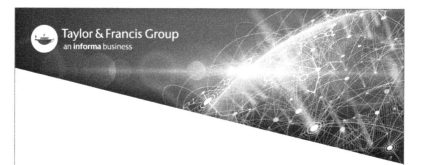

For Product Safety Concerns and Information please contact our EU
representative GPSR@taylorandfrancis.com
Taylor & Francis Verlag GmbH, Kaufingerstraße 24, 80331 München, Germany

www.ingramcontent.com/pod-product-compliance
Ingram Content Group UK Ltd.
Pitfield, Milton Keynes, MK11 3LW, UK
UKHW021451080625
459435UK00012B/451